MULTIPLE IMAGING PROCEDURES

Volume 1

PULMONARY SYSTEM

MULTIPLE IMAGING PROCEDURES

Series Editors: Leonard M. Freeman, M.D.
Jerome H. Shapiro, M.D.

Volume 2: Central Nervous System
Edited by Samuel M. Wolpert, M.D.

MULTIPLE IMAGING PROCEDURES

Volume 1

PULMONARY SYSTEM

Practical Approaches to Pulmonary Diagnosis

Edited by
Stanley S. Siegelman, M.D.

Professor of Radiology
Director of Diagnostic Radiology
Department of Radiology and Radiological Science
Johns Hopkins Medical Institutions
Baltimore, Maryland

Frederick P. Stitik, M.D.

Associate Professor of Radiology
Director Chest Radiology
Department of Radiology and Radiological Science
Johns Hopkins Medical Institutions
Baltimore, Maryland

Warren R. Summer, M.D.

Associate Professor of Medicine
Environmental Health Sciences and Anesthesiology
Clinical Director Respiratory Division
Director of Medical Intensive Care Unit
Johns Hopkins Hospital
Johns Hopkins Medical Institutions
Baltimore, Maryland

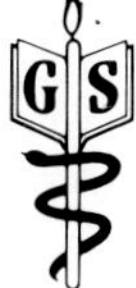

GRUNE & STRATTON
A Subsidiary of Harcourt Brace Jovanovich, Publishers
New York San Francisco London

Library of Congress Cataloging in Publication Data
Main entry under title:

Pulmonary system.

(Multiple imaging procedures; v. 1)
Includes bibliographical references and index.
1. Lungs—Diseases—Diagnosis. 2. Mediastinoscopy.
I. Siegelman, Stanley S., 1932– II. Stitik,
Frederick P. III. Summer, Warren R. IV. Series.
RC733.P86 616.2′4′075 78-31980
ISBN 0-8089-1143-0

Grune & Stratton, Inc.
111 Fifth Avenue
New York, New York 10003

Distributed in the United Kingdom by
Academic Press, Inc. (London) Ltd.
24/28 Oval Road, London NW1

Library of Congress Catalog Number 78-31980
International Standard Book Number 0-8089-1143-0
Printed in the United States of America

CONTENTS

PREFACE

The physician caring for a patient with pulmonary disease at a modern hospital will find that the professional staff includes a group of consultants capable of performing a wide range of sophisticated examinations for the diagnosis of pulmonary disorders. Each consultant internist specializing in lung disease, radiologist, otolaryngologist, thoracic surgeon, or pathologist will generally be well trained and experienced in the performance of a particular study. Conditioned by many successful applications of his or her own special skills, the consultant becomes an *advocate* of a particular technique. In this setting, a physician who is primarily responsible for the patient's management is often faced with the problem of choosing an *appropriate* series of diagnostic tests for the patient. Physicians in this position should be familiar with the preparation of the patient for the testing, the nature of the examination, the anticipated results, and the potential complications of each procedure. Each of the authors in this volume has spent a number of years actively engaged in managing patients with chest diseases at The Johns Hopkins Hospital. Dr. Carter has departed to assume a position in the Department of Pathology at Yale University, but the other principal authors remain. In Chapters 1–10 the authors were asked to provide a practical description of their own specific techniques of examination for the benefit of the general medical reader. They were also directed to detail the advantages and limitations of their diagnostic modality. In many instances the authors have provided data on their personal experiences in the delivery of health care to the patients at The Johns Hopkins Hospital.

After assimilating the material in Chapters 1–10, physicians may be troubled by uncertainties in choosing the proper sequence of tests for each patient. How shall they guide the evaluation of the middle-aged man with a solitary pulmonary nodule? What are the roles for cytology, bronchoscopy, needle biopsy, and mediastinoscopy? What are the roles for nuclear medicine and pulmonary angiography in the work-up of the patient with possible pulmonary infarct? What approach is indicated for the young female with newly discovered diffuse lung disease? In complicated clinical situations, it is apparent that the best patient care is provided by a team approach with appropriate contributions from each specialist. At The Johns Hopkins Hospital, the authors have repeatedly discussed these questions in joint consultations and in conferences over the past several years. As the result of the ongoing dialogue, a Johns Hopkins' approach to several key problems of pulmonary disease has evolved. These current ideas are provided in the concluding chapters of this volume.

Stanley S. Siegelman, M.D.
Frederick P. Stitik, M.D.
Warren R. Summer, M.D.

CONTRIBUTORS

Philip O. Alderson, M.D.
Associate Professor of Radiology
Associate Director, Division of Nuclear Medicine
The Johns Hopkins Medical Institutions
Baltimore, Maryland

R. Robinson Baker, M.D.
Professor of Surgery
Professor of Oncology
Department of Surgery
The Johns Hopkins Medical Institutions
Baltimore, Maryland

William R. Bell, M.D.
Associate Professor of Medicine
Assistant Professor of Radiology
Division of Hematology
Department of Medicine
The Johns Hopkins Medical Institutions
Baltimore, Maryland

Darryl Carter, M.D.
Professor of Pathology
Director of Diagnostic Pathology
Yale University School of Medicine
New Haven, Connecticut
(Formerly Associate Professor of Pathology and Oncology, The Johns Hopkins Medical Institutions)

Yener S. Erozan, M.D.
Associate Professor of Pathology
Division of Cytopathology
Department of Pathology
The Johns Hopkins Medical Institutions
Baltimore, Maryland

Bob W. Gayler, M.D.
Associate Professor of Radiology
Department of Radiology and Radiological Science
The Johns Hopkins Medical Institutions
Baltimore, Maryland

Stephen L. Kaufman, M.D.
Assistant Professor of Radiology
Department of Radiology and Radiological Science
The Johns Hopkins Medical Institutions
Baltimore, Maryland

Bernard R. Marsh, M.D.
Associate Professor of Laryngology and Otology
Director, Broyles Bronchoscopic Clinic, The Johns Hopkins Hospital
The Johns Hopkins Medical Institutions
Baltimore, Maryland

Stanley S. Siegelman, M.D.
Professor of Radiology
Director, Diagnostic Radiology
Department of Radiology and Radiological Science
The Johns Hopkins Medical Institutions
Baltimore, Maryland

Toby L. Simon, M.D.
Assistant Professor of Pathology and Medicine
Departments of Pathology and Medicine
University of New Mexico School of Medicine and United Blood Services
Albuquerque, New Mexico

Frederick P. Stitik, M.D.
Associate Professor of Radiology
Director, Chest Radiology
Department of Radiology and Radiological Science
The Johns Hopkins Medical Institutions
Baltimore, Maryland

Warren R. Summer, M.D.
Associate Professor of Medicine, Environmental Health Sciences, and Anesthesiology
Clinical Director, Respiratory Division
Director of Medical Intensive Care Unit, The Johns Hopkins Hospital
The Johns Hopkins Medical Institutions
Baltimore, Maryland

Peter B. Terry, M.D.
Assistant Professor of Medicine
Assistant Professor Environmental Medicine
Department of Medicine
Respiratory Division
The Johns Hopkins Medical Institutions
Baltimore, Maryland

Ko Pen Wang, M.D.
Assistant Professor of Medicine
Assistant Professor of Laryngology and Otology
The Johns Hopkins Medical Institutions
Baltimore, Maryland

Robert I. White, Jr., M.D.
Professor of Radiology
Director, Cardiovascular Diagnostic Laboratory
Department of Radiology and Radiological Science
The Johns Hopkins Medical Institutions
Baltimore, Maryland

Bob W. Gayler, M.D.

1

Chest Technique

INTRODUCTION

Chest radiographs are the most frequent general medical radiographs taken in the United States, accounting for 40 to 50 percent of radiographic examinations, or some seventy million examinations annually.[1] These radiographs may be taken as part of the evaluation of a specific complaint, to follow a previously demonstrated abnormality, or as a screening evaluation. Because of the range in anatomic densities in the thorax, the change in some of these densities which disease processes may cause, and the variations in size of patients, chest radiography is technically more demanding than radiographic examination of other parts of the body. Unfortunately it is frequently assumed that chest radiography is simple and that its performance may be relegated to minimally trained personnel. That which we call a chest radiograph can be produced under a variety of conditions, and we shall here consider how some of these conditions will affect the end product.

POSITIONING AND TUBE–FILM DISTANCE

For the patient with a chest complaint, erect posterior-anterior (P-A) and lateral films are standard. Variations include a posterior-anterior only, stereo P-A, or stereo P-A and lateral views. Historically, photofluorography has been widely used[2] with the production of a 70-mm- or 100-mm-wide film, but this system has fallen into disfavor because of the amount of radiation involved.[3] Other useful positions include the anterior-posterior (A-P) apical lordotic, an A-P angle view to see the posterior costophrenic sulci, shallow (15- to 20-degree) P-A obliques for lung detail, and 45-degree P-A obliques for cardiac characterization. These films are typically taken with the x-ray tube 72 inches (1.83 m) from the film and the patient positioned close to the film. This configuration of tube, patient, and film may be used whether or not a lead grid is used to reduce scattered radiation. The distance of 72 inches results in from 10–15 percent magnification of structures farthest away from the film in a normal-sized person. To reduce this magnification to 5–8 percent would require an approximate doubling of the focal spot–film distance. In those instances in which an air space is used between the patient and the film to reduce scattered radiation[4–6] without a lead grid, focal spot-to-film distances of 9 feet to 12 feet are generally used.

Although most disease processes visible on a chest radiograph may be seen on the single P-A view, it is well accepted that the lateral view may be helpful in defining the abnormality better or may clarify questionable findings; in some instances an abnormality may be seen only on the lateral view.[7–9] The lateral view does generally involve more radiation than the P-A view and considering limited silver reserves and steadily increasing radiographic film cost, it is reasonable to question the appropriateness of the lateral chest film in every case. A recent article by Sagel et al.[8] supports the omission of the lateral chest film in true screening situations of people under the age of 40. These authors also recommend that routine chest films not be taken of people under the age of 20 as part of the hospital admissions procedure when there is no clinical or historical evidence of chest disease.[8] Sagel et al. emphasize that their suggestions apply to a situation where the P-A film is taken with moderately high kilovoltage and there is therefore good mediastinal, cardiac, and diaphragmatic penetration.

NONINVASIVE SPECIAL PROCEDURES

Tomography has long been used to provide better definition of questionable lung densities and to characterize recognized abnormalities in the lungs and adjacent structures. This tomography generally has been done with a linear movement. The parasite shadows of linear tomographic motion are usually not as much of a problem in the thorax as they may be elsewhere in the body because of the horizontal orientation of the ribs. Linear tomography may be done with a short exposure time, frequently less than one second, so there is not as much vascular motion and unsharpness as with pluridirectional tomographic units, which require from 2 to 6 seconds of exposure time. Problems with linear tomography of the chest include incomplete blur of prominent costochondral junctions and the posterior rib–vertebral body junction. Immediate subpleural lesions may not be seen as discrete lesions by linear tomography unless some manipulation of patient position is done. Nonetheless, linear tomography is a satisfactory method in the evaluation of lung lesions for which tomography is typically used. Ravin et al.[10] review some aspects of lung tomography in their 1977 article, and Littleton emphasizes the advantage of pluridirectional tomography in his recent book.[11] A common problem encountered in chest tomography is that different technical factors may be needed for good visualization of the hilum, mediastinum, and lungs. A practical solution to this has been the use of an aluminum filter that is thinner centrally than it is laterally. This device can be used when both hilar regions are to be imaged.[12] A simpler wedge filter may be used when only one lung and its adjacent hilum are to be imaged.

Fluoroscopy of the chest has gone through a period of decline, but with the advent of high-resolution image intensifiers, the usefulness of chest fluoroscopy may well increase. Fluoroscopy can resolve questionable masses more efficiently than tomography in some instances.[13] Lesions near the lung periphery appear to be particularly suited to this modality, with or without spot films.

EQUIPMENT

Abrams et al.[14] in 1971 made a number of recommendations concerning the equipment for chest radiography. Their recommendations included a three-phase, 12-pulse, 1,000 mA generator; automatic exposure termination; and an x-ray tube with 0.6-mm small focal spot, and 1.0- to 1.3-mm large focal spot (30 kw to 85 or 100 kW); for magnification, a 0.3-mm focal spot was listed. This equipment will permit an exposure time of less than 50 msec on most patients and will allow use of 150 kilovolt peak. If very high kVp is desired, special equipment is available.

TECHNICAL FACTORS

Perhaps the most controversy about the specifics of chest radiography involves the technical factors chosen. For convenience, these may be thought of as low kVp (70–80 kVp), medium kVp (90–110 kVp), high kVp (125–150 kVp), and very high kVp (300–350 kVp). These will be considered individually.

Low kVp

Chest radiographs were taken in the low kVp range when most generators would not exceed 90 kVp. Such films have a pleasing appearance with good definition of bony structures; a sharp, clean appearance of the pulmonary vascularity; and a good balance of contrast. For adequate film density, from 10 to 20 mAs may be required for a medium-speed system (medium-speed screens and medium-speed film) for the P-A exposure. The standard rule of thumb is that the lateral film requires 3 times the mAs required for the

P-A view. One can produce very acceptable radiographs using this technique with either single-phase or three-phase equipment, although the lateral view may be borderline where motion is concerned. Historically and from a radiation-exposure standpoint this is a sound technique. From a film-appearance standpoint on small- and medium-sized patients, it is also a sound technique, but there is a problem when one encounters the larger-than-normal patient. The increased scatter in larger patients will compromise the film quality unless a scatter-reducing system, generally a grid, is used. (It is recognized that the air-gap technique may be used as an alternative to a grid. This is further considered in a separate section, "Air-Gap Films," later in this chapter.) The use of a grid will triple or quadruple the mAs required for adequate film density, depending on the grid ratio selected. The use of a scatter-reducing grid will increase the radiation to the patient substantially and will increase the mA required of the machine if the exposure time is to be kept short, or it will introduce longer exposure times if the mA cannot be further increased. Use of a grid in low kV ranges will also enhance the contrast more than one may wish, so that areas near the chest wall and in the mediastinum may be very light and the central lung regions too dark.

Because of the problems with larger patients, it is difficult to recommend this technique for new installations. However, if use of low kVp seems to be the most reasonable technique for a particular room, the following techniques are recommended: With medium-speed screens and film, use 5 mAs and variable kVp for children up to 15 cm A-P diameter and 10 mAs and variable kVp for those between 15 and 25 cm. For patients measuring 25 cm, use of a grid with a fairly low ratio (e.g., 6 to 1) is suggested, 20 to 30 mAs, and variable kVp. If possible, use of a somewhat faster screen-film system will help keep the exposure times short. If faster than medium-speed screens are used for all patients, appropriate mAs adjustments can readily be made.

Medium kVp

At the 80–110 kVp level, the contrast between bone and adjacent soft tissue will be slightly less than that obtained at the lower kVp level. In spite of this reduced contrast, calcification should still be readily distinguishable, and there will be somewhat more penetration of the heart and other mediastinal structures. In the small- and medium-sized patient, between 2 and 5 mAs will be needed without grid for a medium-speed, medium-screen film system, permitting short exposure times. The overall appearance of the films will reflect rather wide latitude and low contrast, which in larger patients will be objectionable. Therefore, a grid will be used to reduce scatter with a relatively smaller patient than at the lower kVp ranges (Fig. 1-1).

Without a grid, the radiation to the patient at this energy level is low and generally will work out to be the lowest possible in chest radiography. If a

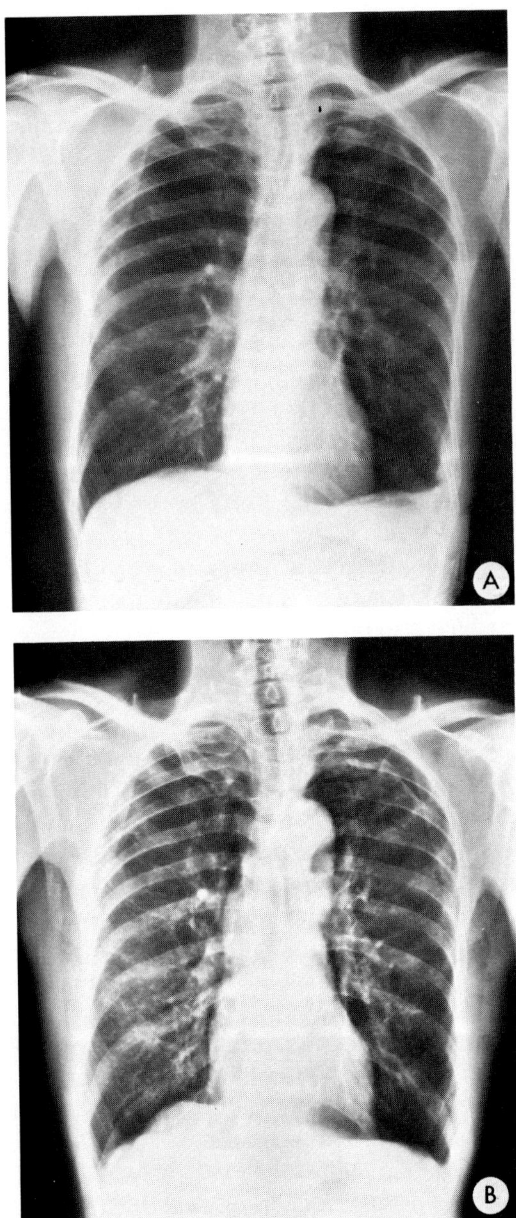

Fig. 1-1. Male, left pneumothorax. (A) 100 kVp, no grid, (B) 110 kVp, with 8:1 grid.

grid is used the radiation will be almost as high as when a grid is used in the low kVp range. Chest films made with a grid at this kVp will again be quite high in contrast, with the result that there will be difficulty in penetrating the bones and mediastinal structures. On average, I think the best results will be obtained in this kVp range using approximately 100 kVp without a grid unless the patient exceeds 24 cm, in which case an 8:1 fine-line stationary grid should be employed. A 6:1 grid will probably be satisfactory. With this system the changeover patients, that is those who measure from 22 to 28 cm, will have the poorest quality films, but it is a workable arrangement if the technologist is careful in measuring the patient.

High kVp

At the 125–150 kVp level a grid is generally used for all patients. One might think that a high-ratio grid, such as a 16:1 would have to be used, but a 10:1 grid is satisfactory for 95 percent of patients (Figs. 1-2, 1-3, and 1-4). Since it is usually very inconvenient to change grids, the 5 percent of patients who are quite large may be studied with a suboptimal appearance to the film. To use a high grid ratio for everyone would require an unnecessary amount of radiation for a great many people as well as producing somewhat higher contrast than one might like to see on small patients. With about 140 kVp, reasonably short exposure times can be obtained with anywhere from 200 to 500 mA, allowing some choice in equipment characteristics. There is sufficient latitude in the upper portions of this kVp range to provide some tolerance for failure to measure the patient, but the film quality will suffer greatly if the technologist's eye is used as the only measuring instrument. Automatic exposure termination can be used very successfully in conjunction with a grid as long as one remembers that the response time of the x-ray generating equipment is finite; thus, there will be a variable continuation of the exposure for a few milliseconds after the phototimer has instructed the generator to terminate production of x-rays. A special comment must be made about equipment used consistently at high kVp. Many x-ray tubes that are perfectly satisfactory at 125 kVp and below will not stand up to higher kVp use. It is essential that the tube supplier be aware of the intended use of the tube. The high-tension cables may also develop problems more frequently at high kVp than at the lower kVp levels. The output of the generator should be calibrated frequently when high kVp levels are used so that the rated capacity of the cables or tube is not unwittingly exceeded.

Radiologist acceptance of films taken with this technique has been good.[15–17] It must be recognized that the rib detail is not as distinct as with lower kVp ranges, and one must become accustomed to the normal appearance of the lung parenchyma and calcifications at this kVp. Very large patients will have films that appear gray. The use of an aluminum wedge filter

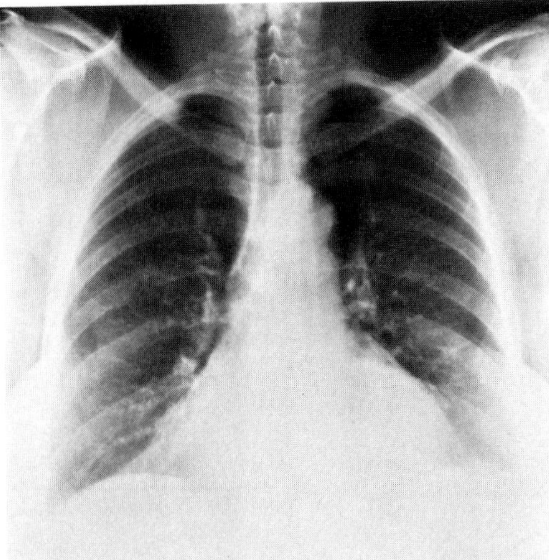

Fig. 1-2. Female patient, quite obese, 140 kVp, 10:1 grid.

in patients whose A-P diameter is markedly different over the upper chest than it is over the lower chest can contribute to improved film quality by compensating for some of the difference in tissue absorption.[18]

Very High kVp

For the last several years, the Field Emission Corporation, and subsequently the Hewlett-Packard Company, have marketed a 350-kVp field-emission-type of x-ray generating unit. This can be used with conventional

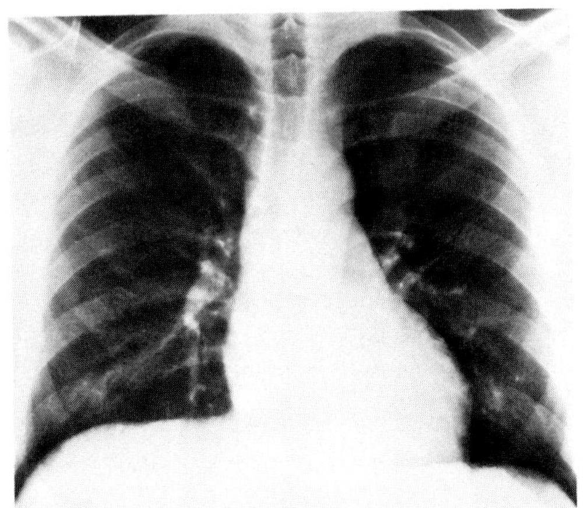

Fig. 1-3. Male patient, normal 140 kVp, 10:1 grid.

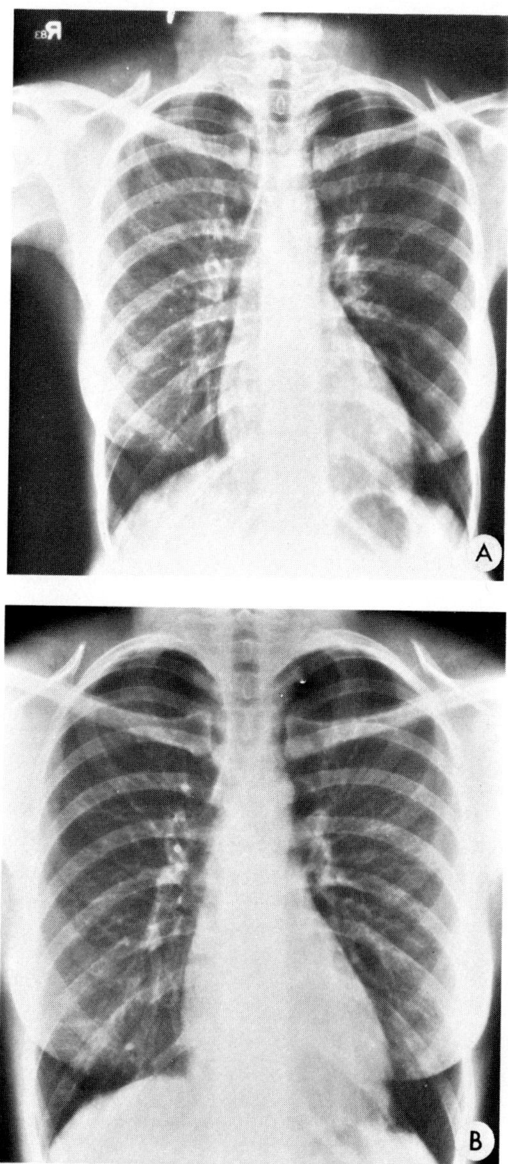

Fig. 1-4. Female patient. (A) 95 kVp, 8:1 grid; (B) 140 kVp, 10:1 grid This patient is slender, and both films are satisfactory. The skeleton is better visualized in the 95 kVp film, whereas lung detail is better seen in the 140 kVp film.

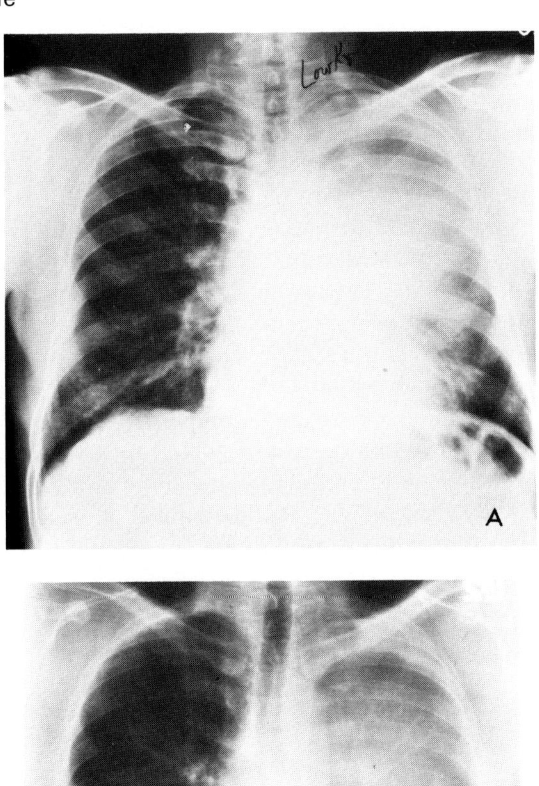

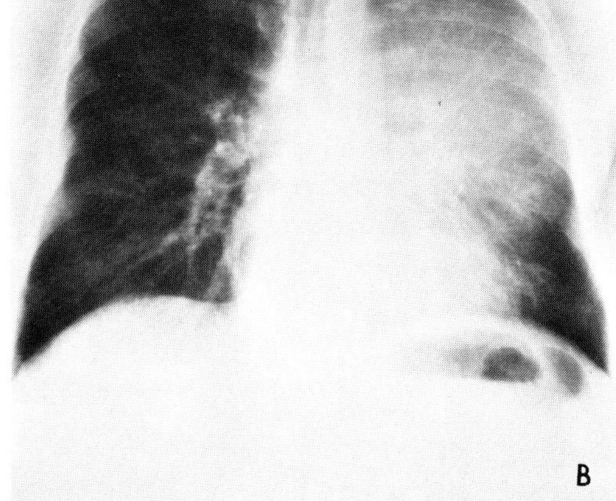

Fig. 1-5. Male patient with obstructing cancer of the left upper lobe bronchus. (A) 70 kVp, no grid; (B) 350 kVp, 12:1 grid. The 350 kVp film shows the airway to the point of obstruction. (Published through the courtesy of John De-Carlo, M.D., St. Joseph's Hospital, Baltimore, Maryland.)

cassettes and screens, although DuPont has a special screen that may be better suited for the very high (300–350) kVp level. A high-ratio grid, such as a 16:1, seems to be slightly preferable to lower-ratio grids, and very short exposure times, typically 1/70th of a second, and acceptable radiation levels are produced with this type of unit. One of its major drawbacks at this point seems to be that the unit cannot be used for other areas of the body than the chest, although for most multi-room departments that is not a severe problem. There is very wide latitude for soft tissue shadows, so that the mediastinum and cardiac silhouette are well penetrated. Overlying ribs are seldom a problem. Bone detail is not good, so that a lower kVp chest or rib film may be required for visualization of bone tissue (Figs. 1-5, 1-6, and 1-7). Calcification is very difficult to distinguish from soft tissues, so that the evaluation of masses detected with this technique may include a lower kVp film to check for calcification. Interpretation of these films does require some reorientation on the part of the radiologist, but the characteristics of these films generally are learned quickly.[19] The very large patient appears to be better studied with this kVp than with any of the lower ones. At this time, reliability and price appear to be quite competitive with any of the 125–150 kVp systems. This unit can be readily mated to most of the high-volume chest changers. Some additional comments about this type of unit are noted in a recent article by Dyke et al.[20] Tuddenham et al. suggested the potential usefulness of very high kilovoltage in 1954.[21]

CASSETTES

The unsatisfactory durability of many cassettes has done much to stimulate cassetteless radiography and to promote the development of new types of cassettes. Several cassetteless systems, generally called automatic chest changers, are on the market and have had a significant positive impact on chest film quality. With any system it is essential to have good film-screen contact without light leaks. When cassettes are used, film-screen contact tests should be done as part of the acceptance procedure on new cassettes, and this contact test should be repeated at least annually but preferably at six-month intervals for 14 × 17 in. (35 × 43 cm) cassettes.

FILM-SCREEN COMBINATIONS

As recently as six years ago, one could make a fairly simple compilation of available intensifying screens and films and note their relative compatibility and speed. With the availability of rare earth intensifying screens and their varying light-emission characteristics, this has become considerably more complicated. The elements used in the rare earth screens include gadolinium, lanthanum, terbium, and yttrium. When appropriately used these screens may result in resolution similar to that obtained with calcium tungstate screens, but with less radiation required. There have been various types of screens produced, some of which are much faster than calcium tungstate screens and which involve some loss of detail. Articles by Rossi et al.[22] and by Thompson et al.[23] are suggested for further reading. In gen-

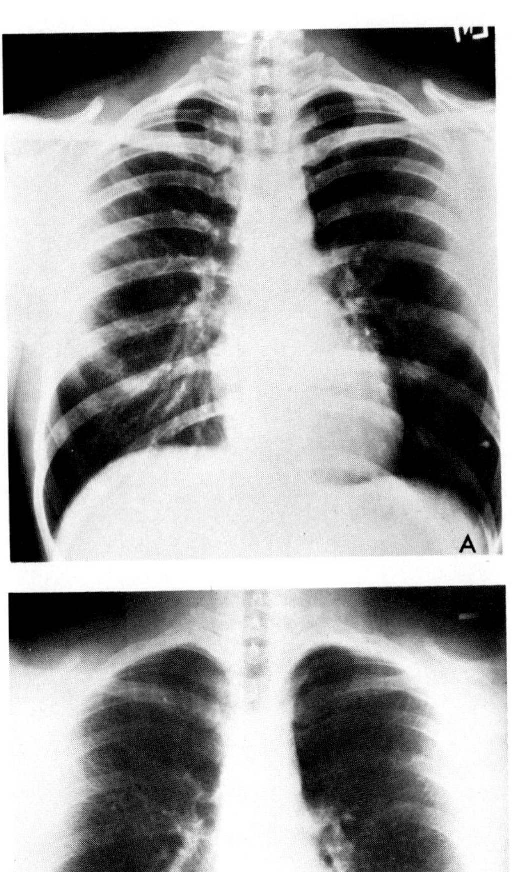

Fig. 1-6. Male with small calcified granuloma, left lower lobe and left hilum. (A) 70 kVp, no grid; (B) 350 kVp, grid. The calcification is better seen in the 70 kVp film, but the overall lung visualization is better with the 350 kVp film. (Published through the courtesy of John DeCarlo, M.D., St. Joseph's Hospital, Baltimore, Maryland.)

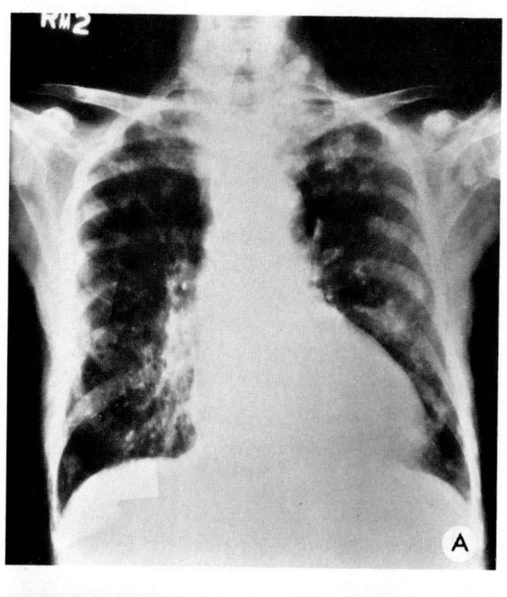

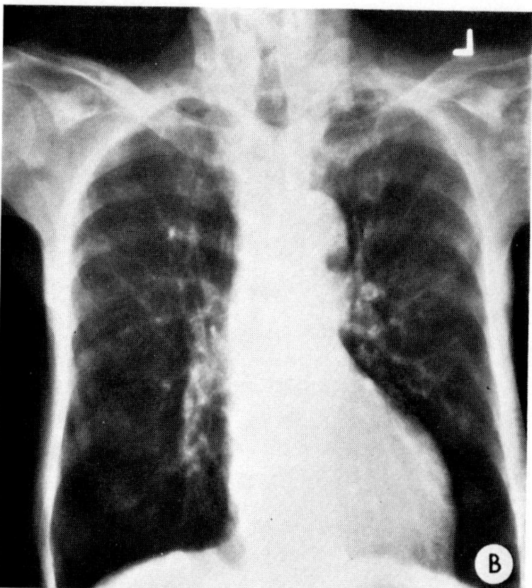

Fig. 1-7. Male with diffuse blastic lesions, metastatic from cancer of the prostate. (A) 70 kVp, no grid; (B) 350 kVp, 12:1 grid. The bony lesions were very difficult to see in the 350 kVp film. (Published through the courtesy of John De Carlo, M.D., St. Joseph's Hospital, Baltimore, Maryland.)

eral, as radiation levels are decreased, the quantum mottle will increase. The point at which this becomes objectionable seems to be an individual matter. This writer's impression is that one can accept chest films made at twice the speed of the usual medium-speed screen–medium-speed film combination most of the time. At this time it does not seem appropriate to generalize about systems faster than this. It should be noted that accuracy of technical factors becomes more important with increasing speed of a system. It should also be noted that the optimal range for realizing the increased speed of the rare earth systems is between 80 and 120 kVp. Their relative speed in comparison to calcium tungstate falls off below and above these levels. From a practical standpoint, resolution capability of a film-screen system is not the most important factor in total image quality as ordinarily experienced. Film-screen contact, processing, collimation, the care of the technologist in selecting technical factors, and the characteristics of the x-ray generating equipment combine to have a greater impact on the image quality of a film than the resolution of the film–screen system.

PROCESSING

There are a number of good automatic processors available today. The filmmaker's recommendations concerning temperature and processing cycles must be carefully followed. Changes in developer temperature do not have to be very great to result in significant overdevelopment or underdevelopment of the film. Periodic use of a separate thermometer (the thermometers built into the processors tend to be unreliable) or use of sensitometric strips is recommended. A regular program of processor cleaning is essential to good film quality. Manual film processing is still fairly widely used, despite the availability of automatic processors for about a quarter of a century. Manual processing is probably done in smaller installations where volume is not great. Manual processing requires considerably more skill; poor temperature control, exhausted solutions, inadequate agitation, and artifacts will be visually apparent when care is not taken in processing. There is nothing inherently wrong with manual processing, but it must be done correctly.

VIEWBOXES

The rules for maintaining viewboxes are simple but often overlooked. Fluorescent tubes should be replaced in an entire set, not one at a time, since tubes from the same manufacturer may have slightly different colors. When they are replaced, they should be visually checked for color after a warm-up, and any that are mismatched should be replaced. Light sources of different colors in adjacent viewboxes are disconcerting and may distract the radiologist from concentrating on the image. Suboptimal tubes should either be discarded or used for illuminating something other than radiographs. The diffusing plates should be cleaned regularly. Peripheral light and glare should be minimized. People with blue or green eyes should be particularly attuned to this since they seem to be bothered more by glare than people with brown eyes.

SPECIAL COMMENTS

Grids

As noted above, grids are used to reduce scattered radiation in larger patients, or in all patients in the upper kVp ranges. The structure of grids, the relative efficiency of various types, and the details of their performance will not be gone into here. The general practice is that as one increases the kVp, the grid ratio also is increased. Because of the relatively large volume of air in the thoracic region, it is not necessary to use as high a grid ratio in the chest as in the abdomen to get acceptable films.[24] It is common practice to use a medium ratio grid, such as an 8:1, with a grid-moving device in an upright filmholder. This device may be used for erect abdomen films and erect chest films. In such a unit it is essential to use a medium- or low-ratio grid, since the focal spot–film distances will vary between 40 and 72 inches. This type of device represents a compromise, therefore, and tends not to be ideal for either abdomen work or chest work. It should also be remembered that with any grid-moving device there is finite time required for grid travel, and at very short exposure times, the grid lines may be visualized. Grids made for a bucky device (which moves the grid during the exposure) do not have lines as fine as those on grids made to be stationary. Visualized grid lines in a bucky device are normally objectionable. High-quality stationary grids require rather close inspection before the grid lines can be seen. The efficiency of a grid in reducing scattered radiation is related to the total amount of lead in the grid. Usually this is directly related to the grid ratio but will not have a precise relationship to the number of lines per inch.

Air-Gap Films

Moving the patient six to nine inches from the film can be used as an alternative to use of a grid for reducing scattered radiation. Trout et al.[6] have recently reviewed a number of aspects of this air-gap maneuver. With the air-gap method there is an increase in film contrast. This increased contrast results because (1) the scattered radiation, which comes off at an acute angle to the incident beam, may miss the film as the film is moved away from the patient; and (2) there is a reduction of the intensity of the scattered radiation due to the inverse square law.

An advantage of this system over the use of a grid is that the primary beam is not attenuated by a grid, so that the usual increase in "technique" needed when a grid is used is not required. Technical factors must be increased due to the increase in focal spot–film distance, but the patient dosage turns out to be lower than with other techniques. Trout et al.[6] found the skin dose with this technique to be comparable to that of a 70 kVp chest film taken without a grid. When a regular 0.6- or 1.2-mm focal spot is used at a 72-inch focal spot–film distance and the patient–film distance is increased, there is some loss of sharpness due to the so-called penumbra effect. As the focal spot–film distance is increased, sharpness also increases.

This procedure does not appear to be widely used, perhaps because of the altered configuration of the filmholder, the slightly higher x-ray tube output, or the size of the room required.

Portable Chest Films

The term "portable chest x-ray" is interesting in that it consists of but three words, two of which are inappropriately used, and yet it is perfectly understandable to radiologists, primary care physicians, and most health service professionals. Although no radiologist would use "x-ray" in place of film or radiograph (a misnomer as well, according to some) in formal discourse, many use it in conversation. The films made by x-ray exposure are all portable, whether they are made with a fixed installation or with a mobile x-ray-producing device. The mobile device itself may be fairly easy to move, but it is not strictly speaking, portable. However, the term "mobile unit chest radiograph" is unlikely to replace "portable chest x-ray" in U.S. conversational usage.

Films made with portable units historically have suffered from electrical outlet limitation. Getting 100 kVp is usually possible, but unless special circuits have been run, mA limits of 15–25 are the rule. One can easily work this through, given a 115–120-volt, 15-amp outlet, full wave rectification, and some slight heat loss. Exposure times of 0.2 sec are quite common with this equipment. In many of the newer installations outlets with 220 volts and 50 amps have been installed at regular intervals. These may permit 200 mA with acceptably short exposure times for chest radiographs. Since this extra circuitry is expensive, these outlets generally have been installed in operating rooms and intensive care units but are lacking in regular patient wards. Another potential problem with the plug-in unit is that, with an increase in monitoring equipment, electrical safety requirements have become quite stringent, and the standard plug-in unit may not meet some of these requirements. Recent developments which get around the limitations of the wall circuitry to some degree are the condensor-discharge unit and the battery-energized x-ray unit. Both these types of units appear to be capable of acceptable mA with short exposure times, but they have both suffered from significant reliability problems, which will probably be resolved in the near future.

Film Size

The most frequently used film size for the adult P-A projection is 14 inches wide by 17 inches high (35 × 43 cm). Some departments have used a 14 × 14 in. size, which is somewhat less costly. Almost all women will fit on a 14-inch-wide film, but a significant number of men will be either too wide to fit on the film or will have sufficient soft tissue thickness of the chest wall that the technologist will be concerned about a non-fit.

Audsley et al. in 1970[25] studied a group of 714 men and found that only 66 percent fit conveniently on a 14-inch-wide film, whereas 99+ percent fit on a 15.7-inch (40 cm) film. Our own experience suggests that 70 percent of men will fit easily on a 14-inch (35 cm) film, approximately 15 percent are borderline, and another 15 percent are slightly wider than 14 inches (35 cm). For the wider patient, a 14 × 17 in. cassette may be used transversely in almost all instances, since the vertical height of the lung fields in these very wide patients is usually not as great as the transverse width. An occasional patient will require separate exposures of each side of the chest. Use of a 40-cm-wide film seems to be increasing somewhat in Europe, but is not likely to become widespread in the United States very quickly because viewing devices, film jackets, and filing spaces are set up for the 14 × 17 in. film.

For the lateral view, an 11 × 14 in. (28 × 35 cm) film will frequently suffice. This does require care in positioning but can result in a monetary saving.

Radiation Dosage

The skin dose for a single P-A chest film with any of the kVp values mentioned will be under 100 millirads for a 25-cm patient. Using the same screens and films, the relative dosage will be higher for grid techniques at 100 kVp or less, somewhat lower with higher kVp and use of a grid, and lowest with non-grid techniques.[6,26]

Film Interpretation

Tuddenham in an article in *Radiologic Clinics of Noth America*[27] over ten years ago discussed in depth some problems with the observational abilities of the radiologist. His comments remain pertinent. He urged the use of a minification lens in chest work, as well as double reading and directed search for abnormalities. It is apparent from reading the article that he assumes a high-quality film. It remains the responsibility of the radiologist to work very closely with the technologist to produce the best possible films and then to do his best in interpreting them. The recurring features of sub-optimal films, including processing problems, over- or under-exposure, poor film–screen contact, positioning problems, patient movement, and failure to use a grid when appropriate account for almost all of the remediable negative features of chest radiographs. Ideally the film-taking process should be set up to minimize the opportunities for these problems to occur. This requires that appropriate procedures be set up and followed through continuously. The problems of reliability of interpretation require considerable attention as well, but I feel that one must begin with a high-quality radiograph.

REFERENCES

1. Lindheim R: Uncoupling the radiology system. Chicago, Hospital Research and Educational Trust, 1971
2. Deasy JB: Mass radiography. Br Med J 3:48, Letter to the Editor, 1970
3. United States Department of Health, Education, and Welfare: The chest x-ray as a screening procedure for cardiopulmonary disease. Publication No. (FDA) 73-8036, US Govt Printing Office, Washington, DC
4. O'Donnell EB: Concerning high voltage technique and accessories. X-ray Tech 36:71–75, 1964
5. Ardran GM, Crooks HE: The reduction of scatter fog in chest radiography. Br J Radiol 37:477–479, 1964
6. Trout ED, Kelley JP, Larson VC: A comparison of an air gap and a grid in roentgenography of the chest. Am J Roentgenol 124:404–411, 1975
7. Vix VA, Klatte EC: The lateral chest radiograph in the diagnosis of hilar and mediastinal masses. Radiology 96:307–316, 1970
8. Sagel SS, Evens RG, Forrest JU, Bramson RJ: Efficacy of routine screening and lateral chest radiographs in a hospital based population. N Engl J Med 291:1001–1004, 1974
9. Pfister RC, Oh KS, Ferrucci JT: Retrosternal density. Radiology 96:317–324, 1970
10. Ravin CE, Wallin K, Sorenson J: Chest tomography. A practical approach. Appl Radiol 6: 119–126, 1977
11. Littleton JT: Tomography, Physical Principles and Clinical Applications. Baltimore, Williams & Wilkins, 1976
12. Edwards FH, Pfeil CE: Use of compensating filter in lung hilus tomography. Radiology 121:745–746, 1976
13. Forrest JV, Sagel SS: Special procedures in pulmonary radiology. In Current Concepts in Radiology, Vol 2, St. Louis: C. V. Mosby, 1975, pp 157–212
14. Abrams HL, Adelstein SJ, Elliott LP, Ellis K, Greenspan RH, Judkins MP, Viamonte M: Optimal radiologic facilities for examination of the chest and cardiovascular system. Circulation 43:A125–A136, 1971
15. Christensen EE, Dietz GW, Murray RC, Moore JG, Stokely EM: Effect of kilovoltage on detectability of pulmonary nodules in a chest phantom. Am J Roentgenol 128:789–793, 1977

16. Jacobson G, Bohlig H, Kiviluoto R: Essentials of chest radiography. Radiology 95:445–450, 1970
17. Roberts SR, Clements JL, Weens HS, Rogers JV, Shuford WH, Sprawls Jr P: The 350 kV chest x-ray. Exhibit at American Roentgen Ray Society Meeting, Washington, DC, September 1976
18. Lynch PA: A different approach to chest roentgenography: Triad technique (high kilovoltage, grid, wedge filter). Am J Roentgenol 93:965–971, 1965
19. Hallenbeck GS: Clinical evaluation of the 350 kV chest radiography system. Radiology 117:1–4, 1975
20. Dyke WP, Barbour JP, Charbonnier FM: Depth resolution: A mechanism by which high kilovoltage improves visibility in chest films. Radiology 117:159–164, 1975
21. Tuddenham WJ, Gibbons JF, Hale J, Pendergrass EP: Supervoltage and simultaneous roentgenography—New technics for roentgen examination of the chest. Radiology 63:184–190, 1954
22. Rossi RP, Hendee WR, Ahrens RT: An evaluation of rare earth screen/film combinations. Radiology 121:465–471, 1976
23. Thompson TT, Radford EL, Kirby CC: A look at rare-earth and high-speed intensifying screens. Appl Radiol 6:71–72, 129, 1977
24. Trout ED, Kelley JP: A phantom for the evaluation of techniques and equipment used for roentgenography of the chest. Am J Roentgenol 117:771–776, 1973
25. Audsley WP, Latham SM, Rossiter CE: Film sizes for radiography of the chest. Radiology 36:70–72, 1970
26. Gayler BW: Toward optimizing chest x-ray technique. In Potchen EJ (Ed.): Current Concepts in Radiology, Vol 2. St. Louis, CV Mosby, 1975, pp 131–156
27. Tuddenham WJ: Problems of perception in chest roentgenology: Facts and fallacies. Radiol Clin North Am 1:277–289, 1963

Frederick P. Stitik, M.D.

2

Contrast Studies of the Airways

Radiologic contrast studies of the airways have undergone wide swings in popularity over the past forty years. At present, there is considerable disagreement about which type of patient may benefit from this procedure and when it should be performed. The former indications for Dionosil bronchography included bronchiectasis, hemoptysis, chronic pulmonary disease, chronic infiltrates and atelectasis, the solitary pulmonary nodule, congenital abnormalities, outlining bronchopleural fistula, and bronchial mapping prior to bronchoscopy. With the advent of new techniques (fiberoptic bronchoscopy, catheter bronchial brushing, and percutaneous lung biopsy) that establish a definitive histologic, cytologic, or microbiologic diagnosis of pulmonary disease, many of the previous indications for bronchography have been eliminated. In addition, with the routine immunization against pertussis and the liberal use of antibiotics, bronchiectasis is less frequently encountered. In this chapter, we shall review each of the indications for bronchography as well as current indications for performing Dionosil bronchography.

INDICATIONS FOR DIONOSIL BRONCHOGRAPHY

Bronchiectasis

Bronchiectasis is the only common disease that is definitively diagnosed by bronchography. Furthermore, bronchography is the only means of establishing the diagnosis short of histologic examination. The incidence of clinically recognizable bronchiectasis has decreased. The decrease is probably due to the liberal use of broad-spectrum antibiotics and widespread immunization against pertussis. The current trend is toward medical management for bronchiectasis, with fewer pulmonary resections being performed. In the young patient, particularly below twenty years of age, and in the older patient with severe symptoms not responding to medical treatment, resection still merits consideration. Sanderson et al.[1] have compared the mortality and morbidity of 393 patients treated by surgical or medical therapy. The results of this study suggested that the current prejudice toward medical management may be unjustified. The authors advocate resection or partial resection of the involved segments; resection, however, is not justified without a bilateral bronchogram demonstrating the exact extent of disease. Should the observation of these investigators become substantiated, bronchography with Dionosil may become a more frequently used procedure in the future.

A patient with recurrent pneumonia, especially in the same segment, may have significant, localized bronchiectasis that requires resection. Bronchoscopy should be performed to exclude an endobronchial obstruction. In the patient with recurrent pneumonia, bronchography should not be performed until at least four months after the pneumonia has subsided. This delay is necessary to avoid misdiagnosing the reversible bronchiectasis that occurs with an acute pneumonia.[2]

Hemoptysis

Hemoptysis is listed by the American College of Chest Physicians review of bronchography as the second most common indication for bronchography.[3] Forrest et al.[4] have reviewed 196 patients undergoing bronchography with hemoptysis as the major indication. Ninety-two patients had normal P-A and lateral chest radiographs. The bronchogram demonstrated localized bronchiectasis in two patients and benign broncho-occlusive disease presumably due to healed granulomatous disease in another two patients. The total yield in this group of 92 patients was 4.5 percent. Thirty-three patients, or 36 percent, had bronchographic evidence of bronchitis, though this information was not useful in clinical management. No cases of radiologically occult cancer were detected. It is apparent that in a patient with a single episode of hemoptysis, a normal chest radiograph, and normal bronchoscopy, bronchography adds little significant clinical information.

In the remaining 104 patients with hemoptysis and an abnormal chest x-ray, the bronchogram frequently did not provide useful clinical information. Seven cases of bronchiectasis, not suspected by routine chest radiographs, were diagnosed. There is a role for selective bronchography in two clinical situations. First, the major role of the bronchogram is in demonstrating patent bronchi in an infiltrate outside the reach of the fiberoptic bronchoscope. In a patient with a localized area of consolidation, carcinoma can usually be excluded by fiberoptic bronchoscopy with brushing and biopsy.

If further confirmation is necessary a selective bronchogram demonstrating widely patent bronchi adds further information. Needle aspiration biopsy may also confirm that the infiltrate is a chronic pneumonia and not a bronchogenic carcinoma. Second, selective bronchography may also be of value in a patient in whom blood has been localized to one segment but in whom no definite diagnosis has been established by bronchoscopy (Fig. 2-1). It is preferable to wait four to five days after the hemoptysis has subsided, as the clots in the bronchial tree may give the false appearance of an obstructed bronchus or a luminal filling defect.

Chronic Pulmonary Disease

The bronchographic abnormalities in patients with chronic bronchitis and emphysema have been described in great detail.[5] The bronchographic demonstration of these diseases frequently does not add useful information to that already obtained by history and physical examination, chest radiographs, and pulmonary function tests. One possible exception is the patient with an unexplained chronic, severe, productive cough. Seven percent of patients with bronchiectasis will have a normal chest x-ray even in retrospective review.[6] If bronchiectasis is demonstrated in such a patient, the clinician may be inclined to use more prolonged courses of antibiotics or continuous doses of antibiotics as well as postural drainage.

Chronic Infiltrates and Atelectasis

Bronchoscopy in these patients has clearly replaced bronchography as the major means of evaluation. Central carcinoma can be easily diagnosed by bronchoscopy. (See Chapter 8.) If the chronic infiltrate and atelectasis are due to a foreign body or mucus plug, bronchoscopy is often diagnostic and therapeutic. If the bronchi are patent, suppuration due to pneumonia is easily identified. Transbronchial biopsy is likely to establish a definitive histologic diagnosis of lipid pneumonia or alveolar cell carcinoma.

Bronchography with liquid contrast agents still plays a significant role in the management of children with chronic right middle lobe collapse. Exact bronchoscopic visualization of the right middle lobe bronchus distal to the orifice is difficult in children. The obstruction is frequently 0.5 to 1.0 cm beyond the orifice. Billig and Darling[7] evaluated 11 children with right middle lobe collapse by bronchoscopy and bronchography. In six children with the bronchographic findings of bronchial stenosis, bronchiectasis, or nonfilling of the middle lobe bronchus despite selective catheterization, all showed scarred pulmonary parenchyma at surgery. Of the other five children, all of whom had normal bronchi at bronchography, four responded to medical treatment. The other went on to surgical resection. At surgery this child's bronchi and pulmonary parenchyma were well preserved despite six episodes of collapse. The authors recommend that every effort be made

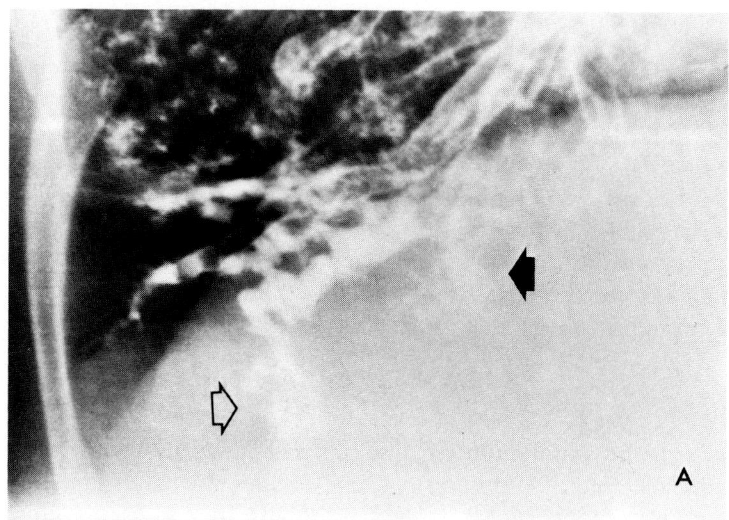

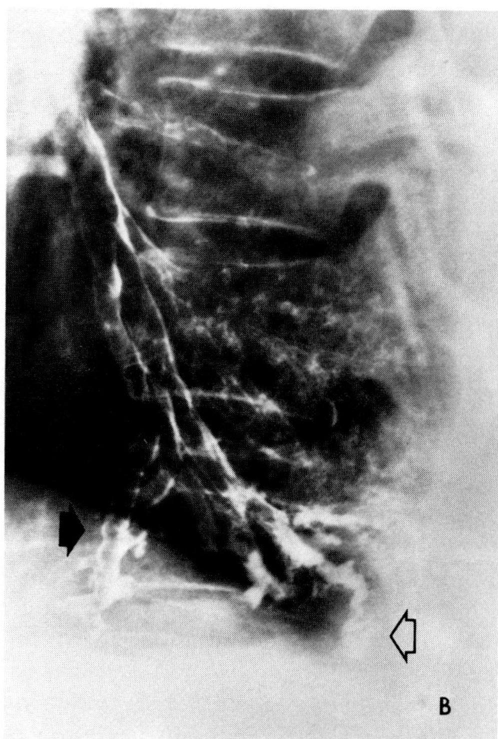

Fig. 2-1. *Bronchiectasis.* A 65-year-old black male had hemoptysis. His P-A and lateral chest radiographs were normal except for signs suggestive of chronic obstructive pulmonary disease. Fiberoptic bronchoscopy localized the source of bleeding to the posterior basal segment of the right lower lobe. Washings and brushings from this area showed no evidence of cancer or tuberculosis. Selective bronchogram of the posterior basal segment showed cylindrical (solid arrow) and saccular (open arrow) bronchiectasis. (A) P-A view; (B) Lateral view.

to use medical rather than surgical treatment in children with right middle lobe atelectasis and normal bronchi at bronchography.

Solitary Pulmonary Nodule

In previous years, bronchography has been used extensively to differentiate between benign and malignant pulmonary masses. In some centers the diagnostic accuracy for bronchogenic carcinoma has been reported to be as high as 94 percent.[8] Despite these enthusiastic reports, bronchography has not been widely used in the evaluation of the solitary pulmonary nodule. The bronchographic findings of narrowed, obstructed, and displaced bronchi are strongly suggestive of bronchogenic carcinoma but may also be seen in tuberculosis. In the inoperable patient, these bronchographic findings are frequently considered insufficient evidence of bronchogenic carcinoma to treat the patient with radiotherapy. Conversely, crowded dilated bronchi in or near a solitary pulmonary nodule are strongly suggestive of inflammatory disease but do not exclude a scar carcinoma and do not give the clinician the exact bacteriologic etiology. Bronchoscopy, catheter bronchial brushing, or needle aspiration biopsy often give the exact histologic or cytologic diagnosis of malignant disease. These techniques can also give the exact microbiologic diagnosis in the patient with a solitary pulmonary nodule of infectious etiology.

Congenital Abnormalities

Bronchography can be of value in carefully delineating the anatomy prior to surgery. In the rare anomaly of atresia of the left upper lobe bronchus, the chest radiograph often demonstrates oligemia and a peripheral collection of mucus (Fig. 2-2). In these cases a bronchogram that shows the absent or atretic bronchus is virtually diagnostic. Congenital bronchial cysts, though rare, are also easily diagnosed with Dionosil bronchography (Fig. 2-3).

Bronchopleural Fistula

In patients with an empyema secondary to a suspected bronchopleural fistula, we can generally delineate the communication between the bronchus and pleural space with an injection of Dionosil. Dionosil is usually introduced through a chest tube that has been placed in the patient to drain the empyema. Topical anesthesia is injected via the chest tube prior to the injection of the contrast agent. Frequent spot films are obtained while the contrast agent is injected, as the patient may cough once the Dionosil reaches an unanesthetized bronchus. Attempting to delineate a bronchopleural fistula with conventional transnasal bronchography is often unrewarding, as the communication is frequently from a small distal bronchus and therefore does not become filled with Dionosil.

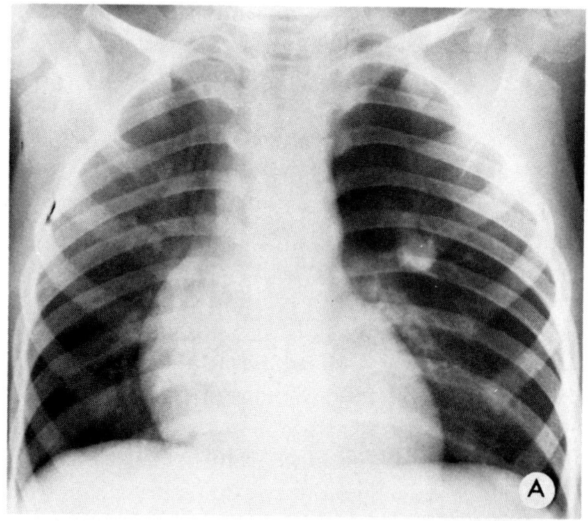

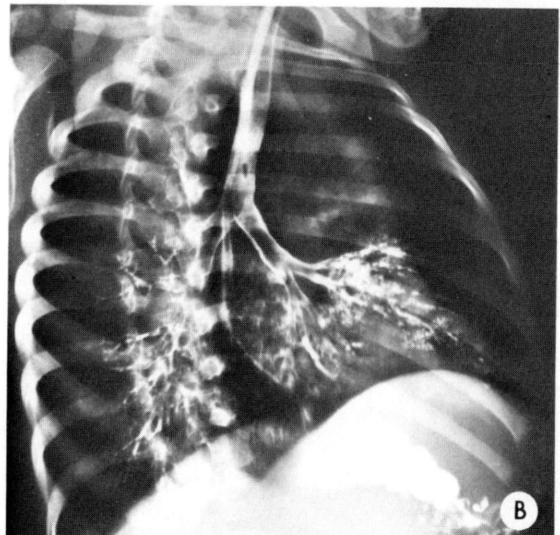

Fig. 2-2. *Segmental Bronchial Atresia.* A 3-year-old white male with an abnormal chest radiograph since birth. (A) AP chest radiograph demonstrates oligemia of the left upper lobe. The mass in the midportion of the left lung is due to pooling of mucus behind the obstructed (absent) bronchus; (B) An oblique bronchogram shows absence of the apical posterior bronchus.

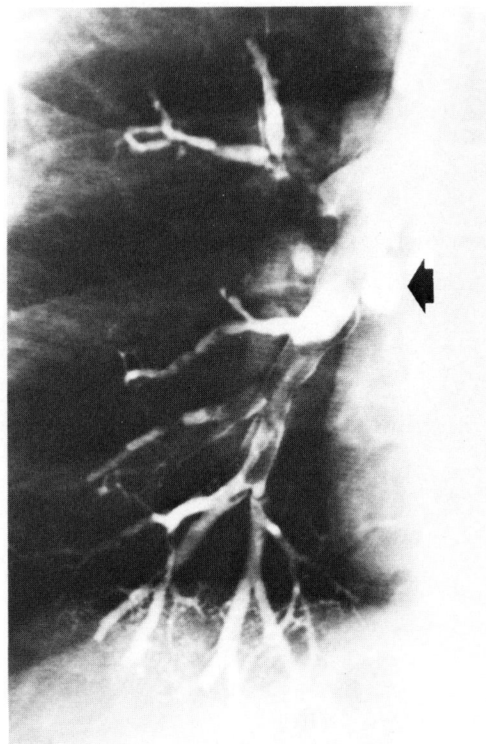

Fig. 2-3. *Bronchial Cyst.* A 32-year-old white female with repeated episodes of coughing. P-A and lateral chest radiographs were normal. Dionosil bronchogram shows a congenital cyst of the bronchus intermedius (arrow).

Bronchial Mapping

Obtaining a bronchogram solely for the purposes of establishing a "road map" for subsequent fiberoptic bronchoscopy or bronchial brushing is a common practice in Japan.[9] In the United States, however, bronchography is seldom performed for this purpose. In rare cases when there is a contraindication to needle aspiration biopsy and surgery, selective bronchography has been performed prior to a repeat fiberoptic bronchoscopy (Fig. 2-4).

Several centers combine selective bronchography with selective bronchial brushing. This has been reported to increase the rate of accurate diagnosis of bronchogenic carcinoma.[10] If the bronchogram is performed first, the contrast agent often obscures the material sent for cytologic and microbiologic evaluation. Bronchography done after bronchial brushing may give the false appearance of bronchial obstruction and irregularity due to bleeding and mucosal trauma. We rely on our knowledge of the anatomy of the

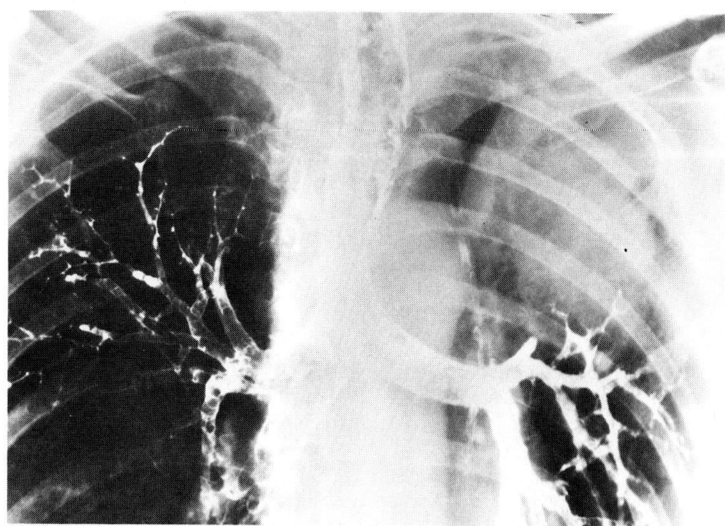

Fig. 2-4. *Bronchogenic Carcinoma.* A 67-year-old white female with a twenty-pound weight loss. A large left upper lobe mass was present on her chest radiograph. Sputum cytologies and fiberoptic bronchoscopy were inconclusive. A bronchogram demonstrated complete occlusion of the apical posterior segment. Also note moderate lateral and inferior displacement of this segment. Repeat fiberoptic bronchoscopy, with the abnormal origin and course of the apical posterior segment having been delineated, demonstrated squamous carcinoma (contrast agent—tantalum powder).

tracheobronchial tree and its variants, as well as biplane fluoroscopic localization of the brush in the pulmonary density when we perform selective catheter bronchial brushing.

TANTALUM

Dionosil is the only contrast agent available for general bronchographic use today, and it has a number of disadvantages which are discussed in the section that follows. Different contrast agents (sterile barium, aqueous Dionosil, and fluorocarbons) have been tried, but at present tantalum powder is the only agent that holds promise for replacing Dionosil. In 1968, Nadel first described the experimental use of tantalum powder as a contrast agent.[11] Since 1970, we have been co-investigators in the clinical evaluation of this material.

Disadvantages of Dionosil

Dionosil, an iodinated peanut oil, is moderately toxic. After bronchography the mucosa of the airways will show signs of acute inflammation,[12,13] and systemic toxicity is manifested by fever. A one-degree temperature rise over the prebronchogram state will be seen in approximately 30 percent of patients after a bronchogram with oily Dionosil.

After a Dionosil bronchogram, chemical pneumonias are not infrequent. Rare cases of iodism,[14,15] fatal anaphylaxis,[16] and lobar atelectasis[17] have also been reported. Even though the iodinated portion of the Dionosil is hydrolyzed off and excreted by the kidneys, the oily portion may remain behind and cause granulomas and other manifestations of chronic inflammation.[18] Long-term retention of both the iodinated and oily portions of conventional bronchographic contrast agents is a rare, though reported complication.[19]

With conventional contrast agents, large volumes are used to fill the airways. The average amount of oily Dionosil instilled during a bilateral adult bronchogram is 30–40 cc. With the volume of the airways below the carina being only 65 cc,[20] it is not surprising that pulmonary function is moderately decreased in a patient undergoing conventional bronchography. Changes in pulmonary function occurring after Dionosil bronchography were extensively studied in the 1960s. Christoforidis et al., reported a decrease in vital capacity of 30–40 percent and a decrease in $FEV_{1.0}$ of 23 percent in patients undergoing bilateral bronchography.[21] These changes usually resolved within 24 hours after the study. Bhargava and Woolf showed that the diffusing capacity is also reduced by an average of 47 percent.[22] The diffusing capacity may not return to normal until 72 hours after the bronchogram.

Thus, in seriously ill patients with decreased pulmonary function, and in patients with narrowed airway diameters, it is often too hazardous to perform contrast studies of the airways using these conventional contrast agents. Unfortunately, it is this group of patients who often would benefit the most from an accurate radiologic assessment of their anatomic abnormalities.

Properties of Tantalum

Tantalum is a very radiodense, inert metal. There is substantial evidence for the lack of toxicity of tantalum. Tantalum has been used extensively in many surgical procedures for over thirty years. For example, tantalum is used in certain, orthopedic prosthetic devices and sutures; it is also used in the mesh implanted in the abdominal wall for hernia repairs and in plates for cranioplasties. Furthermore, direct application of powdered tantalum has been made onto the dura to aid in detection of postoperative intracranial bleeding.[23] Follow-up of patients in whom tantalum has been used has failed to demonstrate any toxic effect; also, there is no evidence of any toxic effect in industrial workers exposed to powdered tantalum, even though a small amount of this metal can often be seen on their chest radiographs.[24] A large quantity of tantalum fed to rats failed to demonstrate any gastrointestinal absorption or systemic toxicity.[25] Large amounts of tantalum instilled into the lungs of guinea pigs did not cause any pulmonary fibrosis.[26]

Controlled studies by Nadel et al. in both dogs and humans undergoing tantalum bronchography, have failed to demonstrate any local or systemic toxicity;[27] our experience confirms this work. Febrile reactions to tantalum are rare. In Nadel's and our combined experience with over 400 adult patients, we have encountered only two with a temperature elevation after a tantalum study. In both of these, bronchoscopy was performed either the day before or concomitantly with the bronchogram. In one patient, a pneumonia was demonstrated radiologically in an area that was not insufflated with tantalum. In the other patient, the temperature returned to normal limits without specific therapy eight hours after the combined bronchoscopy and tantalum bronchography.

Tantalum is cleared rapidly via the mucociliary blanket. In an intact animal with surgically exposed trachea, tantalum particles can be seen clearing under direct vision.[28] Table 2-1 gives the average clearance times for different portions of the airways. If tantalum is insufflated distal to the effective mucociliary blanket, it may remain there indefinitely. In animal experiments when tantalum was purposely insufflated into the periphery of the lung, sacrifice of the animal two years later showed no evidence of inflammation or other histologic abnormalities around the retained tantalum.[27] In our clinical population, every effort is made to keep tantalum out of the more distal non-ciliated airways by proper catheter placement, appropriate insufflating pressures, and careful monitoring of the deposition of tantalum under fluoroscopic control.

Coughing and other vigorous respiratory movements will not dislodge the tantalum from the mucosal surface. On the other hand, such maneuvers during a Dionosil bronchogram will result in rapid alveolarization making the study difficult to interpret.

When tantalum powder is properly administered, long-term retention is not a problem. Our experience in both animals and humans has not confirmed the claims of Upham et al., and Morrow et al., who demonstrated long-term retention of a tantalum isotope in animals.[29,30] Their results are probably explained by filling of the alveoli. The published postmortem radiographs show most of the tantalum in the alveoli. In 1972 Friedman demonstrated alveolarization of tantalum powder in areas of pneumonia.[31] We consider pneumonia to be the only absolute contraindication to a tantalum study.

Tantalum powder coats the airways, giving excellent mucosal detail. The fine tantalum cloud is deposited on the mucosal striations rendering a double-contrast appearance even in small airways 1–2 mm in diameter. Oily contrast, because of its high surface tension, tends to fill the airways and coalesce into aggregates, thus giving poor mucosal detail.

The fine mucosal coating and ability to detect small submucosal lesions with tantalum was well demonstrated by Dodds et al. They were able to detect small intramural gelatin masses that were surgically implanted in the wall of feline stomachs.[32]

Pulmonary function tests, including lung volumes, flow rates, and dif-

Table 2-1
Clearance of Tantalum

Trachea	6 hr
Major bronchi	24 hr
Normal smaller bronchi	48 hr
2 mm bronchi	4 days
<2 mm bronchi	7–28 days
Alveoli	Unknown

fusing capacity in humans and dogs undergoing bilateral tantalum bronchography, have demonstrated little or no significant change. In dogs, the more sensitive parameters of dynamic pulmonary compliance and total lung resistance have confirmed the lack of significant change in pulmonary function.[27] Since pure powdered tantalum is approximately 15–20 times more radiodense than the iodine suspensions, a study can be performed with surprisingly small amounts of tantalum. The very radiodense tantalum powder coats, rather than fills, the airways, and therefore only 0.5 to 1.5 cc are necessary to perform an adequate bilateral bronchogram. The small amount of tantalum necessary is the major reason for the lack of alteration in pulmonary function. There is no outpouring of edema fluid into the airway lumen and no swelling of the airway mucosa such as occurs with conventional bronchography. This lack of local toxicity also plays an important role in maintaining pulmonary function.

In summary, contrast studies of the airways with tantalum overcome the major objections of conventional contrast agents. Tantalum is very radiodense, nontoxic, and rapidly cleared from the airways. It coats the airways, giving superior mucosal detail without significantly altering pulmonary function.

Clinical Use of Tantalum Powder

In our institution, there are two major indications for a tantalum powder study of the airways. The first is in any patient with suspected upper airway obstruction. The second is localization of radiologically occult bronchogenic carcinoma in the patient with a positive sputum cytology and a normal chest radiograph.

GENERAL CONSIDERATIONS

The tantalum powder used is the commercially available 5 μ fraction (Fansteel Corporation). It does not support any bacterial or fungal growth; therefore, sterilization is not required. Prior to clinical use 2 or 3 cc are placed in the reservoir of a modified Devilbiss model 175 powder blower and dried by constant suction for 24 hours in a 250-cc desiccator containing anhydrous calcium sulfate crystals. The next day, the power blower is assembled and dried in the desiccator for an additional 24 hours. Immediately before the study, the suction is discontinued and the sealed desiccator is brought into the radiologic site. The vacuum is not broken until we are ready to insufflate the tantalum.

We used compressed air as the insufflating gas in patients undergoing tracheography and a 90 percent nitrogen–10 percent oxygen mixture in patients undergoing bronchography. The usual insufflating pressure for tracheography is 8 to 10 pounds per square inch. For bronchography, the insufflating pressure is varied between 8 and 25 psi, depending on the catheter position and the region of the lung to be coated. For tracheography, the insufflation is performed as the catheter is slowly withdrawn, whereas at bronchography, short, 3–5 second bursts are delivered into different regions of the lung after selective catheterization of lobes or segments.

One hundred percent oxygen should never be used because of the danger of combustion. When performing tracheography in patients who are receiving supplemental oxygen, the oxygen is discontinued during the 20 to 30 seconds of insufflation and restarted as soon as the insufflation is completed. There is no hazard of explosion or combustion once the tantalum powder is deposited on the mucosal surface. The patient and the tantalum generator should be electrically grounded to a common ground during the insufflation as an additional precaution to prevent combustion.

Pneumonia is an absolute contraindication and is excluded by a posterior-anterior and lateral chest radiograph and physical examination. For at least 6 hours prior to the study, the patient should have nothing by mouth. The patient is carefully questioned to determine any contraindications to atropine or topical anesthetic agents. We administer atropine intravenously in 0.2–0.3 mg increments until the peripheral pulse reaches 120 or a maximum of 2 mg have been injected. The usual dose ranges from 1.0–1.5 mg delivered slowly in three to five minutes. This thorough atropinization is necessary to dry the secretions completely and to block potential vagal reactions to the catheter and the powder. We do not use sedation routinely for tracheography, but when indicated, 50–100 mg of phenobarbital are given intramuscularly. Codeine, in appropriate dosages, is used routinely in all patients undergoing bronchography as a sedative and antitussive.

CINE LARYNGOTRACHEOGRAPHY IN THE ADULT PATIENT

Technique

Following our routine preparation, posterior-anterior, lateral and both oblique scout films of the larynx and entire trachea are obtained. It is important to document the exact length and location of the tracheal or laryngeal abnormality. In every patient we obtain a "measurement series" to determine the exact dimensions of the abnormal segment. After appropriate topical anesthesia, the catheter is placed into the trachea via the nasal tracheal approach and positioned above the carina under fluoroscopic control. The first half of our "measurement series" is obtained by taking posterior-anterior and lateral spot radiographs of the catheter in the patient by rotating the patient in a cradle and maintaining the spot film device in a fixed position. Tantalum is insufflated through the same catheter into the main stem bronchi, trachea, and larynx. Once the catheter is removed, the patient is rotated back into the initial position where identical posterior-anterior and lateral spot radiographs are obtained, thus completing the second half of the "measurement series." The usual magnification is 1.4 in the posterior-anterior projection and 1.6 in the lateral projection.

Immediately after the "measurement series" the larynx is studied by spot filming and a cine recording in deep inspiration, expiration, and phonation. The larynx is studied before the trachea as it clears the tantalum powder more rapidly than the trachea. The trachea is then studied with posterior-anterior, lateral, and both oblique spot radiographs, with the spot film device moved as close to the patient as possible to maximize the fine mucosal detail. Finally, the trachea is studied with a cine recording in deep inspiration, deep expiration, as well as deep inspiration and expiration against a closed glottis (Müller and Valsalva maneuvers). These multiple maneuvers done both in the posterior-anterior and lateral projection are necessary to detect tracheomalacia, a pathologic weakening of the tracheal wall due to destruction of the supporting cartilaginous rings.

Additional precautions are taken with the patient who has severe upper airway obstruction. Instead of the routine Metras catheter (Roche Incorporated), a grey Kifa catheter (outer diameter 2.8 mm, inner diameter 1.8 mm—United States Catheter and Instrument Corporation) with 2-mm metallic rings spaced 5 cm apart is used for the "measurement series" and insufflation. In patients presenting with a tracheostomy, the tracheostomy tube is not removed until the first half of the "measurement series" has been completed. It is replaced immediately at the end of the cine recording, or if the patient becomes dyspneic. Spot radiographs of the trachea with the tracheostomy tube reinserted then should be taken. This is to guarantee that the tracheostomy tube bypasses the tracheal lesion (if present) and to insure that the tracheostomy tube is not angulated against the posterior or lateral tracheal wall, which would subsequently produce tracheal injury.

Etiology of Upper Airway Obstruction

Most of our patients had tracheal lesions caused by endotracheal intubation or prolonged tracheostomy required to deliver positive pressure respiration during respiratory failure. In many cases, it was difficult to decide whether the endotracheal tube or the tracheostomy tube was the major cause of the tracheal abnormality. In these cases, both were recorded as probable etiologies. Surgery was also a common etiologic factor in this se-

Table 2-2
Probable Etiologies
(94 initial studies)

Tracheostomy tube	44
Endotracheal tube	39
Surgery	25
Other	27

ries, as many of the patients were referred to The Johns Hopkins Hospital after initial unsuccessful attempts to correct laryngeal and tracheal abnormalities. The probable etiologies are presented in Table 2-2.

Results

Using the above techniques, we have performed 120 tantalum cine laryngotracheograms in 94 adult patients. Twenty-six patients had repeat studies after operative correction. No patient needed a repeat study because the initial examination was unsatisfactory. The results are tabulated in Table 2-3. Tracheal stenosis, a well-recognized complication of endotracheal tube intubation and tracheostomy, was our most common finding, being found in 58 of our initial 94 studies (62 percent) (Fig. 2-5). Tracheal stenosis was found both at the tracheostomy site and at the site of the balloon cuff (Fig. 2-6). Tracheomalacia, occurring in 35 percent of our patients was the second most common finding. This was found more frequently at the site of the balloon cuff, although occasionally it was evident at a previous tracheostomy site. The overexpanded balloon cuff of an endotracheal tube or a tracheostomy tube causes a pressure necrosis of the tracheal wall with subsequent destruction of the cartilaginous rings. This insult is frequently

Table 2-3
Findings (initial 94 studies)

Normal		9
Tracheal stenosis		58
Minimal	21	
Moderate	24	
Marked	13	
Tracheomalacia		33
Minimal	20	
Moderate	10	
Marked	3	
Tracheal stenosis and tracheomalacia		21
Glottic involvement		25
Granulation tissue		9
Other		15

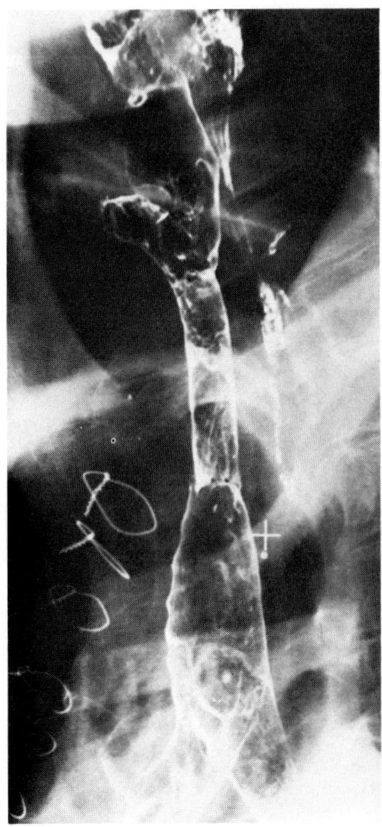

Fig. 2-5. *Acquired Tracheal Stenosis.* A 20-year-old white male with moderate dyspnea on exertion two months after cardiac surgery complicated by postoperative tracheostomy. The oblique tantalum tracheogram shows a long remarkably uniform segment of tracheal stenosis in the mid trachea.

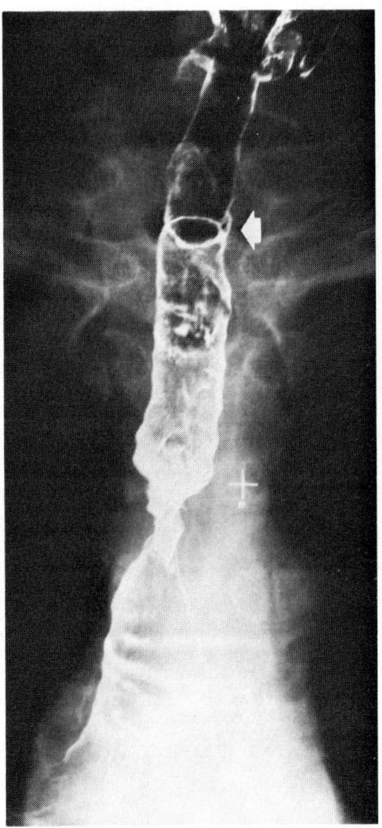

Fig. 2-6. *Multifocal Tracheal Stenosis.* A 59-year-old black female had moderate dyspnea three months after abdominal surgery. The postoperative course was complicated by aspiration pneumonia requiring endotracheal tube intubation and a tracheostomy. Two areas of tracheal stenosis are seen on the P-A tantalum tracheogram: Minimal tracheal stenosis at the site of previous tracheostomy (arrow) and marked tracheal stenosis in the lower trachea, presumably due to an overexpanded balloon cuff or endotracheal tube tip.

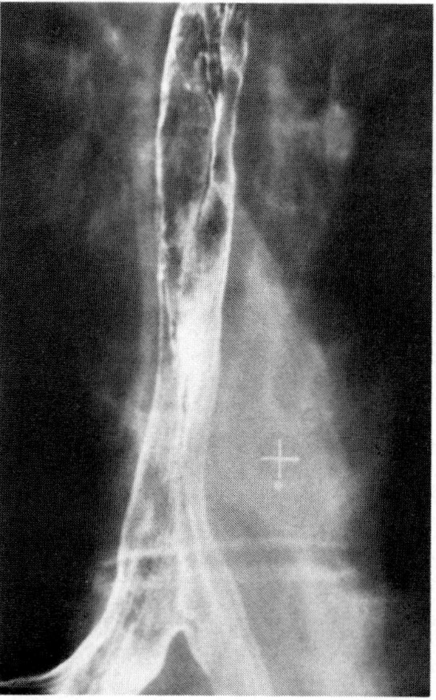

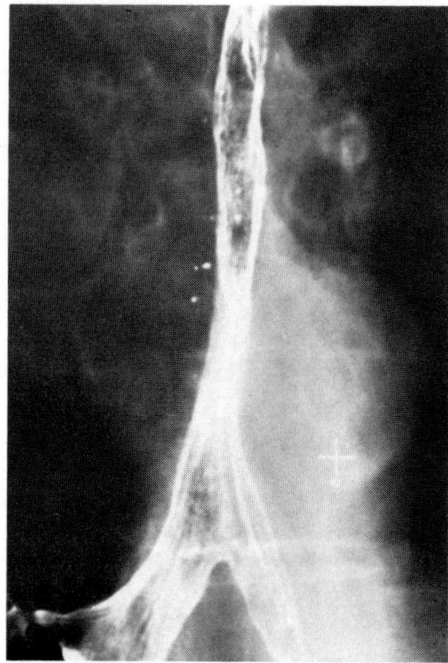

Fig. 2-7. *Tracheomalacia.* A 63-year-old white male had moderate dyspnea on exertion, three months after mediastinal irradiation for an oat cell carcinoma. P-A spot radiographs done in inspiration (left) and expiration (right) showed marked tracheomalacia.

compounded by superimposed infection and friction associated with mechanical respiration. We believe that this focal area of weakened trachea is as aerodynamically significant as a fixed tracheal stenosis. It should be distinguished from the minimal mobility of the lateral and anterior walls of the trachea in patients with chronic obstructive pulmonary disease and should be distinguished from the normal movement of the posterior membrane. Severe tracheomalacia can be recognized by spot filming in forced inspiration and forced expiration (Fig. 2-7); or if the malacic segment is located in the upper trachea by flexing and extending the neck. A cine recording is frequently necessary to recognize moderate and minimal degrees of tracheomalacia (Fig. 2-8). Reliance on a few spot radiographs done in deep inspiration and deep expiration may not give the true extent of disease when compared to a complete cine recording of many respiratory cycles done with different respiratory maneuvers. We do not use coughing as part of our evaluation, since the trachea may collapse 50 percent or more in patients with chronic obstructive pulmonary disease.[33,34]

Twenty-seven percent of our patients had vocal cord or other laryngeal injuries (Fig. 2-9). The larynx is frequently overlooked as a cause of upper airway obstruction and should be carefully studied in all patients with dyspnea. Usually a patient will have endotracheal tube intubation for two or three days and then assisted respiration through a tracheostomy tube for a longer time. With decannulation of the tracheostomy tube and the subse-

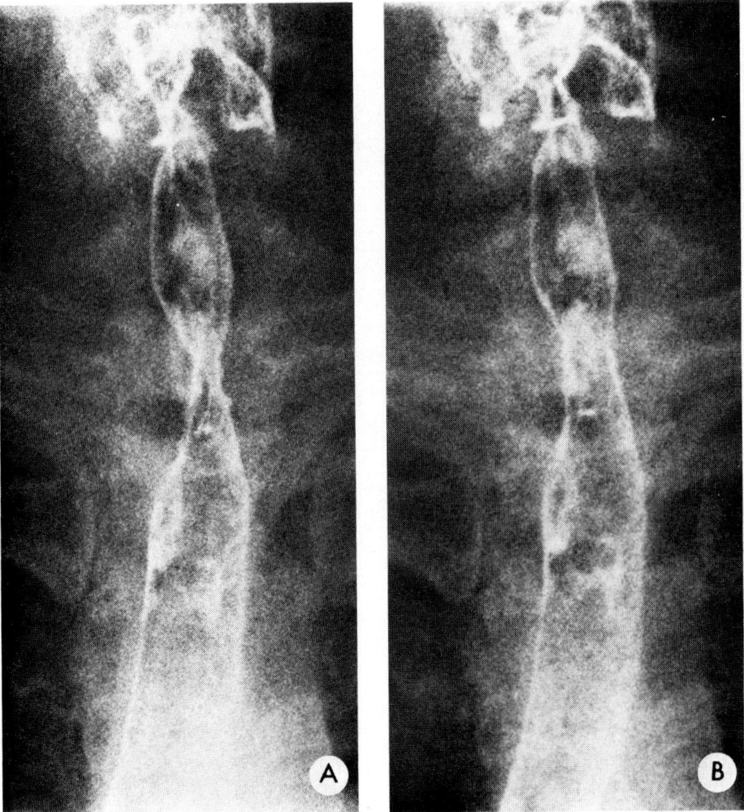

Fig. 2-8. *Tracheomalacia.* A 32-year-old black female with mild dyspnea on exertion. Three months earlier a tracheostomy had been performed for respiratory support after a drug overdose. Cine recordings in inspiration (A) and expiration (B) show moderate extrathoracic tracheomalacia at the site of previous tracheostomy.

quent development of respiratory distress, often the previous endotracheal intubation and possible damage to the glottis are forgotten.

Once the stenotic or malacic segment has been confirmed as the cause of the patient's dyspnea, surgical resection is the procedure of choice. The exact length, location, and degree of tracheal obstruction are important to the surgeon, who has the option of freeing the trachea at the larynx, or, if more length is necessary for the reanastomosis, entering the mediastinum and mobilizing the lower trachea and main stem bronchi. Accurate morphologic detail and a reliable physiologic assessment are obtained easily and safely with the tantalum study. Measurements provided by the tantalum tracheogram have proved exceptionally accurate when compared to the surgical specimen. In our institution the tantalum cine laryngotracheogram has become the major, and often the only, diagnostic procedure in evaluating

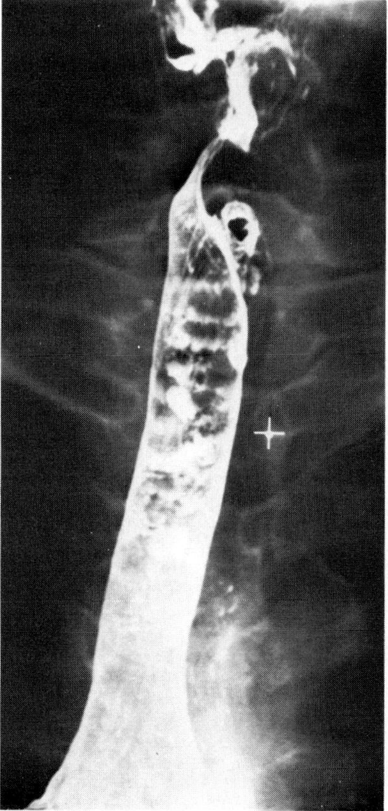

Fig. 2-9. *Transglottic Stenosis.* A 40-year-old white female who sustained head trauma three months earlier. The patient required several weeks of assisted respiration with an endotracheal tube and a tracheostomy. Attempts to decannulate the patient were unsuccessful. The tantalum study shows marked transglottic stenosis.

these patients, replacing the standard work-up of mediastinal tomography and bronchoscopy.

Complications of Tantalum Tracheography

There have been no serious or fatal reactions in our experience. Five patients had minor complications resulting from the procedure.

Three patients have retained a small amount of tantalum in the lung parenchyma. Two patients have retained tantalum powder because higher than necessary insufflating pressures were used and the tip of the catheter was not localized accurately. Follow-up at 3 and 6 years, respectively, in each of these two patients has shown no toxic effects from this minimal amount of retained tantalum. A third patient probably coughed or aspirated tantalum-coated mucus into the peripheral non-ciliated airways. In this patient no toxic effect has been demonstrated in a one-year follow-up.

Two patients developed mucus plugs in a main stem bronchus the evening following the tantalum tracheogram. Both of these responded to routine suction procedures. Presumably the fasting prior to the procedure, the atropine, and the tantalum, or a combination of these factors increased the viscosity of the tracheobronchial secretions, thus causing the mucous plugs.

CINE LARYNGOTRACHEOGRAPHY IN THE PEDIATRIC PATIENT

Technique

Older children, after sedation, can occasionally be studied with topical anesthesia. The methods employed for studying an infant vary considerably from the adult patient. Close cooperation between the radiologist and the pediatric anesthesiologist is mandatory. The infant is kept NPO for at least 6 hours. Intravenous infusion of 5 percent dextrose in 0.2 normal saline is started and delivered slowly. Thorough atropinization is also necessary in the pediatric age group. The doses given are generally greater than those used for other endoscopic procedures. Three doses of atropine are given at 30-minute intervals. Each dose consists of 0.03 mg/kg. The last dose is given 5 minutes before the procedure. The first two doses are administered intramuscularly; the last, intravenously. As in the adult population, four scout films are obtained. After study of the scout films, an appropriate endotracheal tube is selected. The child is then temporarily paralyzed with a small intravenous dose of Succinylcholine 0.5 mg per kg. The endotracheal tube is inserted, and the child is ventilated with 100 percent oxygen. After 60–90 seconds of assisted ventilation, a radiopaque angiography catheter (2.7 mm in diameter[35]) is inserted through the endotracheal tube and positioned immediately above the carina. The insufflating pressure is adjusted so that only a small amount of tantalum exits from the catheter tip. As the child resumes spontaneous respiration, the tantalum is insufflated under careful fluoroscopic control as the endotracheal tube and catheter are slowly withdrawn over a period of 15 to 30 seconds. Spot radiographs are obtained in the P-A, lateral, and both oblique projections. Then a cine recording in the same four projections is obtained. Careful monitoring of the child's vital signs is mandatory during and after the procedure. As infants may clear the tantalum powder within a few minutes, occasionally the temporary paralysis, intubation, and insufflation may have to be repeated.

Table 2-4
Children with Upper Airway Obstruction

Patient	Presumptive Diagnosis	Diagnosis after Tantalum Study
3 mo WM	Subglottic hemangioma	Tracheomalacia
9 yr WF	Tracheo-esophageal fistula	Tracheal stenosis
13 mo WM	Tracheal stenosis	Tracheomalacia
9 mo BM	Uncertain	Tracheomalacia
4 mo WM	Uncertain	Tracheomalacia
2 yr WF	Tracheomalacia	Established presumptive diagnosis
7 mo WM	Tracheomalacia	Established presumptive diagnosis

Results

We have performed 20 tantalum cine laryngotracheograms in 16 pediatric patients. Four examinations were repeated solely to evaluate surgical correction. The patients ranged in age from 3 months to 11 years. Seven patients initially had upper airway obstruction. The tantalum tracheogram established the diagnosis in all seven. In three of these patients, the tantalum tracheogram changed the presumptive diagnosis, which had been made on the basis of history and physical examination, high kVp films and often laryngoscopy and bronchoscopy (Table 2-4, Fig. 2-10). The other nine patients were studied because of an inability to decannulate the child after tracheostomy tube placement. Again the tantalum tracheogram established the etiology of the upper airway obstruction in all nine. In four of these patients the tantalum tracheogram changed the presumptive diagnosis (Table 2-5, Fig. 2-11).

Before we began using the experimental contrast agent tantalum powder, establishing a precise diagnosis in infants and children with upper airway obstruction was frequently difficult and hazardous. Two of the patients

Table 2-5
Children Presenting with Decannulation Problems

Patient	Presumptive Diagnosis	Diagnosis after Tantalum Study
19 mo WF	Tracheal stenosis and tracheomalacia	Granuloma ball
1 yr WF	Subglottic cyst	Normal
3 yr WF	Tracheomalacia	Tracheal stenosis
4 yr WM	Tracheal stenosis	Tracheomalacia
2 yr WF	Uncertain	Granuloma ball and tracheomalacia
2 yr BF	Granuloma ball	2 Granuloma balls
4 yr BM	Tracheal stenosis	Established presumptive diagnosis
11 yr BM	Tracheal stenosis	Established presumptive diagnosis
11 yr WF	Tracheal stenosis	Established presumptive diagnosis

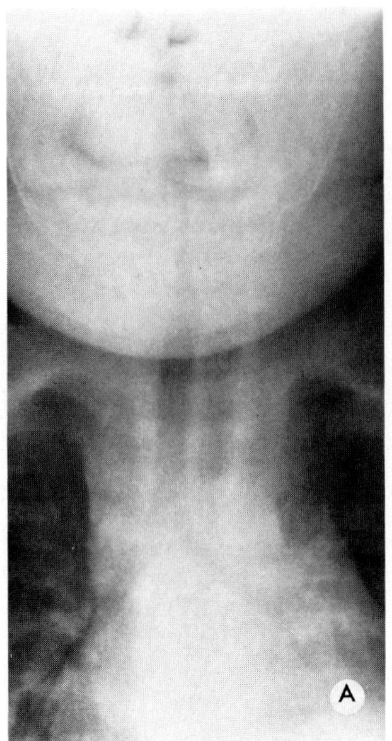

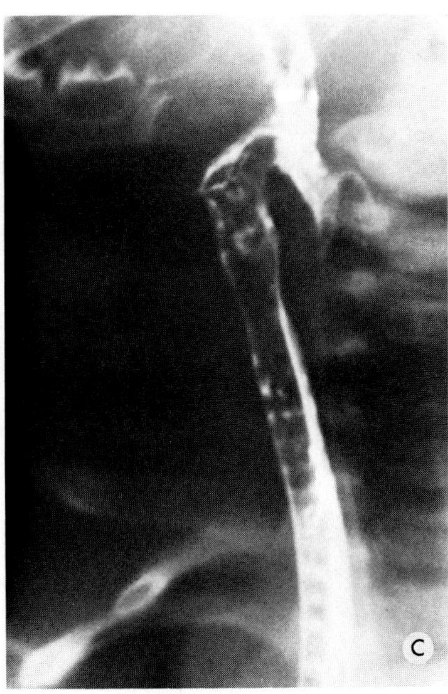

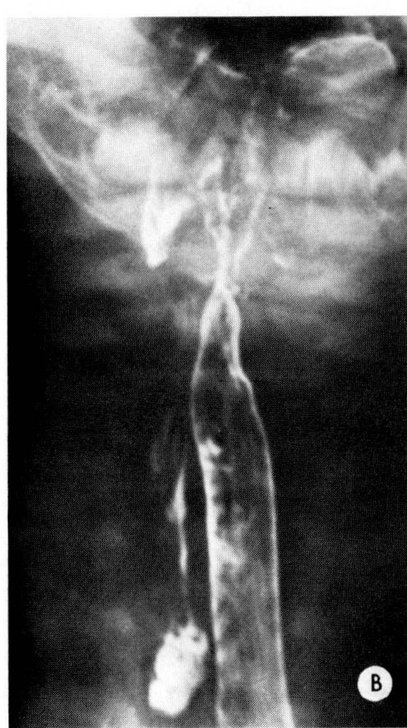

Fig. 2-10. *Normal Study in Suspected Upper Airway Obstruction.* A 3½-month-old white male with stridor since birth. Hemangiomata were present on the scrotum and buttocks. (A) High kVp films of the neck suggested a subglottic hemangioma. Tantalum tracheography done after a preliminary inspection of the subglottic area shows the upper trachea to be normal with normal kinking and tracheomalacia in the subglottic area; (B) P-A view; (C) Lateral view.

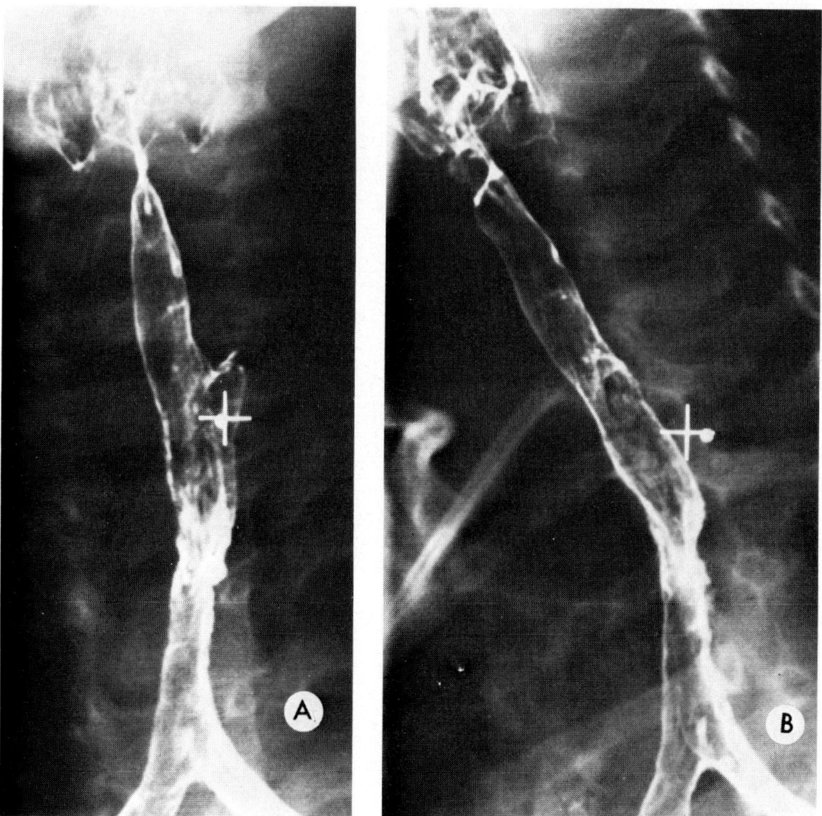

Fig. 2-11. *Tracheal stenosis*. A 3-year-old white female who had repeated tracheostomies for respiratory failure with recurrent pneumonias. Attempts at decannulation were unsuccessful. The working diagnosis after endoscopy was tracheomalacia. Tantalum tracheography demonstrated tracheal stenosis in the lower trachea. No evidence of tracheomalacia was demonstrated on the cine study. (A) P-A view; (B) Oblique view.

had previously been evaluated by Dionosil tracheography. During the Dionosil studies, one child suffered a cardiopulmonary arrest, and the other child developed a chemical pneumonia.

Complications

In the 16 patients, the only complication was a small amount of retained tantalum in the pulmonary parenchyma of one child. Follow-up of this child at one year showed no untoward effects. A few infants developed a one-degree temperature elevation after the study. This was probably related to the atropine. No specific therapy was required, and the temperature returned to normal within 8 hours after the study. Anterior-posterior and lateral chest radiographs done 24 hours after the study showed no evidence of pneumonia in any child and complete clearance of the tantalum powder in all but one child.

TANTALUM BRONCHOGRAPHY

Early squamous bronchogenic carcinomas may shed malignant cells into the sputum years before they become radiologically apparent.[36] Prompt and accurate localization of these very early malignancies for the surgeon is mandatory. Fiberoptic bronchoscopy in a patient with a positive cytology and a negative chest radiograph is a long and tedious procedure. Meticulous search of all lobes, segments, and subsegments with repeated washings and brushings usually requires two or three hours. Even if a lesion is located early in the search, it is desirable to examine for a second cancer. Tantalum bronchography does not establish a tissue diagnosis, but it does allow the bronchoscopist, when confronted with a patient with a positive cytology and a negative chest radiograph, to concentrate his efforts on an area or areas of suspicion. The time of bronchoscopic search for radiologically occult malignancy can be significantly shortened by careful evaluation of the tantalum bronchogram and subsequent clearance films.

Results

Tantalum bronchography has been used to localize these early lesions by identifying morphologic abnormalities on the initial bronchogram and abnormal bronchial dynamics on the cine study, and by delayed clearance on serial daily radiographs. We have studied nine patients with radiologically occult bronchogenic carcinoma. In these nine patients, eleven bronchogenic carcinomas have been documented. Four were localized by delayed clearance, three by delayed clearance and morphologic abnormalities, two by morphologic abnormalities alone, and one by a dynamic abnormality on the cine study (Fig. 2-12).

Delayed clearance is the major, and frequently the only, way the small early lung cancers were localized. Delayed clearance from airway malignancies has been described in a number of publications.[37–39] Tantalum powder is cleared solely by mucociliary action, therefore, early bronchogenic carcinomas, which interrupt mucociliary flow, demonstrate delayed clearance. Many other factors beside bronchogenic carcinoma alter mucociliary clearance. These include: (1) impaired ciliary function and altered mucus secretion, (2) obstruction, (3) trauma, (4) local inflammation, and (5) pharmacologic agents.

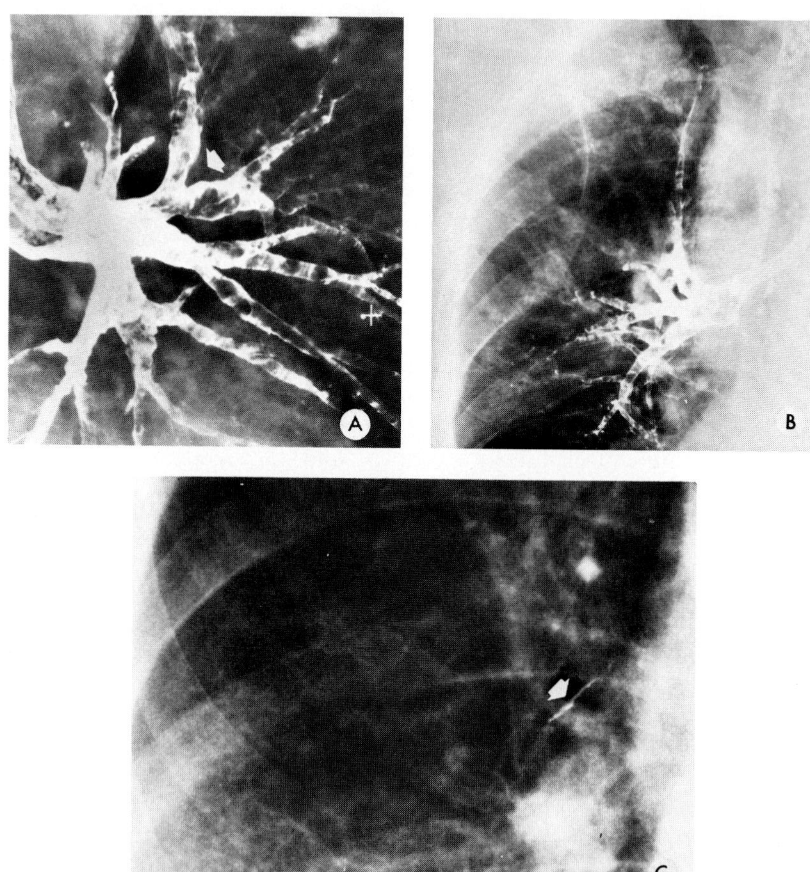

Fig. 2-12. *Tantalum bronchography for the localization of radiologically occult cancer.* A 67-year-old white male had a positive sputum cytology. His chest radiograph and full chest tomography showed no evidence of bronchogenic carcinoma. (A) Tantalum bronchogram of the left lung (oblique view) shows thickening of the left upper lobe spur (arrow). Cine study demonstrated abnormal dynamics of the inferior portion of the lingula. Both sites were confirmed as bronchogenic carcinoma; (B) Selective right upper lobe bronchogram in the same patient. No morphologic or dynamic abnormalities are demonstrated; (C) Coned down view of the right upper lobe 48 hours later shows linear delayed clearance characteristic of a bronchogenic carcinoma (arrow). The presence of carcinoma at this third site was also confirmed at bronchoscopy.

MUCOCILIARY CLEARANCE AND ALTERED MUCUS SECRETION

In carcinoma in situ there is a small, sharply defined contiguous area where cilia disappear and airway secretions are altered. When this area becomes large enough, prolonged retention of a surface material such as tantalum will occur. Bronchiectasis, which destroys a large contiguous area of epithelium, has also been shown to exhibit delayed clearance.[38] Bronchiectasis, however, can be easily differentiated from an early bronchogenic carcinoma by the bronchial dilatation on the initial tantalum bronchogram. The mucosal destruction in bronchitis is often spotty, ill-defined, and noncoalescent. Clearance from focal areas of bronchitis occasionally can be delayed, but usually it is normal. These very small areas do not appear to alter mucociliary clearance. The tantalum is probably removed by adjacent mucous streams.

OBSTRUCTION

Partial obstruction of the airways due to non-malignant causes is frequently associated with a delay in mucociliary clearance. The tantalum powder delivered distal to the narrowing is cleared slowly. This form of delayed clearance is usually seen as tantalum-coated mucus distal to the obstruction. The fine, linear area of delayed clearance caused by early bronchogenic carcinoma is easily differentiated from the tantalum-coated mucus. To evaluate further the role of obstruction in delayed clearance by carcinoma, we compared the clearance in a patient with subglottic carcinoma of the trachea, to that of a patient with a similar degree of obstruction due to tracheal stenosis. The carcinoma of the trachea shows no significant clearance at 6 hours, whereas the surrounding normal mucosa has completely cleared the powder. In the patient with subglottic tracheal stenosis there is minimal retained tantalum. This retained tantalum is primarily tantalum-coated mucus distal to the tracheal stenosis (Fig. 2-13).

TRAUMA

Wood's observations,[40] indicated that trauma produced by catheter techniques can significantly alter mucociliary clearance of tantalum in dogs. All of our patients are studied without prior localization of their cancer. Subsequently, trauma from catheter repositioning to ensure a complete bilateral bronchogram was performed in all of these patients. The trauma therefore was presumably identical in all regions of the major bronchi.

LOCAL INFLAMMATION

Pneumonia has been shown to alter mucociliary clearance significantly.[31] We feel that infection was not a cause of delayed mucociliary clearance in our patients. None had radiologic or clinical evidence of pneumonia before the procedure or in the subsequent follow-up. The delayed

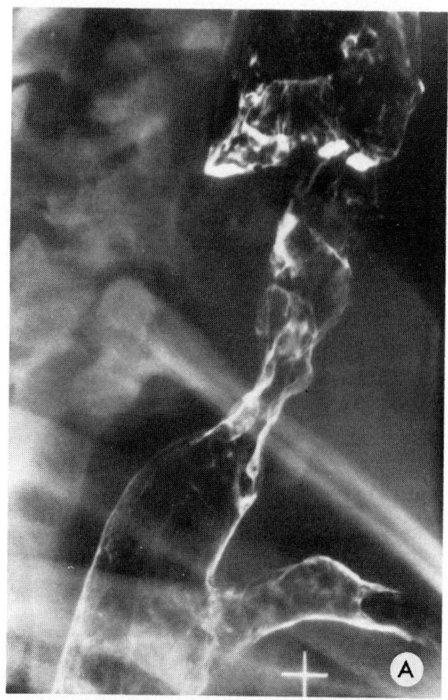

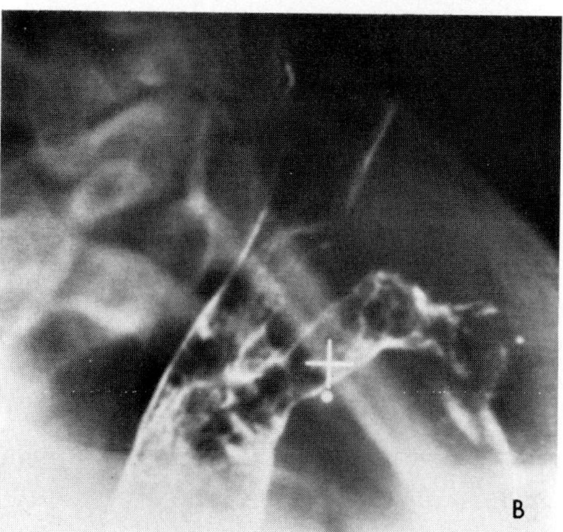

Fig. 2-13. Comparison of delayed clearance due to carcinoma versus mechanical obstruction. (A) Oblique tantalum tracheogram in patient with carcinoma of the upper trachea; (B) Oblique tantalum tracheogram in another patient with stenosis of the upper trachea due to a previous tracheostomy; (C) Six hour lateral clearance film shows marked retained tantalum which is delineating the mucosal extent of this carcinoma; (D) Six hour lateral clearance film shows only a few small flecks of tantalum-coated mucus distal to the partial obstruction. (Reprinted with permission from: Stitik FP, Proctor DF: Delayed Clearance of Tantalum by Radiologically Occult Cancer. *Ann Otol Rhinol Laryngol* 84:589–595, 1975.)

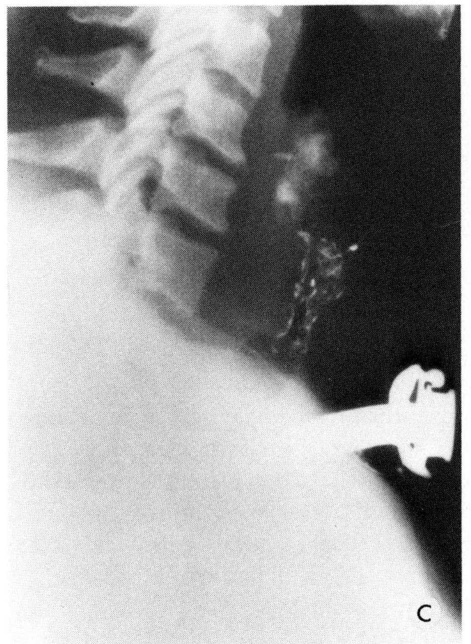

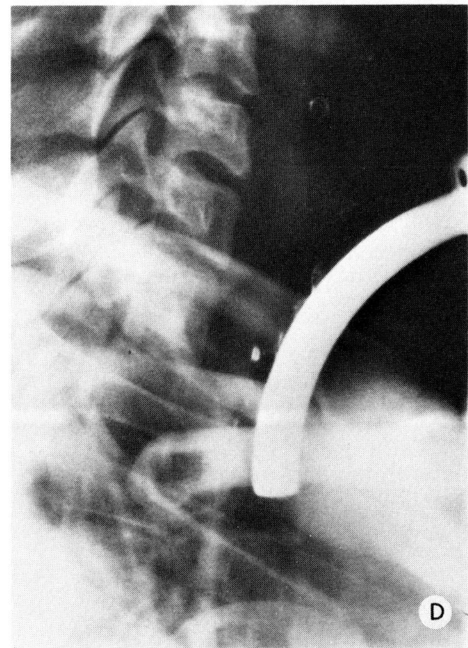

Figs. 2-13C and D.

clearance demonstrated with pneumonia is an "alveolarization" of the contrast material rather than a focal linear area of delayed clearance caused by the destroyed mucociliary epithelium.

PHARMACOLOGIC AGENTS

Pharmacologic agents play a role in slowing the mucociliary clearance. These agents, however, should have a diffuse effect and should not cause the focal delayed clearance as shown by our patients.

SUMMARY

Bronchography with the conventional contrast agent Dionosil is being used less frequently in current medical practice. Dionosil bronchography still has a place in the infrequent situation of localized bronchiectasis severe enough to consider resection, select patients presenting with hemoptysis, chronic right middle lobe atelectasis in children, congenital abnormalities, and in delineating bronchopleural fistula. Although we have tantalum available, we believe that liquid Dionosil is the contrast agent of choice in studying these patients.

Tantalum bronchography can effectively localize radiologically occult cancer in the patient with a positive cytology and a negative chest radiograph. The value of sputum cytology as a screening procedure in the detection of early squamous cell carcinoma has been documented.[41–43] As more centers employ sputum cytology as a routine screening procedure in patients with a high risk of developing lung cancer, more patients will be discovered in this early stage, before the radiograph shows the site of the lesion. In this situation, careful evaluation of the tantalum bronchogram and subsequent clearance films will significantly reduce the time necessary for bronchoscopic localization and confirmation.

The value of tantalum tracheography in children and adults has been stressed in a number of publications.[44–47] When properly performed, tantalum cine laryngotracheography is a safe, simple technique. It gives a highly accurate morphologic and physiologic assessment of the trachea and larynx. When tantalum is released by the U.S. Food and Drug Administration, we believe it will be the major, and frequently the only, diagnostic test in evaluating patients with upper airway obstruction.

REFERENCES

1. Sanderson JM, Kennedy MCS, Johnson MF, et al: Bronchiectasis: Results of surgical and conservative management. A review of 393 cases. Thorax 29:407–416, 1974
2. Nelson SW, Christoforidis A: Reversible bronchiectasis. Radiology 71:375–382, 1958

3. American College of Chest Physicians: Bronchography. Dis Chest 51:663–668, 1967
4. Forrest JV, Sagel SS, Omell GH: Bronchography in patients with hemoptysis. Am J Roentgenol 126:597–600, 1976
5. Freimanis AK, Molnar W: Chronic bronchitis and emphysema at bronchography. Radiology 74:194–205, 1960
6. Gudbjerg CE: Bonchiectasis. Radiological diagnosis and prognosis after operative treatment. Acta Radiol [Diagn] (Stockh) 143:11–20, 1957
7. Billig DM, Darling DB: Middle lobe atelectasis in children. Clinical and bronchographic criteria in the selection of patients for surgery. Am J Dis Child 123:96–98, 1972
8. Rinker CT, Garrotto LJ, Lee KR, et al: Bronchography. Diagnostic signs and accuracy in pulmonary carcinoma. Am J Roentgenol 104:802–807, 1968
9. Wong P: Personal Communication, 1978
10. Genoe GA: Diagnosis of bronchogenic carcinoma by means of bronchial brushing combined with bronchography. Am J Roentgenol 120:139–144, 1974
11. Nadel JA, Wolfe WG, Graf PD: Powdered tantalum as a medium for bronchography in canine and human lungs. Invest Radiol 3:229–238, 1968
12. Light JP, Oster WF: A study of clinical and pathologic reaction to the bronchographic agent hytrast. Am J Roentgenol 92:615–622, 1964
13. Light JP, Oster WF: Clinical and pathological reactions to bronchographic agent Dionosil aqueous. Am J Roentgenol 98:468–473, 1966
14. Scadding JG: Acute iodism following lipiodol bronchography. Br Med J 2:1147–1148, 1934
15. Summer J, Lichter AI, Nassau E: Fatal acute iodism after bronchography. Thorax 6:193–199, 1951
16. Mahon GS: Reaction following bronchography with iodized oil. JAMA 130:194–197, 1946
17. Pentogalos GH, Avgoustiniatos JE: Middle lobe syndrome following pneumonitis due to retention of contrast material. Ohio State Med J 64:928–932, 1968
18. Bjork L, Lodin H: Pulmonary changes following bronchography with Dionosil oily (animal experiments). Acta Radiol [Diagn] (Stockh) 47:177–180, 1957
19. Teates CD, Hunter JG: Unusual retention of iodized oil. Am J Roentgenol 109:562–564, 1971
20. Weibel ER: Morphometry of the human lung. New York, Academic Press, 1963, p. 139
21. Christoforidis AJ, Nelson SW, Tomashefski JF: Effects of bronchography on pulmonary function. Am Rev Respir Dis 85:127–129, 1962
22. Bhargava RK, Woolf CR: Changes in diffusing capacity after bronchography. Am Rev Respir Dis 96:827–829, 1967
23. Victh RG, Tindall GT, Odem GD: The use of tantalum dust as an adjunct in the post-operative management of subdural hematomas. J Neurosurg 24:514–519, 1966
24. Sax NI: Dangerous Properties of Industrial Materials, 2d ed. New York, Reinhold, 1963
25. Cochran KW, Doull J, Mazur M, et al: Acute toxicity of zirconium, columbium, strontium, lanthanum, cesium, tantalum, and yttrium. Arch Indust Hyg (Chicago) 1:637–650, 1950
26. Schepers GWH: The biological action of tantalum oxide: Studies on experi-

mental pulmonary histopathology. Arch Indust Health (Chicago) 12:121–123, 1955
27. Nadel JA, Wolfe WG, Graf PD, et al: Powdered tantalum: A new contrast medium for roentgenographic examination of human airways. N Engl J Med 283:281–286, 1970
28. Edmunds LH, Graf PD, Sagel SS, Greenspan RH: Radiographic observations of clearance of tantalum and barium sulfate particles from airways. Invest Radiol 5:131–141, 1970
29. Upham T, Graham LS, Steckel RJ, et al: Determination of in vivo persistence of tantalum dust following bronchography using reactor-activated tantalum and total body counting. Am J Roentgenol 3:690–694, 1971
30. Morrow PE, Klipper RW, Beiter EH, Gibb FR: Pulmonary retention and translocation of insufflated tantalum. Radiology 121:415–421, 1976
31. Friedman PJ, Tisi GM: "Alveolarization" of tantalum powder in experimental bronchography and the clearance of inhaled particles from the lung. Radiology 104:523–535, 1972
32. Dodds WJ, Goldberg HI, Kohatsu S, et al: Insufflation of tantalum powder into the stomach, new approach to gastrography. Invest Radiol 5:30–34, 1970
33. Rayl JE: Tracheobronchial collapse during cough. Radiology 85:87–92, 1965
34. Hodges FJ, Whitehouse WM, Kittleson AC, et al: Video tape recording of tracheobronchial dynamics. Am J Roentgenol 96:944–946, 1966
35. Heller RM, Galvis AG, Oh KS: Angiographic catheters for tracheobronchial procedures in infants and children. Radiology 106:702–703, 1973
36. Carbone PP, Frost JK, Feinstein AR, et al: Lung cancer; perspectives and prospects. Ann Intern Med 73:1003–1024, 1970
37. Stitik FP, Proctor DF: Delayed clearance of tantalum by radiologically occult cancer. Ann Otol Rhinol Laryngol 84:589–595, 1975
38. Gamsu G, Weintraub RM, Nadel JA: Clearance of tantalum from airways of different caliber in man evaluated by a roentgenographic method. Am Rev Respir Dis 107:214–224, 1973
39. Gamsu G, Nadel JA: New technique for roentgenographic study of airways and lungs using powdered tantalum. Cancer 30:1353–1357, 1972
40. Wood PB, Nagy E, Pearson FG, et al: Measurement of mucociliary clearance from the lower respiratory tract of normal dogs. Can Anaesth Soc J 20:192–206, 1973
41. Baker RR, Marsh BR, Frost JK, et al: The detection and treatment of early lung cancer. Ann Surg 179:813–818, 1974
42. Melamed M, Flehinger B, Miller D, et al: Preliminary report of the lung cancer detection program in New York. Cancer 39:369–382, 1977
43. Fontana RS, Sanderson DR, Miller E, et al: The Mayo Lung Project: Preliminary report of "early cancer detection" phase. Cancer 30:1373–1382, 1972
44. Gamsu G, Platzker A, Gregory G, et al: Powdered tantalum as a contrast agent for tracheobronchography in the pediatric patient. Radiology 107:151–157, 1973
45. Hinchcliffe WA, Zamel N, Fishman NH, et al: Roentgenographic study of the human trachea with powdered tantalum. Radiology 97:327–330, 1970
46. Stitik FP, Proctor DF: Tracheography with the experimental contrast agent tantalum. Ann Otol Rhinol Laryngol 82:838–843, 1973
47. Stitik FP, Bartelt D, James AE, et al: Tantalum tracheography in upper airway obstruction: 100 experiences in adults. Am J Roentgenol 130:35–41, 1978

Philip O. Alderson, M.D.

3

The Role of Radionuclide Studies in the Diagnosis of Pulmonary Disease

Radionuclide studies aid diagnosis of pulmonary diseases by providing information about regional pulmonary ventilation, perfusion, and ventilation–perfusion (V–P) balance which cannot be obtained by other methods. This chapter will review the advantages and limitations of these techniques.

RADIONUCLIDE STUDIES

Perfusion

Pulmonary perfusion is usually assessed following the intravenous injection of radio-labeled particles. The most commonly used radio-pharmaceuticals for assessing perfusion are ^{99m}Tc-labeled macroaggregates of albumin (MAA) or human albumin microspheres (HAM). The physical characteristics of several pulmonary perfusion tracers are given in Table 3-1. Technetium-99m-labeled particles lodge in the pulmonary arterioles or capillaries, and allow the *relative* distribution of pulmonary perfusion to be assessed by imaging. The particles are biodegraded but remain in the lung with a half-life of 6 hours (MAA) to 8 hours (HAM).[1]

Perfusion lung scanning is usually a safe procedure, but several deaths have been attributed to the injection of lung-scanning particles.[2,3] Since pulmonary perfusion imaging is actually a form of iatrogenic microembolism, one should be aware of the safety margins that exist. If a standard lung-imaging dose of 500,000–600,000 labeled particles of MAA (diameter 10–60 microns) is injected, approximately 1:1000 pulmonary vessels will be temporarily blocked.[4] This results in no subjective discomfort or pulmonary

Table 3-1
Properties of Perfusion Lung Imaging Agents

Agent	Physical Half-life	Principle Photon Energy (keV)	Particle Size (microns)
^{99m}Tc-MAA	6 hr	140	10–60
^{99m}Tc-HAM	6 hr	140	10–30
^{133}Xe-in-saline	5.2 days	80	—
^{81m}Kr-in-dextrose	13 sec	190	—

function abnormalities in normal patients or in those with most respiratory diseases.[5] However, if pulmonary hypertension is present the internal diameter of the pulmonary vessels may be reduced. Therefore, the vascular blockade that occurs after injection of the particles will occur more proximally, and the safety factor will be markedly reduced. Therefore a reduction in the number of injected particles is suggested when imaging critically ill patients or patients who may have pulmonary hypertension. Heck and Duley[6] have shown that only about 50,000 particles are needed to give a statistically valid perfusion image. It is difficult, in practice, to determine the exact number of particles injected, as some remain in the hub of the needle after injecting. Therefore, when it is desirable to reduce the number of particles injected, it is wise to begin with about 100,000 particles in the syringe. The same considerations apply to perfusion images performed in infants and neonates. Davies[7] has shown that the number of arteriole and capillary vessels is markedly reduced in infants and neonates and that the internal diameter of the vessels that are present is small. Therefore, the number of injected particles should be kept low when performing perfusion imaging in young children. Alternatively, perfusion lung imaging can be performed using nonparticulate agents like ^{133}Xe-saline or ^{81m}Kr-in-dextrose (Table 3-1).

For many years a four-view perfusion imaging series was considered a complete examination. Recent evidence[8–10] suggests that oblique views provide additional information and should be included as part of the examination. Caride et al.[8] showed that significantly more perfusion defects are seen when the left and right posterior oblique views (LPO, RPO) are added to the four standard views (i.e., anterior, posterior, and both laterals). Neilsen et al.[9] have demonstrated that the posterior oblique views provide additional information in roughly 50 percent of cases, whereas anterior oblique views are helpful in about 15 percent of cases. Animal studies of experimental pulmonary embolism[10] support the conclusions of these clinical studies. Six percent of angiographically proven emboli were seen *only* in oblique views. The oblique views were especially helpful when the emboli involved the lateral segments of the lower lobes (Fig. 3-1). Based on the above information, oblique views are now recommended as a routine part of the perfusion lung scan. The posterior oblique views are more helpful than

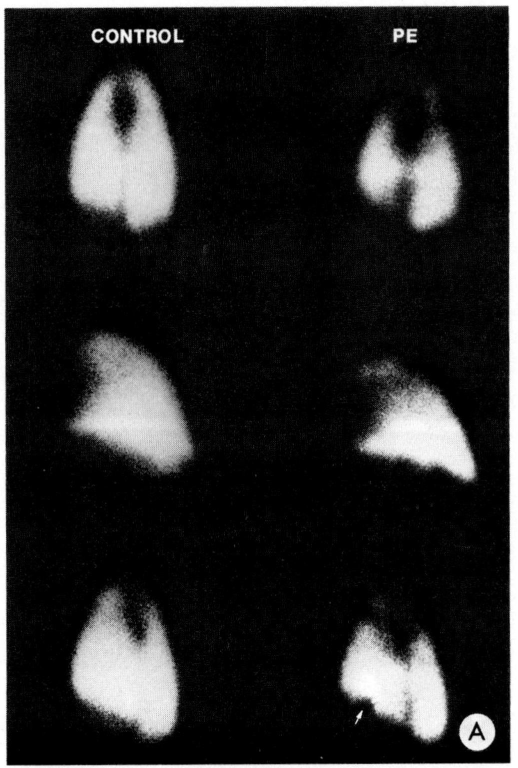

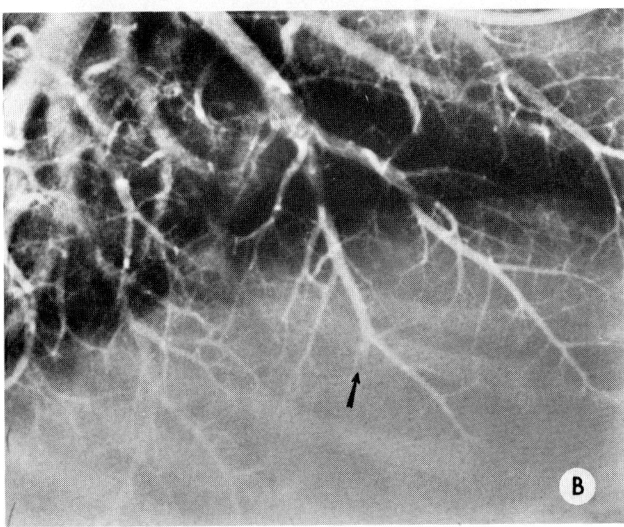

Fig. 3-1. Control and immediate post-embolism perfusion images in a dog with experimentally induced pulmonary emboli are shown. Note the perfusion defect in the lateral segment of the left lower lobe, visualized clearly only in the LPO view. The selective pulmonary angiogram confirms a small, peripheral embolus.

anterior oblique views (in which the heart may cause interpretive problems) and, since more pulmonary emboli are found in the lower lobes, only the posterior oblique views are obtained routinely. A routine perfusion lung scan thus consists of six views—the anterior, posterior, the laterals, and left and right posterior obliques.

Until recently, a diverging collimator was necessary to obtain simultaneous views of both lungs during perfusion imaging. Now the large-field-of-view scintillation camera allows lung imaging to be performed with a high-resolution, parallel-hole collimator. This helps minimize any field distortion that might have been present when imaging in the diverging mode. This improvement, plus the addition of the oblique views, promises to increase even further the ability of perfusion lung imaging to detect perfusion abnormalities in the lung.

Ventilation

There have been two basic approaches to obtaining information about airways disease in man by using radionuclides. One approach involves the inhalation of aerosol particles labeled with a suitable radioactive tracer, usually ^{99m}Tc. These radio-aerosols do not actually depict regional ventilation because most of the particles cannot diffuse freely throughout the lung; instead the majority of them are deposited by impaction or sedimentation on the bronchial mucosa (particles 1–10 microns in diameter) or by random contact with bronchial or alveolar walls during diffusion (particles less than 1 micron in diameter). The fate of the deposited radio-aerosols depends on the nature of the inhaled particles. An ionic aerosol of pertechnetate will be rapidly absorbed across the alveolar mucosa (pulmonary half-time 13 minutes),[11] while a nonabsorbable particulate like ^{99m}Tc-albumin will remain in the lung for much longer times (days to weeks), eventually undergoing mucociliary or lymphatic clearance.[12] In patients with normal airways the radio-aerosol is deposited in a diffuse, homogenous pattern which extends to the periphery of the lung. In disease associated with intrinsically abnormal airways (e.g., chronic bronchitis) the aerosol will tend to be deposited in clumps in larger central airways at sites of turbulent airflow. This pattern of focal central hot spots with decreased peripheral activity is not specific and can be caused by any endobronchial abnormality that results in turbulent airflow. When extrinsic bronchial obstruction is created experimentally, the aerosol is deposited centrally, but without the focal hot spots.[13] This pattern of central deposition without hot spots is also seen in radiation fibrosis[14] and is presumably due to peribronchial fibrosis. Inhalation studies with monodisperse aerosols should improve the clinical utility of this technique.

The predominant method of assessing ventilation in the lung is through imaging using a radioactive inert gas. Studies of this type were introduced by Knipping et al.[15] in 1955. The most widely used tracer since that time has been ^{133}Xe gas. This inert gas has a fairly long physical half-life (5.2 days) and an energy of 80 keV. This relatively low energy is disadvantageous, as the emitted photons undergo a good deal of scatter in the body, and scatter degrades image quality. The 80 keV energy is below that of the perfusion tracer ^{99m}Tc (140 keV). Therefore, most investigators have advocated that ventilation studies with ^{133}Xe precede perfusion lung imaging.

Xenon-133 studies are done with the patient either supine or seated upright in front of a gamma camera. The upright position is preferable, but supine studies are regularly performed in sick patients who cannot sit up. The patient breathes ^{133}Xe gas from a closed delivery system through a plastic mouthpiece. The patient may be asked to begin the study by performing a vital-capacity, single-breath inhalation followed by a breath-hold. The success of a single-breath study is effort-dependent, and the distribution of the tracer is greatly affected by the speed of inhalation and the volume of the lung at the beginning of the single breath.[16] Thus, one must attempt to have patients initiate the single breath from a similar starting volume (e.g., functional residual capacity) and to control the rate of inspiration. If the rate of inspiration can be kept steady and relatively slow (less than 0.5 L/min), the distribution of the tracer will largely reflect the regional mechanical properties of the lung (rather than airway resistance). This slow, steady inhalation comprises the inspiratory capacity test described by Milic-Emili[17] to provide information about regional pulmonary compliance in various diseases.

Following the single-breath study the patient is instructed to breathe at his usual rate and depth. The patient then breathes ^{133}Xe-in-air for several minutes (usually 4–6) from a closed system containing a CO_2 absorber in an attempt to reach "equilibrium" with the rebreathing spirometer. In fact, only normal patients are likely to attain a true equilibrium distribution of ^{133}Xe during this time. Most patients with obstructive pulmonary disease only approach equilibrium, but this approximation is used as the beginning point for the clearance phase. During the clearance phase of the study (washout) the patient breathes room air, and the expired ^{133}Xe is vented from the room or trapped in a charcoal-filled container. Xenon-133 has a physical half-life that is long relative to pulmonary clearance times, so areas of abnormally slow washout (regions of obstructive airways disease) are detected as regions of retained activity during the washout phase. This retention is evidence of two of the hallmarks of obstructive lung disease, uneven ventilation and slow ventilation.

Recently two other inert gas tracers, ^{127}Xe and ^{81m}Kr, have become available.[18–23] Their physical properties are compared with ^{133}Xe in Table 3-2. The energies of these newer gases exceed that of ^{99m}Tc, so ventilation imaging can be performed after the perfusion study. This allows the physician to preselect the view of greatest interest and maximize the yield of the ventilation study. The half-lives of these two new tracers differ markedly; ^{127}Xe has a 36.4-day half-life, whereas ^{81m}Kr has only a 13-second half-life. This leads to several important differences between the two tracers. First, ^{81m}Kr, which is produced from a 4.5-hour half-life ^{81}Rb generator system, must be used quickly. The 30+ day shelf-life of ^{127}Xe, however, means that it can be employed in facilities with a smaller patient load, as it does not

Table 3-2
Physical Properties of Inert Radioactive Gases

Agent	Physical Half-life	Principle Photon Energy (keV)
^{133}Xe	5.2 days	80
^{127}Xe	36.4 days	203, 172
^{81m}Kr	13 sec	190

need to be used rapidly. Second, the physiologic events depicted by the two tracers are different. Like ^{133}Xe, ^{127}Xe has a physical half-life that greatly exceeds the half-time for pulmonary clearance of the gas. Thus, regions of obstructive airway disease are detected as areas of retained activity during the clearance phase. On the other hand, ^{81m}Kr has a physical half-life so short that it literally decays to undetectable levels as the image of ventilation is being made. This rapid decay during ventilation results in an image that is a reflection of the regional distribution of tidal breathing. Abnormal areas must be detected by their lack of activity rather than by the retention of activity during the clearance phase.

Few comparative studies of these tracers have been performed to date. Schor et al.[21] performed ^{99m}Tc-perfusion lung images and both ^{81m}Kr and ^{133}Xe ventilation studies in 30 patients with suspected pulmonary embolism. The results were similar with the two tracers; however, the authors suggested that the abnormal retention of ^{133}Xe during the clearance phase was easier to detect than the absence of ^{81m}Kr in areas of mild obstructive airways disease. Similar ventilation studies with ^{127}Xe and ^{133}Xe demonstrate that the superior physical properties of ^{127}Xe are advantageous. Coates and Nahmias[22] examined the ability of these two tracers to detect voids of certain volumes in a lung phantom. Xenon-127 could detect a smaller void, whether the void was air-filled (to represent a bulla) or oil-filled (to represent lung-density tissue). Atkins et al.[23] used these two tracers in patients and found increased counting rates per mCi of administered activity with ^{127}Xe. They also demonstrated increased resolution with ^{127}Xe, especially during the clearance phase. These early experiences suggest that ^{127}Xe may increase the ability of ventilation studies to detect obstructive pulmonary disease, and ^{81m}Kr may improve detection of the V–P mismatch seen with pulmonary embolism. Further experience is needed to determine which of these tracers is best suited for a particular clinical use.

Ventilation–Perfusion Imaging

The nonspecificity of the defects seen in perfusion lung images has been recognized for several years.[24] Perfusion defects are commonly seen secondary to pulmonary emboli, in areas of parenchymal consolidation or compression, and in regions of obstructive pulmonary disease. The hypoperfusion in regions of airways disease occurs by reflex vasoconstriction of pulmonary vessels entering the hypoxic area and can be considered an attempt by the lung to retain normal ventilation–perfusion balance. The appearance of a perfusion defect does not indicate whether it is caused by emboli or airways disease. Approximately 80 percent of emboli appear as defects conforming to known bronchopulmonary segmental anatomy, but 20 percent are nonsegmental. Conversely, roughly 80 percent of defects secondary to airways disease are nonsegmental, with only 20 percent of defects appearing segmental.[25] The latter defects usually occur in areas of moderate-to-severe obstructive airways disease.

A combined ventilation–perfusion study provides information that allows the etiology of perfusion defects to be more clearly discerned. This is important, as obstructive pulmonary disease may be present in individuals who have normal chest radiographs. This has been demonstrated in a study[26] comparing the sensitivity of chest radiography and ventilation imaging for detecting obstructive pulmonary disease. In a double-blind analysis of the chest radiographs and ventilation studies, radiographs failed to reveal evidence of obstructive pulmonary disease in 35 of 76 patients (46 percent). The pulmonary function test results in 24 patients who had ^{133}Xe ventilation studies, chest radiographs, and routine spirometry are given in Table 3-3. These results demonstrate that the patients with obstructive lung disease detected by ^{133}Xe but not by chest radiographs had less severe abnormalities of pulmonary function than those who were detected by both techniques. It is not surprising that chest radiography is insensitive to mild degrees of obstructive pulmonary disease, as these mild abnormalities are less likely to lead to morphologic derangements in the lung that can be detected radiographically. It is the sensitivity of the ventilation study for detecting obstructive pulmonary disease that makes it a valuable adjunct to the perfusion image.

Combined V–P imaging is more specific for the diagnosis of pulmonary embolism than is perfusion imaging alone. This was demonstrated by Alderson et al.,[25] who studied 40 patients who had ventilation–perfusion imaging and pulmonary angiography. A double-blind analysis of perfusion imaging alone, then ventilation–perfusion images, revealed that the addition of the ventilation image changed the probability of the diagnosis of pulmonary embolism from low to high or vice versa in 10 cases (25 percent) (Fig. 3-2). Some patients who had high-probability perfusion images (i.e., images showing segmental perfusion defects) actually had moderate or severe obstructive lung disease in the regions of the perfusion defects and were reclassified as having a low probability of embolism. Other patients had low-probability nonsegmental perfusion defects but had no ventilation abnormalities and were reclassified as high probability for pulmonary emboli. However, the alteration of the diagnostic category was not correct in every case. One of the patients who had a high-probability perfusion image also

Table 3-3
Pulmonary Function* in Patients with ^{133}Xe Evidence of Obstructive Lung Disease

Chest Radiograph	Vital Capacity	Forced Expiratory Volume (1.0 sec)	Maximum Mid-expiratory Flow (L/sec)
Normal (n = 10)	69 ± 17	59 ± 18	42 ± 23
Obstructive lung disease (n = 14)	49 ± 19	35 ± 14	18 ± 7

* Results expressed as mean percent of predicted normal value ± standard deviation. All values in group with abnormal radiographs significantly ($p < 0.005$) worse than in those with normal x-rays.

had diffuse *and* severe obstructive pulmonary disease. This patient (Fig. 3-3) was placed in the low-probability category because his V–P studies showed matching ventilation–perfusion defects. The pulmonary angiogram of this patient, however, showed small bilateral pulmonary emboli in addition to vascular changes of obstructive lung disease. This case emphasizes one significant limitation of radionuclide imaging in the diagnosis of pulmonary embolism. When a patient has co-existent severe *and* diffuse obstructive pulmonary disease, the probability of detecting pulmonary emboli accurately is small. In *most* cases, however, adding the ventilation image to the perfusion scan increases both the accuracy and the specificity of the radionuclide diagnosis of pulmonary embolism and helps to avoid false-positive perfusion scans.[25]

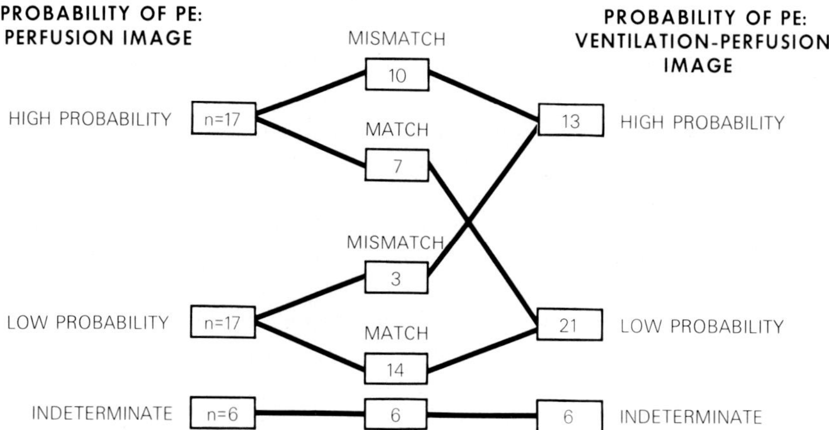

Fig. 3-2. Changes in diagnosis caused by addition of the ventilation image to the perfusion scan in 40 patients are shown.

These data do not necessarily mean that all perfusion images must be accompanied by a ventilation study. Greenspan[27] has stated that the normal perfusion lung scan essentially excludes a clinically significant pulmonary embolus. There are no data to refute this statement; therefore, if one is dealing with a young population not yet exposed to urban pollution or cigarette smoke, perfusion imaging is an excellent screening test. If the perfusion study is abnormal, however, a ventilation study is necessary to elucidate the cause of the perfusion defect.

ADVANTAGES OF RADIONUCLIDE STUDIES

Radionuclide studies have several unique advantages for evaluating pulmonary diseases. The most ovbious advantage is the ability of radionuclide studies to evaluate and quantitate regional lung function. Widespread application of computer techniques to radionuclide studies has resulted in several approaches to quantitating regional lung function. These include the simple determination of the relative distribution of ventilation, the determination of the ^{133}Xe clearance half-time, the determination of the fractional exchange of air,[28] or the analysis of ^{133}Xe clearance as a biexponential function.[29] The fractional exchange of air is an index of the mean rate of change of the downslope of the pulmonary clearance time–activity curve. It is calculated using the H/A technique of Zierler.[30,31] The H of this equation represents the counts within the lung field at ^{133}Xe equilibrium (i.e., the height of the equilibrium curve). The A of the equation is obtained by finding the area under the washout curve. The fractional exchange of air represents the fractional turnover of air containing ^{133}Xe with nonradioactive environmental air inhaled during the washout phase. The predicted normal value of 3%/sec is in good agreement with the known ratio of alveolar ventilation per second to functional residual capacity in man (approx. 80 cc/2400 cc). In patients with lung disease, there is a good correlation ($r = 0.70$; $p < 0.001$) between the fractional exchange of air and standard spirometric tests such as the forced expiratory volume in one second ($FEV_{1.0}$) and the mid-maximal expiratory flow rate (MMEF).

Few direct comparisons of these techniques have been performed. Secker-Walker et al.[30] compared the ability of the fractional-exchange and relative-ventilation methods to separate patients with normal lung function from those with obstructive pulmonary disease; they found the fractional-exchange method more accurate. One of the advantages of the fractional-exchange method is the fact that it takes into account both the early and late phases of clearance, thus including clearance of the pulmonary "slow space" as well as that of the "fast space" in its calculations. In patients with obstructive lung disease the poorly ventilated pulmonary slow space may comprise a large portion of the anatomic lung volume, though it contributes little to the overall function of the lung. Thus, it is important to evalu-

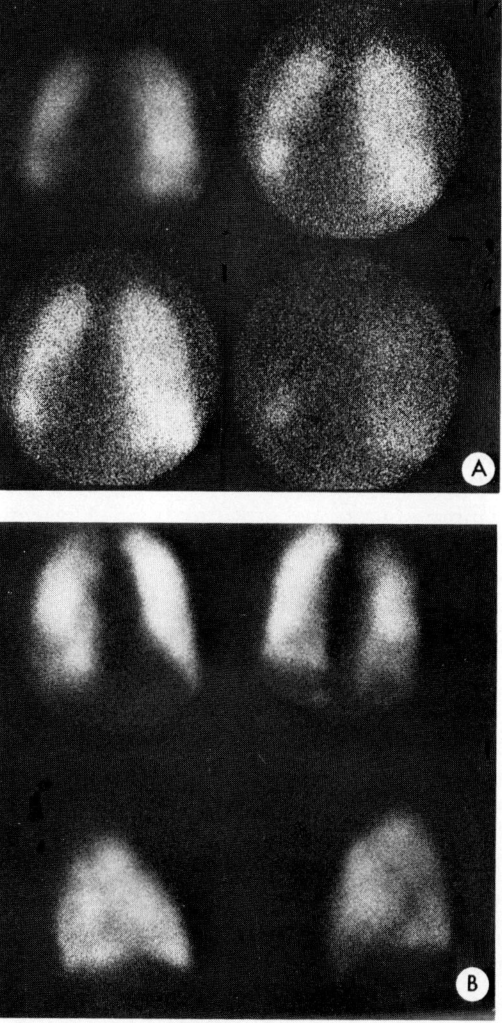

Fig. 3-3. The ^{133}Xe ventilation study (A), perfusion images (B), and pulmonary angiogram (C), of a patient with co-existent PE and severe diffuse COPD are shown. In these patients, accurate diagnosis of emboli by V–P imaging is difficult.

ate the contribution of the slow space when quantitating regional ventilation.

Regional ventilation–perfusion ratios can also be calculated from radionuclide lung studies. The V–P ratio in normal man is greater in the upper portion of the lung than in the middle or lower zones. This is because perfusion is more influenced by the effects of gravity than is ventilation. Therefore, in upright man the lung bases are relatively over-perfused,

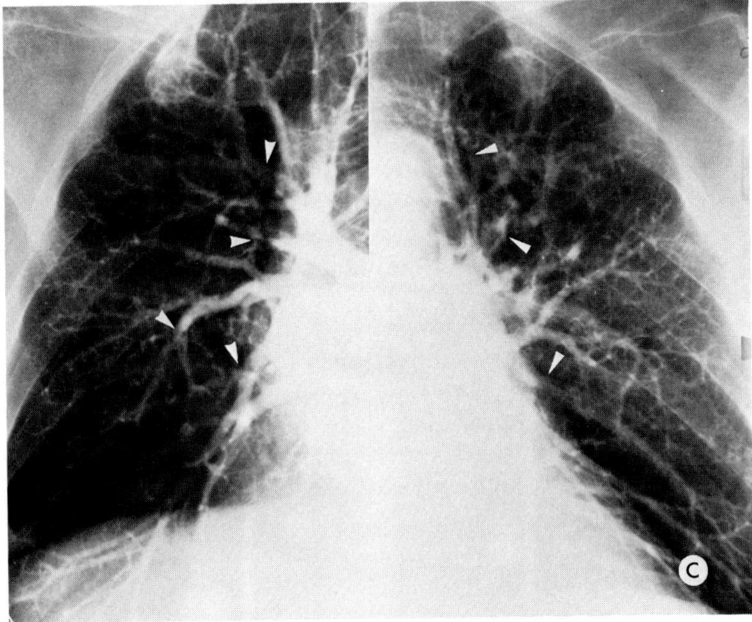

Fig. 3-3C.

whereas the apices are relatively over-ventilated. Several authors[32–34] have attempted to quantitate regional ventilation–perfusion ratios with ^{133}Xe and ^{99m}Tc-labeled perfusion particles. This information can be obtained in two ways. The first is to compare the relative distribution of perfusion to that of ventilation. The relative ventilation–perfusion ratios obtained do not represent true $\dot{V}/\dot{Q}$ ratios, as cardiac output is not known. To obtain these relative V–P ratios the relative regional distribution of a single breath of ^{133}Xe is determined. Next, this figure is divided by the relative distribution of ^{133}Xe at equilibrium (which represents the distribution of lung volume). The quotient represents the relative single-breath distribution per unit lung volume. Similarly, the relative regional distribution of perfusion is determined and also divided by the relative distribution of ^{133}Xe at equilibrium, and the quotient is the perfusion per unit volume. The relative V–P ratio is then obtained by dividing the single-breath distribution per unit volume by the perfusion per unit volume.

A further assessment of V–P ratios, based on regional ^{133}Xe clearance rather than the single-breath distribution is possible. The method used by Secker-Walker et al.[32] serves as an example of this approach. After determining the relative distribution of perfusion and the perfusion per unit lung volume, the clearance rate of ^{133}Xe is determined on a regional basis. This regional index of ventilation, the fractional exchange of air (%/sec), was discussed earlier; it represents ventilation per unit lung volume. Therefore, by dividing the fractional exchange of air by the perfusion per unit lung volume one obtains a ventilation–perfusion ratio based on the dynamics of ventilation rather than on the static distribution of ^{133}Xe and perfusion.

Computers can be used to produce analog images of the regional V–P ratios. These images can be presented as color or grey-scale representations. The normal analog image shows that the apices have a higher V–P ratio than the bases. Patients with abnormal lungs may show a nonhomogeneous mixture of areas of increased (light) or decreased (dark) V–P ratios. Examples of V–P and analog images obtained in a patient with cystic fibrosis are shown in Figure 3-4. Radionuclide lung studies are the only means for quantitating or visually displaying information about regional ventilation–perfusion balance.

The advantages of a regional pulmonary function evaluation are further demonstrated in studies of patients with suspected pulmonary emboli. Before perfusion lung imaging was introduced, Robin[35] suggested that pulmonary embolism could be diagnosed by monitoring the total lung alveolar-arterial CO_2 gradient. Embolized areas of the lung would be ventilated but not perfused, and the air exhaled from these areas would have a low CO_2 concentration. Therefore, the difference between the total lung expiratory CO_2 content and arterial CO_2 would increase. Perfusion imaging has been proved accurate and more specific for the diagnosis of pulmonary emboli than determination of CO_2 gradients.[36] In addition, the localizing information provided by radionuclide perfusion images may be used as a guide for pulmonary angiography. This is particularly important if the angiographer wishes to perform segmental arteriography to maximize his ability to detect emboli.

The advantages of obtaining regional information about pulmonary function can also be seen when evaluating patients with pulmonary masses. In these patients quantitative regional studies of ventilation and perfusion can be obtained preoperatively to assess regional lung function. Olsen et al.[37] demonstrated that quantitative determination of the relative distribution of perfusion preoperatively can be used to predict postoperative pulmonary function in the patient about to undergo pneumonectomy. The relative lung perfusion determined from the quantitative radionuclide study is multiplied by the overall lung $FEV_{1.0}$ and used to predict the postoperative $FEV_{1.0}$. They found a close correlation ($r = 0.72$) between the predicted postoperative $FEV_{1.0}$ and the actual postoperative $FEV_{1.0}$. Quantitative regional lung function studies are also useful in determining preoperative V–P balance in the pulmonary patient. By determining regional V–P balance it is possible to determine whether the area of lung to be resected actually contributes to the patients preoperative pulmonary function, makes no contribution, or is an area of V–P imbalance that is adversely affecting the patient's overall pulmonary function.

Preoperative lung imaging can also be used to assess the probability that a bronchogenic carcinoma or other mass lesion is resectable. Several studies[38,39] have shown that if the lung containing the mass is grossly underper-

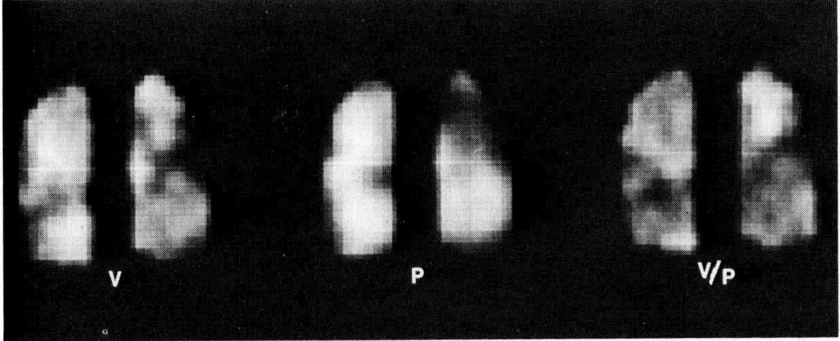

Fig. 3-4. Computer-assisted analog images in a patient with cystic fibrosis. Ventilation (V), perfusion (P), and regional V–P balance are shown. Dark areas in the V–P image are regions where the relative V–P ratio was less than 1.0.

fused (roughly less than $\frac{1}{3}$ of total perfusion), the pulmonary mass is not likely to be resectable. This is obviously true only when the mass is neoplastic. Central masses that are associated with marked reduction in pulmonary perfusion of the involved lung usually are associated with mediastinal spread and/or distant metastases. Centrally located masses are more likely to cause diminished perfusion than ventilation, because the vessels of the low-pressure pulmonary arterial system are more easily compressed than the cartilaginous conducting airways. Although this predictive value of perfusion lung scanning has been demonstrated by several authors, it is still not widely applied.

LIMITATIONS OF RADIONUCLIDE STUDIES

There are several limitations of radionuclide lung studies in diagnosing pulmonary embolism. First, V–P mismatch is not specific for pulmonary thromboembolism. Patients with idiopathic pulmonary hypertension may show V–P mismatch in the absence of angiographically detectable pulmonary emboli.[40] These findings may also be seen in patients with mitral valve disease.[41] Any type of pulmonary vasculitis, especially those found in collagen vascular disease or tuberculosis, can cause V–P mismatch. In addition, radiotherapy can cause decreased perfusion without altering ventilation in the irradiated area. Furthermore, V–P mismatch seen with embolic disease is not specific for any particular type of emboli. Perfusion defects are seen with pulmonary thromboemboli, tumor emboli, fat emboli, air emboli, foreign body emboli (e.g., cottonwool emboli injected by heroin addicts) or something as exotic as Dirofilaria infestation. Thus, although the combination of ventilation and perfusion imaging has significantly improved the accuracy and specificity of lung scanning for pulmonary emboli, definitive diagnosis is not possible.

Another significant limitation of lung scanning in the diagnosis of pulmonary emboli occurs in the patient who has other types of pulmonary disease. In one recent study[25] a segment-by-segment analysis of pulmonary angiograms and ventilation–perfusion studies was made. Although the V–P study demonstrated a true positive rate of 0.92 in 34 patients with suspected pulmonary emboli, the segment-by-segment correlation was poor. In 22 percent of segments showing emboli angiographically, ventilation and perfusion lung images were normal; in an additional 38 percent, the segment showing a perfusion defect also demonstrated a ventilation abnormality and therefore was called a V–P match. In another 17 percent a pulmonary infiltrate, atelectasis, or effusion was present in the region of a perfusion defect, rendering it nondiagnostic. Therefore, only 23 percent of all segments containing emboli showed the characteristic V–P mismatch. The apparent contradiction in a true-positive rate for patient diagnoses of 0.92 and a V–P mismatch rate of 0.23 is clarified by referring to probability theory. Since, on the average, the patients with emboli in this series had 11 embolized segments, probability theory calculates the theoretical rate of patient detection as $1 - (0.77)^{11}$. This calculates to roughly 0.95, greater than the observed 0.92 detection rate. Pulmonary emboli are usually multiple, and this multiplicity assures a high rate of patient detection, even though the segment-by-segment ability of V–P imaging to detect emboli may be limited in patients with co-existent obstructive pulmonary disease or radiographic infiltrates. The problem of co-existent disease is further emphasized by our recent review of 10 patients who had a solitary radiographic infiltrate that corresponded to a single area of decreased ventilation and perfusion. These patients had suspected pulmonary embolism. Segmental pulmonary angiography was performed in these 10 patients and 3 of them (30 percent) were found to have pulmonary emboli. Thus, emboli can occur in a single area, and ventilation–perfusion imaging may not be able to make the diagnosis. This situation occurs infrequently, however, as most patients with pulmonary emboli will have other perfusion defects in addition to the one causing the infiltrate.

Niden et al.[42] have suggested that ^{67}Ga-citrate lung imaging may help differentiate infiltrates caused by emboli from those caused by pneumonitis. In their experience infiltrates caused by emboli do not demonstrate ^{67}Ga avidity, but those caused by pneumonitis show intense ^{67}Ga uptake. Gallium-67 pulmonary uptake is not specific for pneumonitis and has been seen in a wide variety of neoplastic and inflammatory pulmonary diseases (Table 3-4). It may be useful for detecting opportunistic pulmonary infections (e.g., *Pneumocystis carinii*) at a time when radiographs are still normal. Gallium-67 lung imaging has also been used to determine the "activity" of diffuse interstitial lung disease. There is a close correlation between the degree of alveolitis seen pathologically and the uptake of ^{67}Ga.[43]

A third limitation to the diagnosis of pulmonary embolism is the theoretical possibility that pulmonary emboli induce spasm in regional airways and

Table 3-4
Some Causes of ^{67}Ga Pulmonary Uptake

Inflammatory	Iatrogenic	Other
Bacterial, viral pneumonia	Bleomycin toxicity	Pneumoconiosis
Tuberculosis (active)	Radiation pneumonitis	Idiopathic pulmonary fibrosis
Sarcoidosis (active)	Lymphangiography	Lymphangitic carcinomatosis
Opportunistic infections		Primary or secondary neoplasm
Lung abscess		

result in ^{133}Xe retention. Embolic perfusion defects could then be misinterpreted as being secondary to local airways disease. Experimental studies[44] demonstrate that the phenomenon of local bronchial spasm is extremely common in pulmonary emboli. This phenomenon occurs within seconds following embolism, probably due to the bronchial responsiveness to local hypocarbia. Several case reports[45,46] suggest that this phenomenon may also occur in patients. Isawa et al.[47] examined this possibility using a balloon catheter model for pulmonary vascular obstruction. They found ^{133}Xe retention after vascular obstruction in several animals, but the abnormalities were transient, lasting no longer than four to six hours. In a recent study,[10] pulmonary thromboemboli were produced in vivo in dogs. Xenon-133 ventilation abnormalities were induced in segments occluded by only 2 of 136 emboli (1.5 percent). Both these emboli were large, obstructing nearly a whole lower lobe. There was no evidence of ^{133}Xe abnormalities in 21 of 23 animals in this study, though they had, on the average, more than six emboli each. These data suggest that ^{133}Xe-detectable abnormalities induced by pulmonary emboli occur rarely and should not be a major clinical problem. In addition, since other studies have shown these abnormalities to be immediate and transient, the chances of encountering this phenomenon in clinical practice are limited.

Past studies of pulmonary angiography and perfusion lung imaging in animals with experimental pulmonary embolism[48] suggested that perfusion imaging was even more sensitive to small peripheral emboli than routine angiography. However, these angiographic studies were performed by injection at the right atrial or main pulmonary artery level. More recent comparisons between perfusion imaging and selective angiography in animals[10] have revealed that perfusion imaging is not reliable for detecting emboli that completely occlude vessels smaller than one millimeter in diameter (Table 3-5). Partially occluded pulmonary vessels are also detected less readily by perfusion imaging than by selective angiography. Regardless of size, 83 percent of regions containing completely occluded vessels were detected by perfusion imaging, whereas only 26 percent of the partially occluded areas were seen ($p < 0.01$).

To determine the size of lung surface perfusion defects detectable by perfusion imaging, India ink can be injected into embolized dogs prior to sac-

Table 3-5
Radionuclide Imaging and Selective Angiography in Experimental Pulmonary Emboli*

Angiographic Vessel Size Occluded	N	Visualized by Lung Scan
<1.0 mm	9	3 (33%)
1.1–2.0 mm	23	18 (78%)
2.1–3.0 mm	13	12 (92%)
>3.0 mm	24	24 (100%)
	69	57 (83%)

* This table includes only emboli which totally occluded pulmonary vessels.

rifice. India ink stains the perfused segments of the lung black, while leaving pink those vascular segments that are obstructed. Perfusion lung imaging reliably detected surface defects larger than 2 × 2 cm(90 percent) but detected only 29 percent of perfusion defects smaller than 2 × 2 cm. These studies were performed using oblique views in addition to the four standard lung-scan views. Thus, even current lung-imaging techniques that use oblique views have limited ability to detect very small ischemic pulmonary regions.

Ventilation–perfusion lung imaging is also of limited utility in the patient with diffuse lung disease. Most authors would suggest that it is difficult to diagnose pulmonary emboli in a patient with superimposed diffuse lung disease, such as congestive failure or interstitial fibrosis. Putman and Gottschalk,[49] however, studied 25 patients with diffuse radiographic lung disease and were able to exclude pulmonary emboli in 18. This was possible because these patients lacked the characteristic pattern of multiple segmental perfusion defects that would be expected in pulmonary emboli. The possibility that lung imaging may be useful in significantly reducing the probability of pulmonary emboli in patients with diffuse lung disease deserves further investigation.

Regardless of the above limitations, ventilation–perfusion lung imaging has made significant contributions to the diagnosis and management of patients with pulmonary disease. These studies remain the only simple noninvasive method for obtaining regional and quantitative information about pulmonary function. Combination of ventilation and multiple-view perfusion imaging has increased the accuracy and specificity of the diagnosis of pulmonary emboli and has been useful in the preoperative assessment of pulmonary function in patients about to undergo lung resection. Obviously, regardless of the specific application of radionuclide lung imaging (e.g., pulmonary embolism, obstructive lung disease, preoperative evaluation), correlation with the findings of chest radiography is essential. The radiographs should be taken at the time of the scan or should be no more than a few hours old. This close correlation will maximize the ability of the radionuclide study to contribute to patient diagnosis and management. Radionuclide lung studies are well tolerated and expose the patients to only a small radiation dose. The ease with which these studies can be performed, plus the fact that they can be repeated often, places them in an ideal position for evaluating patients prior to more definitive, invasive diagnostic pulmonary procedures.

REFERENCES

1. Alderson PO, Krohn KA, Welch MJ: Radiopharmaceuticals. In Gottschalk A, Potchen EJ (eds): Diagnostic Nuclear Medicine. Baltimore, Williams & Wilkins, 1976, 26
2. Vincent WR, Goldberg SJ, Desilets D: Fatality immediately following rapid infusion of macroaggregates of ^{99m}Tc albumin (MAA) for lung scan. Radiology 91:1181–1184, 1968
3. Child JS, Wolfe JD, Tashkin D., et al: Fatal lung scan in a case of pulmonary hypertension due to obliterative pulmonary vascular disease. Chest 67:308–310, 1975
4. Harding LK, Harsfield K, Singhol SS, et al: The proportion of lung vessels blocked by albumin microspheres. J Nucl Med 14:579–581, 1973
5. Gold WM, McCormack KR: Pulmonary function response to radioisotope scanning of the lungs. JAMA 197:146–150, 1966
6. Heck LL, Duley JW: Statistical considerations in lung imaging with ^{99m}Tc albumin particles. Radiology 113:675–679, 1974
7. Davies G, Reid L: Growth of the alveoli and pulmonary arteries in childhood. Thorax 25:679–681, 1970
8. Caride VJ, Puri S, Slaven JD et al: The usefulness of the posterior oblique views in perfusion lung imaging. Radiology 121:669–671, 1976
9. Nielsen PE, Kirchner PT, Gerber FH: Oblique views in lung perfusion scanning: Clinical utility and limitations. J Nucl Med 18:967–973, 1978.
10. Alderson PO, Doppman JL, Diamond SS, et al: Ventilation-perfusion imaging and selective pulmonary angiography in animals with experimental pulmonary embolism. J Nucl Med 19:164–171, 1978
11. Yeates DB, Aspin N, Bryan AC, et al: Regional clearance of ions from the airways of the lung. Am Rev Resp Dis 107:602–608, 1973
12. Green G: Alveolobronchiolar transport mechanisms. Arch Intern Med 131:101–109, 1973
13. Poe ND: Relation between pulmonary deposition of radioaerosol and ventilation. J Nucl Med 18:606, 1977 (Abstr)
14. Alderson PO, Bradley EW, Bradley ME, et al: Pulmonary ventilation, perfusion, and radioaerosol deposition following hemithorax irradiation with ^{60}Co or fast neutrons. J Nucl Med 18:625, 1977 (Abstr)
15. Knipping HW, Bolt W, Ventrath H, et al: A new method for regional lung function analysis with radioactive ^{133}Xe gas. Deutsch Med Wochenschr 80:1146–1147, 1955

16. Bake B, Wood L, Murphy B, et al: Effects of inspiratory flow rate on regional distribution of inspired gas. J Appl Physiol 37:8–17, 1974
17. Milic-Emili J: Radioactive Xenon in the evaluation of regional lung function. Semin Nucl Med 1:246–261, 1971
18. Fazio F, Jones T: Assessment of regional ventilation by continuous inhalation of radioactive Krypton-81m. Br Med J 2:673–676, 1975
19. Goris ML, Daspit SG, Walter JP, et al: Applications of ventilation lung imaging with ^{81m}Krypton. Radiology 122:399–404, 1977
20. Hoffer PB, Harper PV, Beck RN, et al: Improved Xenon images with ^{127}Xe. J Nucl Med 14:172–174, 1973
21. Schor R, Shames DM, Weber PM, et al: Regional ventilation studies with ^{81m}Kr and ^{133}Xe: A comparative analysis. J Nucl Med 19:348–353, 1978
22. Coates G, Nahmias C: Xenon-127, a comparison with Xenon-133 for ventilation studies. J Nucl Med 18:221–225, 1977
23. Atkins HL, Susskind H, Klopper JF et al: A clinical comparison of ^{127}Xe and ^{133}Xe for ventilation studies. J Nucl Med 18:653–659, 1977
24. Poulouse KP, Reba RC, Wagner HN Jr: Characterization of the shape and location of perfusion defects in certain pulmonary diseases. N Engl J Med 279:1020–1025, 1968
25. Alderson PO, Rujanavech N, Secker-Walker RH, et al: The role of ^{133}Xe ventilation studies in the scintigraphic detection of pulmonary embolism. Radiology 120:633–640, 1976
26. Alderson PO, Secker-Walker RH, Forrest JV: Detection of obstructive pulmonary disease: Relative sensitivity of ventilation-perfusion studies and chest radiography. Radiology 112:643–648, 1974
27. Greenspan RH: Does a normal isotope perfusion scan exclude pulmonary embolism? Invest Radiol 8:97, 1973
28. Secker-Walker RH, Hill RI, Markham J, et al: The measurement of regional ventilation in man: A new method of quantitation. J Nucl Med 14:725–732, 1973
29. Secker-Walker RH: Pulmonary physiology, pathology, and ventilation-perfusion studies. J Nucl Med 19:961–968, 1978
30. Secker-Walker RH, Alderson PO, Wilhelm J, et al: The measurement of regional ventilation during tidal breathing: A comparison of two methods in healthy subjects, and patients with chronic obstructive lung disease. Br J Radiol 48:181–189, 1975
31. Zierler KL: Equations for measuring blood flow by external monitoring of radioisotopes. Circ Res 16:309–321, 1965
32. Secker-Walker RH, Alderson PO, Wilhelm J, et al: Regional ventilation-perfusion relationships. Respiration 32:265–276, 1975
33. Burdine JA, Murphy PH, Alagarsmy V, et al: Functional pulmonary imaging. J Nucl Med 13:933–938, 1972
34. Jones RH, Coulam CM, Goodrich JK, et al: Radionuclide quantitation of lung function in patients with pulmonary disorders. Surgery 70:891–903, 1971
35. Robin ED, Forkner CE, Bromberg PA, et al: Alveolar gas exchange in clinical pulmonary embolism. N Engl J Med 262:283–287, 1960
36. Vereerstraeten J, Schoutens A, Tombroff M, et al: Value of measurement of alveolo-arterial gradient of PCO_2 compared to pulmonary scan in diagnosis of thrombo-embolic pulmonary disease. Thorax 28:306–312, 1973

37. Olsen GN, Block AJ, Tobias JA: Prediction of post pneumonectomy pulmonary function using quantitative macroaggregate lung scanning. Chest 66:13–16, 1974
38. Secker-Walker RH, Provan JL: Scintillation scanning of lungs in preoperative assessment of carcinoma of bronchus. Br Med J 3:327–330, 1969
39. Secker-Walker RH, Alderson PO, Wilhelm J, et al: Ventilation-perfusion scanning in carcinoma of the bronchus. Chest 65:660–663, 1974
40. Wilson AG, Harris CN, Lavender JP, et al: Perfusion lung scanning in obliterative pulmonary hypertension. Br Heart J 35:917–930, 1973
41. Kelley MJ, Elliot LP: The radiologic evaluation of the patient with suspected pulmonary thromboembolic disease. Med Clin North Am 59:3–36, 1975
42. Niden AH, Mishkin FS, Khurana MML, et al: ^{67}Ga lung scan: An aid in the differential diagnosis of pulmonary embolism and pneumonitis. JAMA 237:1206–1211, 1977
43. Line BR, Fulmer JD, Jones AE, et al: ^{67}Gallium scanning in idiopathic pulmonary fibrosis: Correlation with histopathology and broncho-alveolar lavage. Am Rev Respir Dis 113:244, 1976 (Abstr)
44. Hirose T, Yasutake T, Tarabeih A, et al: Location of airway constriction following acute experimental pulmonary thrombo-embolism. J Appl Physiol 34:431–437, 1973
45. Kessler RM, McNeil BJ: Impaired ventilation in a patient with angiographically demonstrated pulmonary emboli. Radiology 114:111–112, 1975
46. Epstein J, Taylor A, Alazraki N, et al: Acute pulmonary embolus associated with transient ventilatory defect. J Nucl Med 16:1017–1020, 1975
47. Isawa T, Taplin GV, Beazell J, et al: Experimental unilateral pulmonary artery occlusion. Acute and chronic effects on relative inhalation and perfusion. Radiology 102:101–109, 1972
48. Moser KM, Harsanyi P, Ruis-Garriga G, et al: Assessment of pulmonary photoscanning and angiography in experimental pulmonary embolism. Circulation 39:663–674, 1969
49. Putman C, Gottschalk A: The effect of diffuse pulmonary parenchymal disease on the diagnosis of pulmonary embolism by perfusion lung scanning. Radiology (in press)

Stephen L. Kaufman, M.D.
Robert I. White, Jr., M.D.

4

Pulmonary Arteriography

The major indication for pulmonary angiography is in the evaluation of pulmonary embolism. This disease represents a significant and prevalent medical problem having been estimated to occur in approximately 2 percent of hospital admissions[1] and to be responsible for 200,000 deaths per year.[2] Yet the mortality for pulmonary embolism, once diagnosed and treated, has been found in two series to be only 8 percent.[3,4] Rapid recognition and treatment of this condition is thus mandatory, and pulmonary angiography is an important tool in the diagnostic armamentarium. Pulmonary angiography is also used in the preoperative assessment of the resectability of bronchogenic carcinoma and in the diagnosis of congenital abnormalities of the pulmonary vasculature such as arteriovenous malformations. The levo phase of the pulmonary angiogram may be employed in the diagnosis of left atrial myxoma. In patients in whom retrograde aortography cannot be performed because of arterial occlusion, the levo phase can be used to diagnose aortic dissections and aneurysms.

This chapter reviews our experience with the technique of pulmonary angiography and with the pre-angiographic and angiographic evaluation of patients suspected of having pulmonary emboli and other conditions amenable to study by pulmonary angiography.

TECHNIQUE

Intracardiac Pressures and Electrocardiographic Monitoring

The two techniques employed in pulmonary arteriography are the upper extremity venous cutdown approach and the percutaneous femoral vein approach. With either technique, electrocardiographic and pressure monitoring are mandatory. Patients with pulmonary emboli frequently have associated cardiac disease, and constant observation of the electrocardiogram is important in early detection of arrhythmias during the procedure. Passage of the catheter through the right ventricle frequently is associated with premature ventricular contractions (PVCs). A few PVCs are of no significance, but runs of PVCs must be recognized quickly and the catheter position changed before ventricular tachycardia develops. Pressure monitoring is important for several reasons. Occasionally, the catheter may seem fluoroscopically to be in the right ventricle but in reality be located posteriorly in the coronary sinus. In this circumstance, continued advancement of the catheter in an attempt to enter the pulmonary artery may result in cardiac perforation. Catheter position in the coronary sinus can be easily recognized by the observation on the monitor of continued right atrial pressure despite the apparent position of the catheter in the right ventricle. The determination of right atrial and ventricular, pulmonary artery, and pulmonary capillary wedge pressure during cardiac catherization also adds important hemodynamic information to the anatomic information obtained by angiography. The mean pulmonary artery pressure shows good correlation with the degree of embolic obstruction in patients without prior cardiopulmonary disease.[5,6] The presence of right ventricular failure has been shown to be a poor prognostic sign in pulmonary embolism.[4] In patients with preexisting cardiac disease and emboli, the resultant hemodynamic status of the patient may be ascertained.[7] The demonstration of pulmonary arterial hypertension in a patient with bronchogenic carcinoma may preclude the possibility of pneumonectomy.[8] Finally, the level of the pulmonary artery pressure is used in deciding the dosage of contrast medium to be injected. This is discussed later in more detail, but in general, with pulmonary arterial hypertension the dosage of contrast material is reduced, and more superselective injections are employed.

Percutaneous Femoral Vein Technique

The development of the pulmonary-artery-seeking catheter by Grollman and associates[9] has made the femoral approach more attractive, and in the past two years we have used it in the majority of cases. The Grollman catheter* is a polyethylene "pigtail" catheter with a small (3 cm) distal secondary curve reversed 90 degrees from the primary curve (Fig. 4-1). This distal curve enables the catheter, once in the right ventricle to pass readily into the pulmonary outflow tract and then into the main pulmonary artery.

There are several advantages to this percutaneous technique. (1) The speed of the procedure is significantly increased by the use of a percutaneous femoral vein puncture as opposed to a venous cutdown. (2) No sutures are required following the procedure. (3) It is relatively easy to posi-

* Cook Inc., Bloomington, Ind.

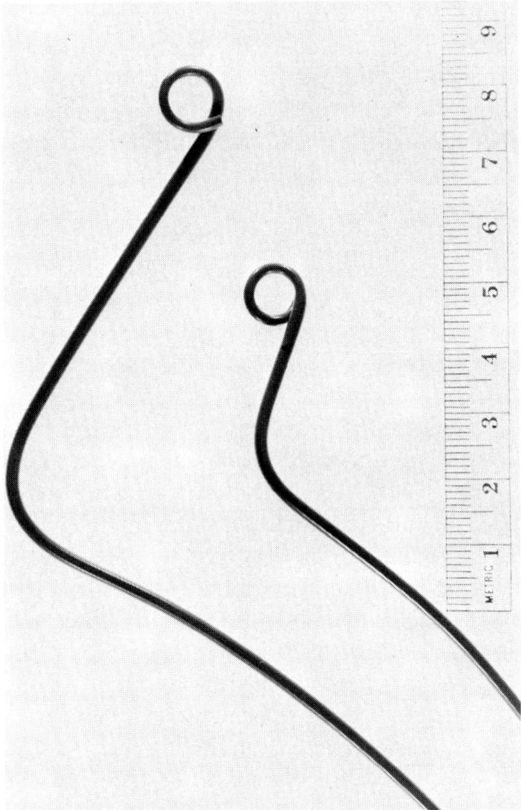

Fig. 4-1. The Grollman catheter (right) used for pulmonary arteriography from the percutaneous femoral vein approach. The catheter on the left with a longer distal curve may be employed in patients with cardiomegaly.

tion the Grollman catheter into either pulmonary artery for selective studies. Using the approach from the arm, it is sometimes impossible to get the catheter into the left pulmonary artery. (4) The soft polyethylene pigtail catheter makes cardiac perforation, a potential though rare complication inherent in other methods, exceedingly unlikely.

A potential disadvantage of the percutaneous femoral vein approach in patients suspected of having pulmonary emboli is the possibility of dislodging unsuspected thrombi in the iliac veins and inferior vena cava with the catheter. Ferris and associates[10] found thrombi in the inferior vena cava in 9 of 65 patients (14 percent) undergoing pulmonary angiography. Our detection of thrombi in the vena cava is less frequent; however, with this possibility in mind, we routinely perform a femoral venogram immediately following puncture of the femoral vein by a rapid 10-cc hand injection and fluoroscopic monitoring of the passage of contrast material up the iliac vein and vena cava. If this appears normal, the guide wire and then the catheter are advanced through the inferior vena cava into the right atrium. If there is any question of abnormality on the femoral venogram, an inferior vena cavogram, with a mechanical injector and filming, is performed. In a patient suspected of having a pulmonary embolus we consider the presence of iliac or inferior vena cava thrombus good presumptive evidence that a pulmonary embolus is present and certainly an indication for therapy in its own right. If direct demonstration of the pulmonary embolus is still desired, the upper extremity cutdown approach can be employed for pulmonary arteriography.

The steps for catheterizing the pulmonary artery in the presence of a normal-sized right atrium are shown in Figure 4-2. The tricuspid valve is crossed by probing with the distal curve of the catheter along the medial portion of the right atrium. Entrance into the right ventricle is marked by a change from atrial to ventricular pressure. Once the right ventricle has been entered, the catheter is rotated until the distal curve is pointing up toward the ventricular outflow tract. The catheter is then advanced into the main pulmonary artery. The catheter usually preferentially enters the left pulmonary artery. The right pulmonary artery may be entered by further manipulation of the catheter. Occasionally with the catheter in the main pulmonary artery, it is necessary to advance a j-tipped guide wire out of the catheter into the right pulmonary artery over which the catheter is then advanced. In patients with right atrial enlargement it is frequently difficult to advance the catheter directly through the tricuspid valve. Various methods of accomplishing this have been suggested, including the use of a j-tipped guide wire in the right atrium, a bend proximal to the distal curve of the catheter, and the use of a tip-deflecting system.[9] The use of the bent back end of the guide wire as a tip deflector has also been advocated.[11] We have been quite successful in entering the tricuspid valve by advancing the catheter tip against the lateral wall of the right atrium and forming a loop in the catheter (Fig. 4-3). The looped catheter is then rotated so that the tip points anteriorly and medially. As the catheter is then withdrawn, the tip "pops" across the tricuspid valve into the right ventricle. A modification of the Grollman shape suggested by Glenn and Ranninger[12] employing a longer distal curve also facilitates passage of the tricuspid valve in the patient with a large right atrium. A variation of this type of catheter is now commercially available* (Fig. 4-1) and may be employed in patients with cardiomegaly.

We have routinely employed superselective pulmonary arteriography in the investigation of pulmonary embolism. The injection of contrast medium is made into the pulmonary artery supplying the area with abnormal perfusion seen on the lung scan. Since pulmonary emboli are most commonly located in the lower lobes,[13,14] the injection is most frequently made in the lower lobe pulmonary arteries. The right middle lobe and lingular arteries are usually branches of the artery supplying the respective lower lobes and

* Cook Inc., Bloomington, Indiana.

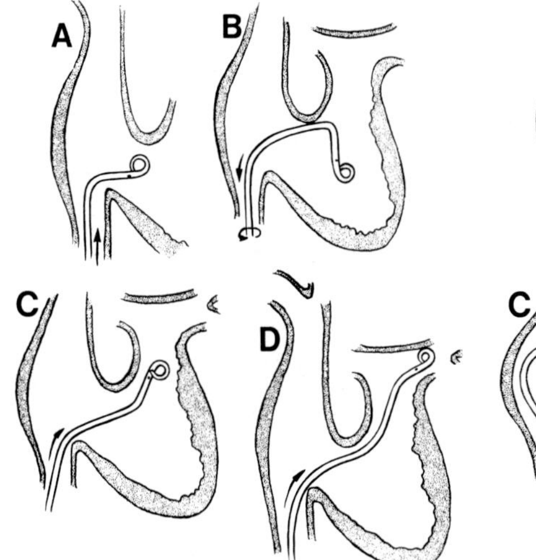

Fig. 4-2. The steps in catheterizing the pulmonary artery using the percutaneous femoral vein approach with the Grollman catheter in the presence of a normal-sized right atrium. The tricuspid valve is crossed by probing the anteromedial portion of the right atrium (A). Once the right ventricle is entered (B), the catheter is rotated and withdrawn slightly until the distal curve points toward the ventricular outflow tract (C). The catheter is then advanced into the pulmonary artery (D).

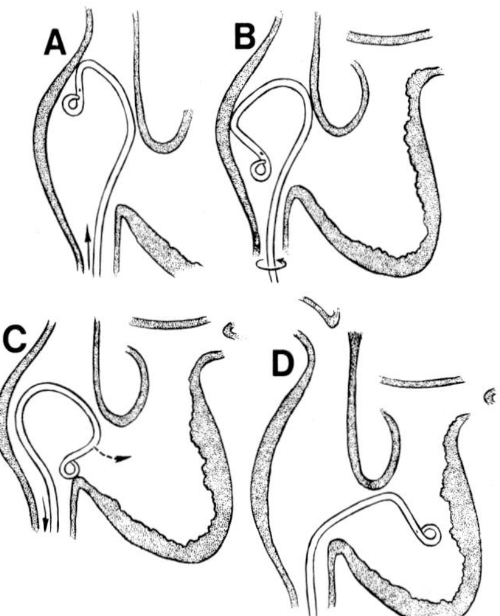

Fig. 4-3. The steps in catheterizing the pulmonary artery using the percutaneous femoral vein approach with the Grollman catheter in a patient with an enlarged right atrium. The catheter tip is advanced against the lateral wall of the right atrium, forming a loop in the catheter (A). The looped catheter is rotated (B) so that the tip points toward the triscuspid valve (C). As the catheter is withdrawn (D), the tip springs into the right ventricle. The pulmonary artery is then entered as in Figures 4-2B through D.

are included in injections in the main lower lobe vessels.[15] In our experience except in patients with congestive heart failure it is unusual for emboli to be located in the upper lobe segments in the absence of associated lower lobe emboli.

When systolic pulmonary artery pressure is normal or slightly elevated (<50 mm Hg), we use an injection rate of 15 cc per second for two seconds selectively in the lower lobe arteries and 20 cc per second for two seconds in the left or right pulmonary artery. If an injection into the main pulmonary artery is performed the injection rate is 30 cc per second for two seconds. If the pulmonary artery systolic pressure is above 50 mm Hg, the injection rates for selective angiography are reduced to 10 cc per second and 15 cc per second, respectively. We do not perform a main pulmonary angiogram in patients with pulmonary artery pressure greater than 50 mm Hg.

The x-ray beam is collimated to cover the area of contrast injection. If selective lower lobe angiography is employed, magnification techniques are

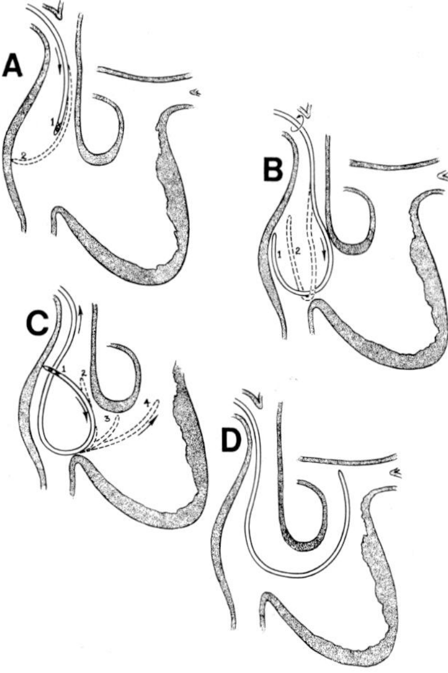

Fig. 4-4. The steps in catheterizing the pulmonary artery using the antecubital vein cutdown approach. The catheter tip is advanced against the right atrial wall (A), forming a loop in the catheter (B). The catheter is then rotated counterclockwise and withdrawn (C). The catheter will then "pop" into the right ventricle, with the tip pointing toward the right ventricular outflow tract. The catheter is then advanced into the pulmonary artery. (Reprinted from White RI Jr: Fundamentals of Vascular Radiology, Philadelphia, Lea & Febiger, 1976, p 112)

often helpful to detect small peripheral emboli (Fig. 4-5). Oblique projections are utilized to reduce superimposition of small lower lobe, middle lobe, and lingular banches.[16] The left posterior oblique projection is used for selective angiography in the right pulmonary artery and the right posterior oblique view, for angiography in the left pulmonary artery (Fig. 4-6C). A satisfactory filming rate is three films per second for three seconds during the pulmonary arterial phase and one film per second for an additional six seconds for visualization of the levo phase.

Venous Cutdown Technic

The venous cutdown technic can be employed from either arm. A medially located superficial vein in the antecubital fossa is selected. Laterally directed superficial veins usually lead into the cephalic system. The cephalic vein enters the axillary vein at approximately a 90-degree angle, preventing passage of the catheter any further. Medially directed veins, how-

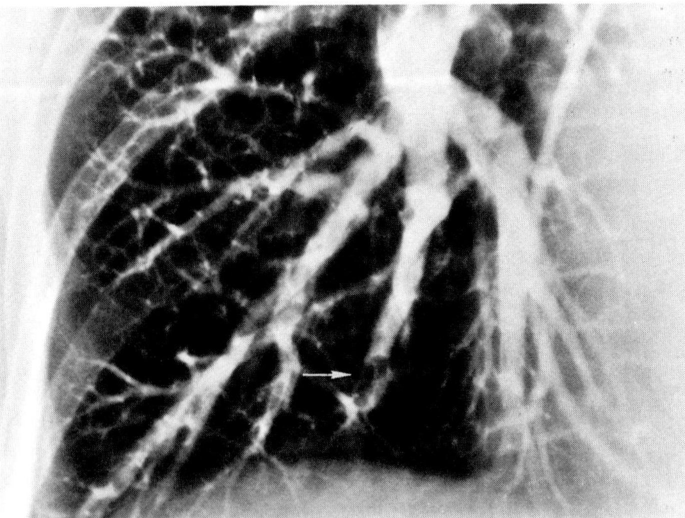

Fig. 4-5. Selective right lower lobe pulmonary arteriogram using magnification technique. A small embolus (arrow) is seen within a peripheral lower lobe branch.

ever, are in direct line with the axillary and subclavian veins. If a superficial vein cannot be found, the cutdown is made over the brachial artery pulse, and one of its vena comitantes selected. A closed-end woven dacron NIH catheter* is employed in this technic. The 7 F size is adequate for any flow rate employed in pulmonary arteriography. The catheter is introduced into the vein and advanced into the right atrium. Occasionally the catheter will enter small branches of the brachial or axillary vein and resistance to further passage will be met. If the catheter is then withdrawn, rotated, and redirected, passage into the right atrium usually can be achieved. Occasionally a small injection of contrast material will be required to map out the course of the brachial or axillary vein. Once the right atrium is entered, the catheter is connected to the pressure manifold and entry into the pulmonary artery accomplished. A loop is formed by advancing the catheter tip against the right atrial wall (Fig. 4-4). Once the loop has been formed, the catheter is rotated counterclockwise and withdrawn. The catheter will then "pop" across the tricuspid valve, with its tip pointing upward toward the right ventricular outflow tract. Entry into the ventricle is confirmed by the observation of ventricular pressure. The catheter is then advanced into the pulmonary artery. Occasionally the catheter will become caught in trabeculae of the right ventricular outflow tract. If the catheter is withdrawn slightly, rotated, and then advanced, the pulmonary artery can usually be entered. It is important in this situation not to try to push the catheter against resistance, as this may result in perforation of the right ventricle. The catheter will usually preferentially enter the right pulmonary artery. Entry into the left pulmonary artery can be difficult, but usually can be accomplished by rotat-

* USCI-Billerica, Massachusetts.

ing the catheter in the main pulmonary artery, so that its tip points to the left, and then advancing it into the vessel. The closed-end configuration of the catheter precludes the use of a guide wire and generally prevents recoil into the right ventricle during the injection. Injection flow rates and filming sequence are identical to those employed with the femoral vein approach.

Complications

Pulmonary arteriography is an invasive technic and complications, though rare, can occur. During the course of The Urokinase Pulmonary Embolism Trial[3] a total of 310 pulmonary angiograms, most using the upper extremity cutdown technic, were performed. One case of cardiac perforation was encountered, and there were five episodes of ventricular arrhythmia requiring treatment. There were no fatalities and no residual morbidity. The incidence of cardiac perforation should be lessened with the use of the Grollman catheter, which is of softer polyethylene material and has a pigtail tip, which should not become lodged in trabeculae.[9,11]

Arrhythmias cannot be avoided completely, but care during passage of the catheter through the right ventricle should decrease their incidence. Indications for pulmonary arteriography in patients prone to ventricular irritability, such as those with digitalis intoxication, should be considered very carefully. *Since right bundle branch block can occur during pulmonary angiography*[17,18] *the procedure should not be performed in patients with pre-existing left bundle branch block without the availability of facilities for ventricular pacing should complete heart block develop.* A defibrillator and emergency cardiac drugs should always be immediately available in the angiography suite in the event serious arrhythmias develop. The potential complication of iatrogenic embolism during catheter passage up the inferior vena cava with the percutaneous technic has been found not to pose a significant problem.[18] Six local complications related to this technic were encountered during 122 catheterizations. These included four hematomas, one minor infection at the puncture site, and one ileofemoral vein thrombosis. Severe pulmonary hypertension occurring after pulmonary arteriography in patients with pre-existing pulmonary hypertension has been described.[19] Superselective technic using the least possible amount of contrast material should be employed in this group of patients.

CLINICAL APPLICATIONS

Suspected Pulmonary Embolism

The clinical recognition of pulmonary embolism is difficult. Symptoms such as dyspnea, pleuritic chest pain, and cough, which are present in the majority of patients with pulmonary emboli,[3] are fairly nonspecific findings.

Table 4-1
Modalities in the Diagnosis of Pulmonary Embolism

Study	Sensitivity	Specificity	Morbidity
Chest radiography	Low	Low	None
Lung scan	High	Intermediate	None
Pulmonary angiogram	High	High	Low

Electrocardiographic changes seen in pulmonary embolism and laboratory findings such as a decreased arterial Po_2 (<80 mm Hg.)[3,20] are also nonspecific. (See Chapter 11.) A high level of clinical suspicion of pulmonary embolism should be maintained in a case of sudden unexplained dyspnea or pleuritic chest pain in a patient who has a predisposing factor such as recent immobilization; prior venous, cardiovascular, or pulmonary disease; or current use of oral contraceptives.[3] The three diagnostic modalities that may be considered in this situation are pulmonary angiography, the routine chest roentgenogram, and perfusion–ventilation lung scanning (Table 4-1). Pulmonary angiography is considered as the definitive procedure for the diagnosis of pulmonary embolism.[13,21] It has a high degree of specificity and with the use of selective technic and magnification is also highly sensitive, although probably not as sensitive as lung scanning. Pulmonary angiography, however, is an invasive procedure with low but definite morbidity and should not be used as a screening test. The chest film has been shown to be abnormal in up to 93 percent of patients with documented pulmonary embolism.[17] The findings most commonly seen on the chest film in pulmonary embolism—consolidation, diaphragmatic elevation, pleural effusion, and atelectasis[3,20]—are nonspecific, and their roentgenographic appearance is occasionally delayed. The chest film, however, is useful in excluding other conditions in the differential diagnosis of pulmonary thromboembolism and is necessary in the interpretation of the lung scan. The perfusion lung scan is a highly sensitive procedure for pulmonary embolism and is essentially noninvasive. It is thus an ideal screening procedure. Its specificity lies between that of the chest film and pulmonary arteriography. A normal perfusion scan excludes the diagnosis of pulmonary embolism.[22,23] Patients exhibiting perfusion defects corresponding to a lobe or pulmonary segment with a normal chest film have a high probability (75 to 80 percent)[17,22,23] of having pulmonary emboli. The addition of a normal ventilation scan significantly raises the probability of pulmonary embolism.[24,25]

Patients with scan defects not corresponding to pulmonary segments or with matching ventilation defects or infiltrates or pleural effusions in corresponding areas on the chest film are in a third intermediate category, having pulmonary emboli in from 12 to 30 percent of cases.[22,23,26]

With these considerations in mind, our recommendations for the work-up of a patient suspected of having pulmonary embolism are as follows: A chest roentgenogram, a perfusion scan, and a ventilation scan should be ob-

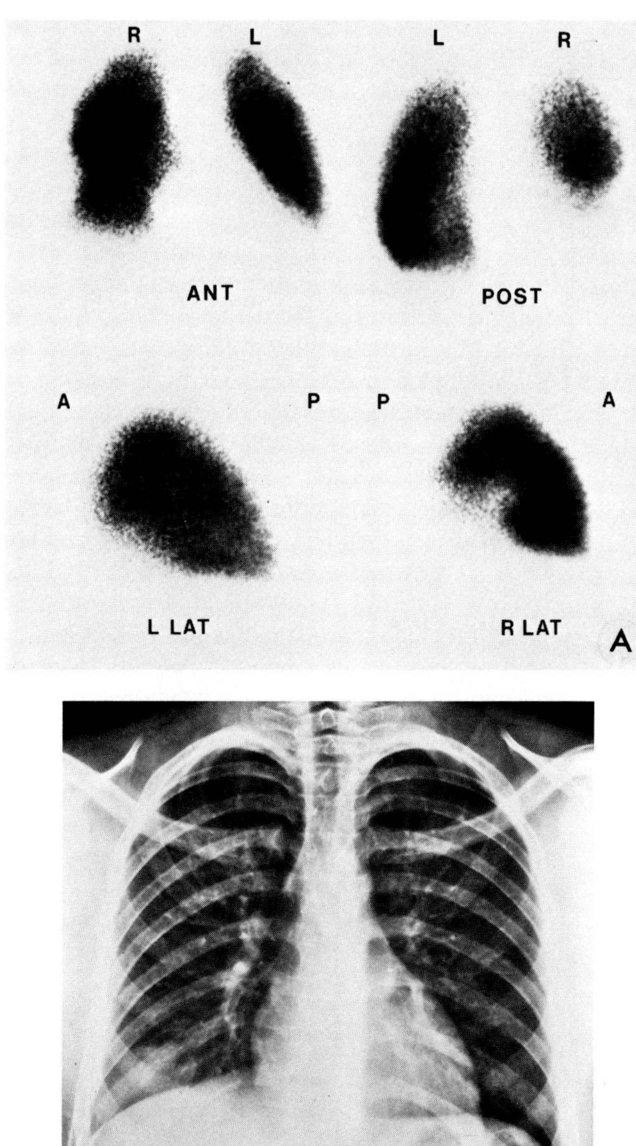

Fig. 4-6. Patient suspected of having pulmonary embolization with nondiagnostic scan and radiographic findings. (A) A four-view perfusion lung scan demonstrates a segmental defect in the right lower lobe; (B) Chest radiograph demonstrates a corresponding right lower lobe infiltrate.

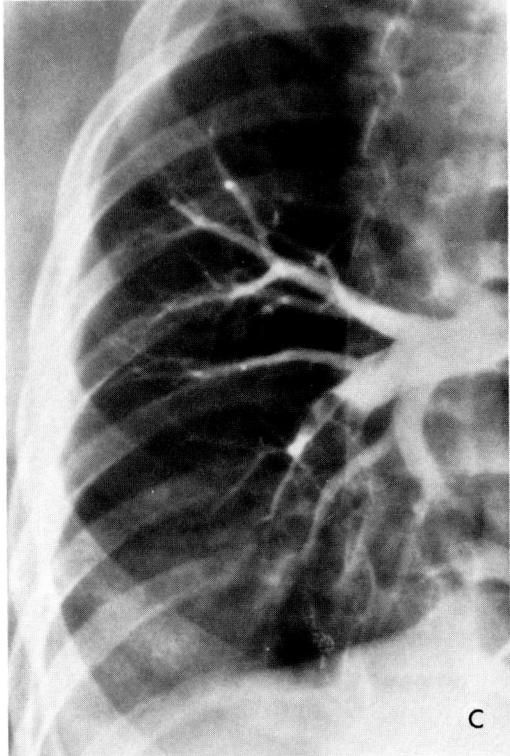

Fig. 4-6. (C) Selective right lower lobe pulmonary arteriogram in the left posterior oblique projection demonstrates an embolus straddling two lower lobe branches.

tained as the initial screening procedures. The possible exceptions are those rare patients with suspected massive pulmonary emboli who are being considered for emergency embolectomy and whose condition requires an immediate definitive diagnosis. A negative lung scan eliminates the possibility of pulmonary embolism, and pulmonary angiography is not necessary. Patients with a high probability of pulmonary embolism also do not ordinarily require pulmonary angiography. The exceptions are those patients, who because of a contraindication to heparinization or recurrent embolism while on heparin, are being considered for inferior vena caval ligation or the placement of an inferior vena cava umbrella. Under these circumstances pulmonary angiography is performed to confirm the diagnosis prior to surgery. The major indication for pulmonary angiography is in the third group of patients with equivocal scan findings. Pulmonary angiography in these cases is required to make the diagnosis (Figs. 4-6 and 4-7). Even when equivocal, scan findings are helpful in localizing the area of abnormality for angiography. Selective pulmonary angiography is performed in the area of

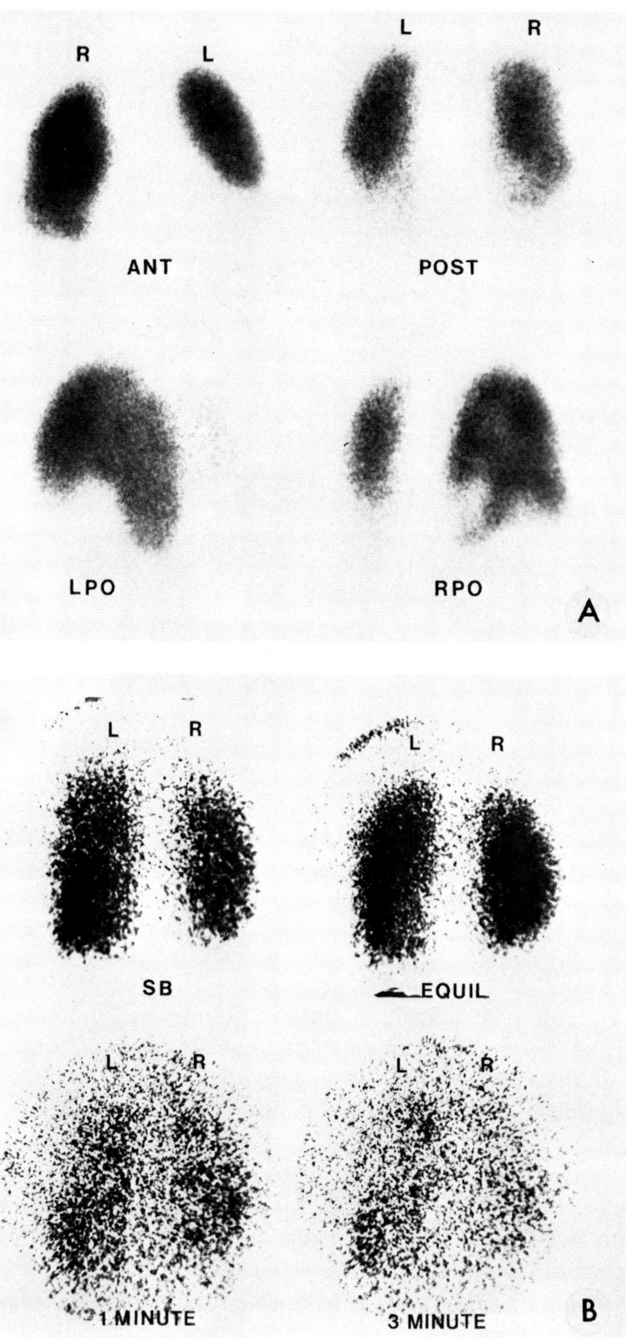

Fig. 4-7. Patient suspected of having pulmonary embolization with nondiagnostic scan and radiographic findings. (A) A perfusion lung scan demonstrates bilateral lower lobe defects; (B) The ventilation scan demonstrates delayed washout at both bases.

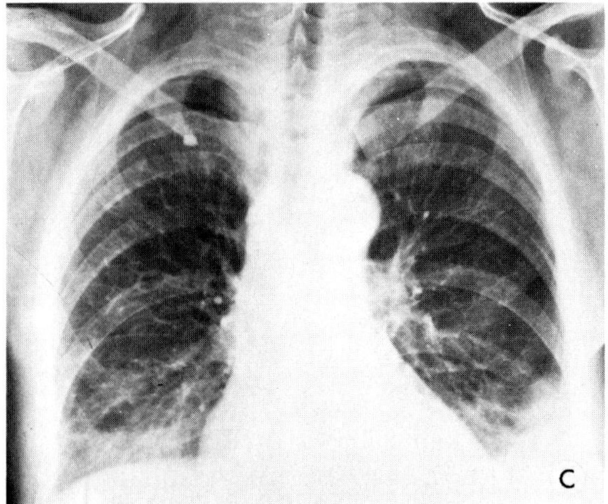

Fig. 4-7. (C) Chest film demonstrates bilateral lower lobe infiltrates corresponding to the scan defects.

abnormality as shown on the scan. Selective technic is more sensitive in detecting small emboli than is a main pulmonary artery injection.[16,27] In addition, the injection of less contrast medium into a smaller area of lung lessens morbidity from the procedure. This is especially important in patients with pre-existing cardiac or pulmonary disease. Once pulmonary emboli are demonstrated, the procedure may be terminated. If no emboli are found in the region of a scan defect, selective injections must be performed in other areas of scan abnormality, if present. There is no need to study areas shown to be normal by scan. In patients in whom pulmonary angiography carries a high risk, such as those with pre-existing pulmonary hypertension, left bundle branch block, or digitalis toxicity, bilateral leg venography is an alternative method of study. The demonstration of thrombi in the veins of the lower extremity or pelvis is sufficient indication for anti-coagulation and good presumptive evidence of pulmonary embolism in a patient in whom there is strong clinical suspicion. Patients with a history of bleeding peptic ulcer or other relative contraindications to anticoagulation, however, usually require definitive diagnosis by pulmonary angiography.

These guidelines for pulmonary angiography have been developed over the past 13 years and are reflected in our changing volume of pulmonary arteriograms performed since 1964. The number of pulmonary arteriograms increased rapidly from 1964 to 1970, reflecting enthusiasm for the procedure and at the time our failure to recognize the value of a normal lung scan in excluding pulmonary embolism. Since 1971, each request for pulmonary angiography has been screened by a member of our cardiovascular radiology staff. Lung scans and chest radiographs are reviewed, and the patient is interviewed. This approach has led to a significant decrease in pulmonary an-

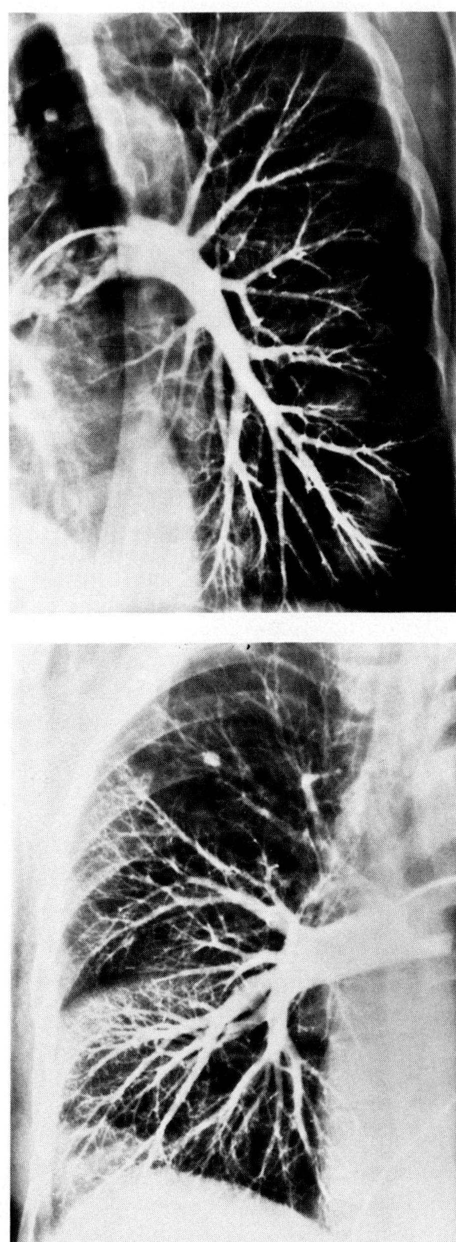

Fig. 4-7. (D,E) Bilateral selective pulmonary arteriograms are normal; the patient was subsequently found to have bilateral lower lobe pneumonias.

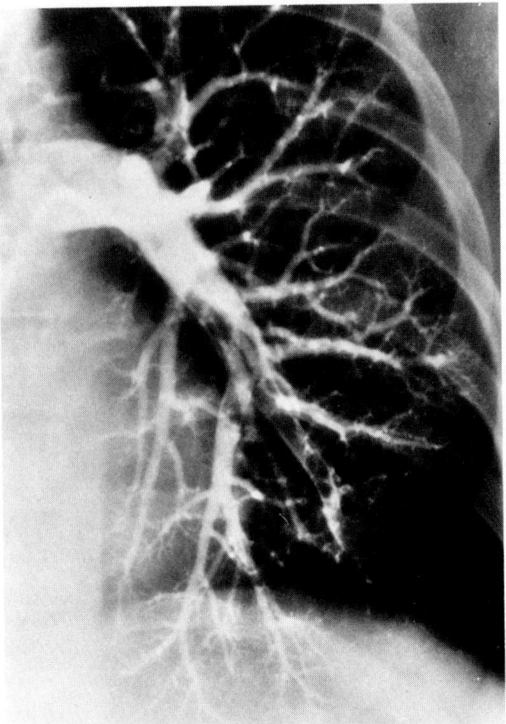

Fig. 4-8. Selective left pulmonary arteriogram. There is an embolus within the artery to the lower lobe extending into several branches. The embolus is seen as an intraluminal filling defect with contrast material around it.

giography, as many patients with either normal lung scans or scans indicating a high probability of pulmonary embolism did not require study. Since 1974 we have increased our number of selective pulmonary angiograms largely as a result of recognizing the nonspecificity of matching ventilation–perfusion scan defects and corresponding pulmonary infiltrates. This approach has been very valuable, as we are now recognizing a significant group of patients (30 percent) with these matching defects who prove to have pulmonary emboli angiographically.[26] It is our feeling, however, that lung scans are necessary in all patients, including those with abnormal chest radiographs, since they are such an effective screening technique and provide an important road map for selective angiography in equivocal cases.

The demonstration of an intraluminal filling defect is essential to the angiographic diagnosis of pulmonary embolus[28–30] (Figs. 4-5, 4-6, and 4-8). If there is complete obstruction to blood flow, the proximal end of the clot must be demonstrated protruding into the lumen of the pulmonary artery (Fig. 4-9). Occlusion of vessels without evidence of a filling defect is not

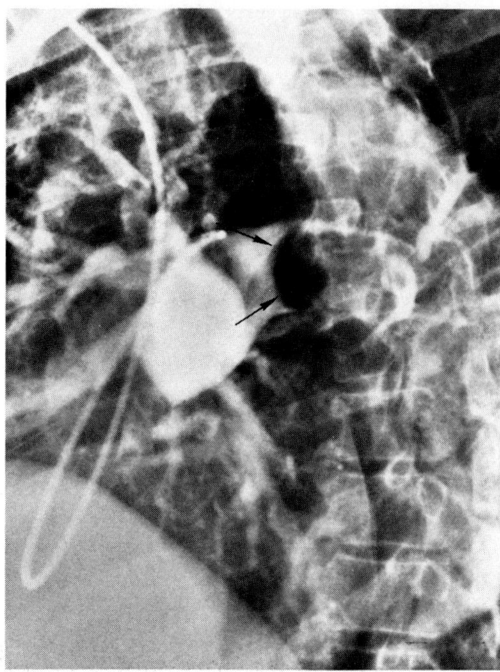

Fig. 4-9. Main pulmonary arteriogram in the right posterior oblique projection. There is nearly complete occlusion of the left pulmonary artery. The trailing edge of an embolus projects into the contrast filled lumen (arrows) permitting the diagnosis of embolization to be made with certainty.

specific evidence of pulmonary embolism and has been seen in pulmonary neoplasms, abscesses, and tuberculosis.[13,30-32] The demonstration of slow or diminished flow in localized areas of the lung is likewise not specific for pulmonary embolism and may be seen in pneumonia, atelectasis, bronchiectasis, or neoplasms.[13,29,30]

Resectability of Bronchogenic Carcinoma

Pulmonary arteriography may be indicated in the preoperative evaluation of certain patients with bronchogenic carcinoma in order to spare patients with nonresectable disease from undergoing thoractomy.[31-34] Pulmonary arteriography is complementary in this regard to mediastinoscopy. Two other angiographic procedures, azygography and superior vena cavography may also reveal vascular invasion. All are employed to determine nonresectability, since vascular occlusion or encasement invariably indicates invasion of vital mediastinal structures by tumor.

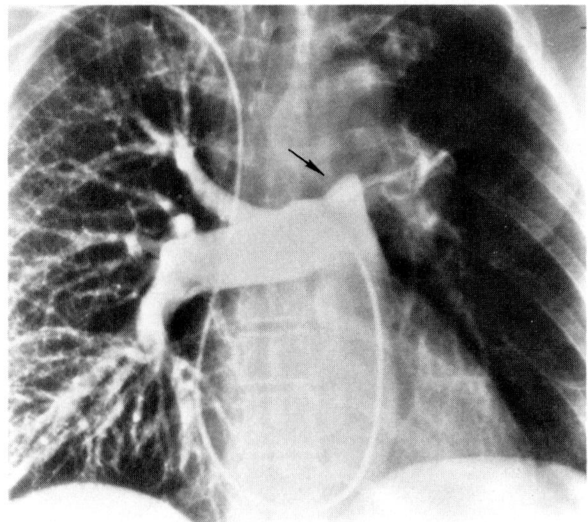

Fig. 4-10. Main pulmonary arteriogram. A mediastinal neoplasm is encasing the proximal left pulmonary artery (arrow). The tumor was unresectable.

Pulmonary arteriography may be considered in a patient with a hilar or mediastinal neoplasm and no evidence of distant metastases or other considerations contraindicating surgery. The angiographic demonstration of occlusion or invasion by tumor of the proximal one to two centimeters of the main left or right pulmonary artery or the intrapericardial pulmonary veins is evidence of nonresectability[31–33] (Fig. 4-10). Catheterization of the azygous vein and retrograde azygography may be performed at the time of pulmonary arteriography. The demonstration of encasement or occlusion of the azygous system by tumor is likewise considered evidence of unresectability.[31,34,35] Superior vena cavography is indicated in patients with clinical signs of superior vena caval obstruction.[34] These studies are accurate in determining nonresectability when positive, but are associated with false-negative rates of from 21 to 46 percent,[31,32] due largely to tumors producing mediastinal involvement in areas not impinging directly on a major vascular structure.

Pulmonary angiography may also be helpful in patients whose tumors are technically resectable but whose pulmonary function leaves doubt about whether they could survive pneumonectomy. Arteriography may reveal whether lobectomy rather than pneumonectomy can be performed.[32,34] Involvement of the lobar vessels distal to the first few centimeters from their origin or involvement of only segmental vessels may indicate the possibility of lobectomy. The presence of pre-existing pulmonary hypertension has been shown to be associated with increased mortality[8] and morbidity[36] fol-

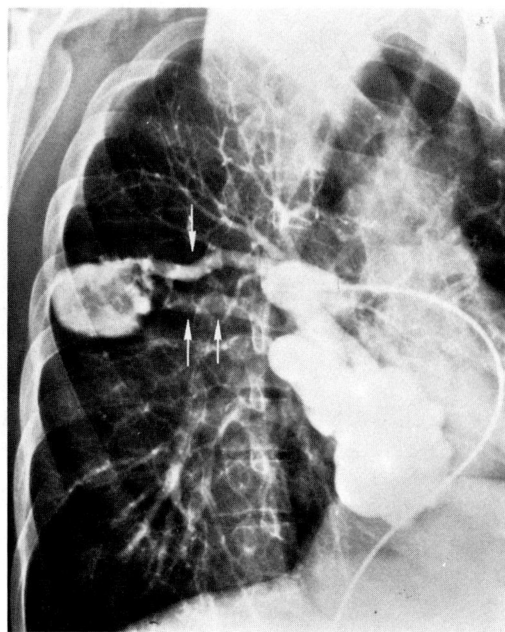

Fig. 4-11. Right pulmonary arteriogram in the left posterior oblique projection. There are two large arteriovenous fistulae present. The feeding artery (single arrow) and an early draining vein (double arrows) from the upper fistula are demonstrated in this projection.

lowing pneumonectomy. This can be determined at the time of pulmonary arteriography. In patients with moderately severe pulmonary function abnormalities and a normal baseline pulmonary artery pressure, temporary balloon occlusion of the pulmonary artery on the side of the tumor may be performed. If this does not result in a mean pulmonary artery pressure of greater than 35 mm Hg proximal to the occlusion, or systemic arterial hypoxemia ($Po_2 < 45$ mm Hg), pneumonectomy is thought to be feasible.[37]

Other Indications

Other conditions amenable to study by pulmonary arteriography include congenital abnormalities such as pulmonary arteriovenous fistula (Fig. 4-11), hypoplasia or aplasia of one of the pulmonary arteries, or anomalous pulmonary venous return. The levo phase of the pulmonary arteriogram may be used in studying left atrial myxoma or thrombosis. Although dissections or aneurysms of the thoracic aorta are optimally studied by direct retrograde aortography, occasionally this procedure will be precluded by occlusion of the femoral or subclavian arteries. In such situations the levo phase of the pulmonary arteriogram may be employed (Fig. 4-12).

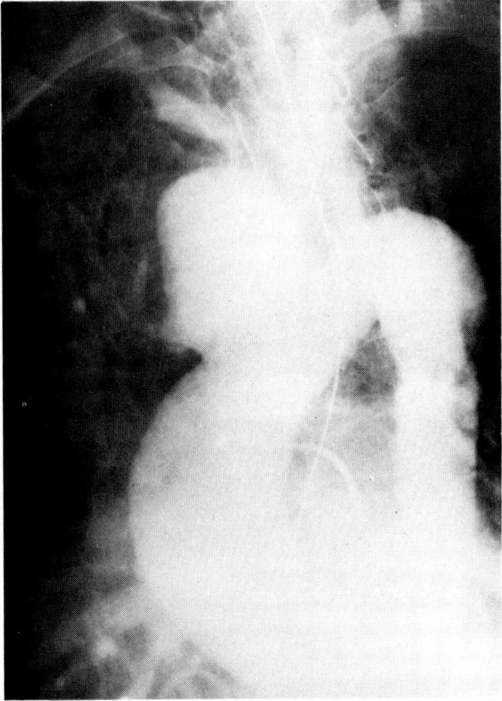

Fig. 4-12. The levo phase of a pulmonary arteriogram demonstrates an aneurysm (mycotic) originating from the aortic arch. Severe atherosclerotic disease precluded a direct retrograde aortogram. (Reprinted from Kaufman SL, White RI Jr, Harrington DP, Barth KH, Siegelman SS: Protean Manifestations of Mycotic Aneurysms. Am J Roentgenol 131:1019–1025, 1978.

REFERENCES

1. Sevitt S: Anticoagulant prophylaxis against venous thrombosis and pulmonary embolism. In Sasahara AA, Stein M (eds): Pulmonary Embolic Disease. Grune & Stratton, Inc., New York, 1965, p 265–276
2. Dalen JE, Alpert JS: Natural history of pulmonary embolism. Prog Cardiovasc Dis 17:259–270, 1975
3. The Urokinase Pulmonary Embolism Trial. Circulation 47 (Suppl. II):1–108, 1973
4. Alpert JS, Smith R, Carlson CJ, et al: Mortality in patients treated for pulonary embolism. JAMA 236:1477–1480, 1976
5. McIntyre KM, Sasahara AA: Hemodynamic alterations related to extent of lung scan perfusion defect in pulmonary embolism. J Nucl Med 12:166–170, 1971

6. McIntyre KM, Sasahara AA: The hemodynamic response to pulmonary emobilism in patients without prior cardiopulmonary disease. Am J Cardiol 28:288–294, 1971
7. Leland OS, Sasahara AA: Hemodynamic observations in patients with pulmonary thromboembolism. In Sasahara AA, Stein M (eds): Pulmonary Embolic Disease. Grune & Stratton, Inc., New York, 1965, p 110–119
8. Rams JJ, Harrison RW, Fry WA, et al: Operative pulmonary artery pressure measurements as a guide to post-operative management and prognosis following pneumonectomy. Dis chest 41:85–90, 1962
9. Grollman JH Jr, Gyepes MT, Helmer E: Transfemoral selective bilateral pulmonary arteriography with a pulmonary-artery-seeking catheter. Radiology 96:202–204, 1970
10. Ferris EJ, Athanasoulis CA, Clapp PR: Inferior venacavography correlated with pulmonary angiography. Chest 59:651–653, 1971
11. Courey WR, de Villasante JM, Waltman AC: A quick, simple method of percutaneous transfemoral pulmonary arteriography. Radiology 113:475–477, 1974
12. Glenn JH, Ranninger K: A variation of the technique of transfemoral pulmonary arteriography. Radiology 117:473, 1975
13. Bookstein JJ: Pulmonary thromboembolism with emphasis on angiographic pathologic correlation. Semin Roentgenol 5:291–305, 1970
14. Smith GT, Dammin GJ, Dexter L: Post mortem arteriographic studies of the human lung in pulmonary embolization. JAMA 188:143–151, 1964
15. Jefferson KE: The normal pulmonary angiogram and some changes seen in chronic non-specific lung disease. Proc R Soc Med 58:677–681, 1965
16. Johnson BA, James AE Jr, White RI Jr: Oblique and selective pulmonary angiography in diagnosis of pulmonary embolism. Am J Roentgenol 118:801–808, 1973
17. Moses DC, Silver TM, Bookstein JJ: The complementary roles of chest radiography, lung scanning and selective pulmonary angiography in the diagnosis of pulmonary embolism. Circulation 49:179–188, 1974
18. Stein MA, Winter J, Grollman JH Jr: The value of the pulmonary artery-seeking catheter in percutaneous selective pulmonary arteriography. Radiology 114:299–304, 1975
19. Watson J: Severe pulmonary hypertensive episodes following angiocardiography with sodium metrizoate. Lancet 2:732–733, 1964
20. Szucs MM Jr, Brooks HL, Grossman W, et al: Diagnostic sensitivity of laboratory findings in acute pulmonary embolism. Ann Intern Med 74:161–166, 1971
21. Sasahara AA, Stein M, Simon M, et al: Pulmonary angiography in diagnosis of thromboembolic disease. N Engl J Med 270:1075–1981, 1964
22. Poulose KP, Reba RC, Gilday DL: Diagnosis of pulmonary embolism. A correlative study of the clinical, scan and angiographic findings. Br Med J 3:67–71, 1970
23. Gilday DL, Poulose KP, DeLand FH: Accuracy of detection of pulmonary embolism by lung scanning correlated with pulmonary angiography. Am J Roentgenol 115:732–738, 1972
24. McNeil BJ, Holman BL, Adelstein SJ: The scintigraphic definition of pulmonary embolism. JAMA 227:753–756, 1974
25. Alderson PO, Rujanavech N, Secker-Walker RH, et al: The role of ^{133}Xe venti-

lation studies in the scintigraphic detection of pulmonary embolism. Radiology 120:633–640, 1976
26. Cavaluzzi JA, Alderson PO, Kaufman SL, et al: The incidence of pulmonary embolism in patients with matching unilateral ventilation-perfusion lung scan defects and corresponding pulmonary infiltrates. Presented at the 78th Annual Meeting of the American Roentgen Ray Society, Boston, Mass., September 26–30, 1977
27. Bookstein JJ: Segmental arteriography in pulmonary embolism. Radiology 93:1007–1013, 1969
28. Weidner W, Swanson L, Wilson G: Roentgen techniques in the diagnosis of pulmonary thromboembolism. Am J Roentgenol 100:397–407, 1967
29. Sagel SS, Greenspan RH: Non-uniform pulmonary arterial perfusion. Radiology 99:541–548, 1971
30. Bookstein JJ, Silver TM: The angiographic differential diagnosis of acute pulmonary embolism. Radiology 110:25–33, 1974
31. Benfield JR, Bonney H, Crummy AB, et al: Azygograms and pulmonary arteriograms in bronchogenic carcinoma. Arch Surg 99:406–409, 1969
32. Sanders DE, Delaure NC, Silverberg SA: Combined angiography and mediastinoscopy in bronchogenic carcinoma. Radiology 97:331–339, 1970
33. James AE Jr, White RI Jr, Cooper M: Pretreatment diagnostic evaluation with reference to pulmonary scans in lung cancer. J Thorac Cardiovas Surg 61:530–540, 1971
34. Baker RR: The clinical management of bronchogenic carcinoma—A progress report. Johns Hopkins Med J 137:208–215, 1975
35. Janower ML, Dreyfuss JR, Skinner DB: Azygography and lung cancer. N Engl J Med 275:803,808, 1966
36. Harrison RW, Adams WE, Long ET, et al: The clinical significance of corpulmonale in reduction of cardiopulmonary reserve following extensive pulmonary resections. J Thorac Surg 36:352–368, 1958
37. Olsen GN, Block AJ, Swenson EW, et al: Pulmonary function evaluation of the lung resection candidate: A prospective study. Am Rev Respir Dis 111:379–387, 1975

Stanley S. Siegelman, M.D.

5

Computed Tomography

TECHNIQUE

Computed tomography (CT) is a sophisticated technique that combines x-rays, an electronic data-acquisition system, and a computer to provide detailed two-dimensional reconstructed images of narrow transaxial sections of the body. The acronym CAT has also been employed, with the letters representing *C*omputerized *A*xial *T*omography or *C*omputer *A*ssisted *T*omography. CT is the product of the union of standard x-ray technology with computer science and the mathematics of image reconstruction. As with standard chest roentgenography, the examination employs an x-ray generator and an x-ray tube. In standard roentgenography, the x-ray beam from a fixed source traverses the patient to strike an intensifying screen. The screen emits quanta of light which react with a film to record an image. Routine roentgenography is very much analogous to photography in which the photographic image is obtained when variable quanta of light impinge upon a sensitive film in a camera. Computed tomography is much more complicated. A source of x-rays rotates in a fixed circle around the patient who is immobilized in the horizontal position within the center of the examining module, which is called a gantry (Fig. 5-1). The x-ray tube emits a highly collimated x-ray beam. The intensity of the attenuated x-ray beam that emerges after traversing a defined pathway through the field of examination is measured at brief, regular intervals by a series of x-ray detectors. In this fashion, a variable-thickness (usually 3 to 13 mm) circumferential section of the body is examined. The detectors consist of an array of scintillation crystals (sodium iodide, bismuth germinate, or calcium fluoride) or a compartmentalized xenon gas ionization chamber. The detectors are de-

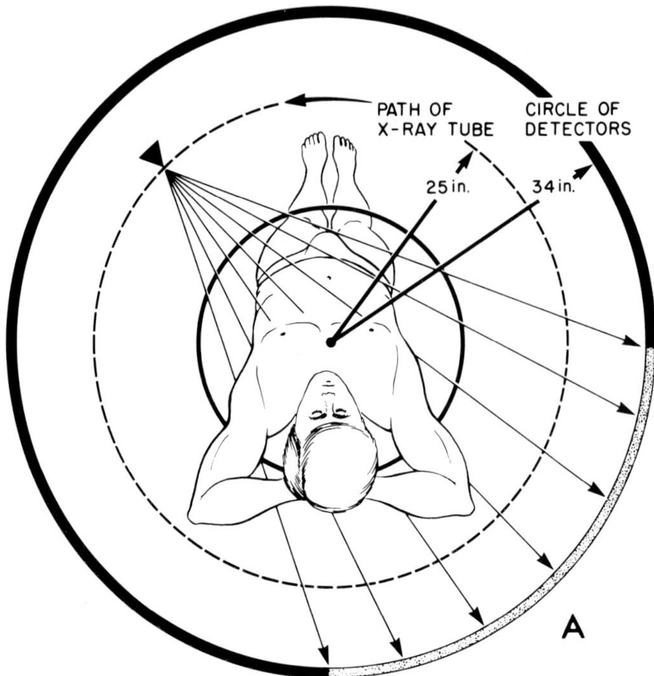

Fig. 5-1. (A) Patient position during CT examination. A fan beam of x-rays traverses the patient to strike a fixed circle of detectors. (B) Side view of patient during examination. Collimation is employed to produce a narrow x-ray beam. The diagram shows a single detector (short arrows) surrounded by tungsten pins (long arrows) for screening scattered radiation.

signed to produce a measurable signal when x-ray photons are intercepted. The crystals emit quanta of light (bismuth germinate emits blue light when it interacts with x-rays), which are amplified by photomultiplier tubes. With gas detectors, the gas is ionized by the x-ray beam. The reactive pulses are electronically amplified to produce a quantifiable electronic current which is a measure of the intensity of the attenuated x-ray beam. The electronic current is transformed by an analog to digital converter into a numerical reading which is stored and processed by a digital computer. The image of the body section provided by the computer is properly called a computed tomogram or CT image. The total examination consists of a series of sequential body sections taken at regular intervals through the appropriate area of interest.

In 1917, Radon, an Austrian mathematician established that a two-dimensional or three-dimensional object can be completely reconstructed if an infinite set of all of its projections is available.[1–3] Computed tomography is the quantitative reconstruction of the internal details of a two-dimensional body section by means of a series of one-dimensional projections. When a beam of x-rays passes through the body, x-ray quanta are absorbed and scat-

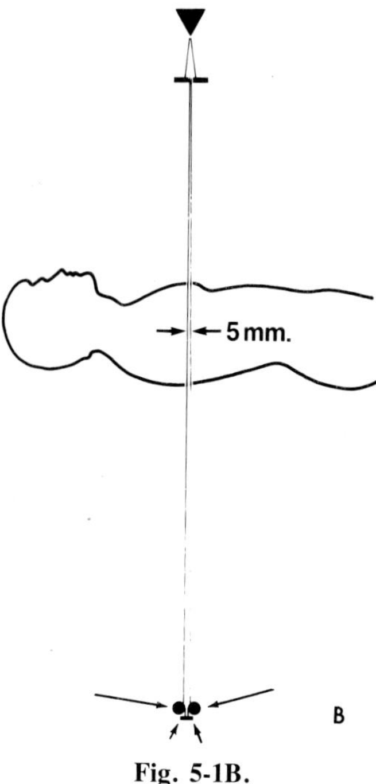

Fig. 5-1B.

tered to a variable degree by body tissues and fluids. The attenuation of x-rays depends upon the physical density and the atomic composition of the tissues in the path of the beam. The x-ray attenuation properties of any tissue may be expressed quantitatively as an effective linear attenuation coefficient. During the CT examination the detectors record the intensity of the x-ray transmissions at various angles. The detector measurements of multiple defined pathways (projections) through the field of examination may be used to calculate the x-ray absorption coefficients of any set of points in the field. With the guidance of an *algorithm* (a detailed mathematical reconstruction formula) the computer processes the data generated to reconstruct a point-by-point array of relative absorption coefficients of the section of the body which has been examined. This array of data points, a *matrix,* (generally 160 × 160, 256 × 256, 320 × 320, or 512 × 512) is highly accurate since it is based upon computer processing of hundreds of thousands of discrete quantitative measurements. Each data point corresponds to a fixed volume of tissue (called a *voxel*) within the area of examination. The pictorialized display of the voxel as a data point is called a picture element or *pixel.* The two-dimensional array of pixels (the matrix) may be conveniently displayed on a cathode ray tube (CRT) or a television monitor using various shades of gray to distinguish the range of effective linear attenuation coefficients. The CRT or TV image is recorded photographically to obtain a permanent record.

CT Numbers

In actual practice CT numbers rather than linear x-ray absorption coefficients are employed to designate the property of tissue which is recorded. Water has been arbitrarily assigned a CT number of zero. For other tissues CT number is determined by the following formula:

$$\text{CT number}_{\text{tissue}} = \text{constant}\ \frac{(\mu_{\text{tissue}} - \mu_{\text{water}})}{\mu_{\text{water}}}$$

In this equation μ represents effective linear attenuation coefficient.

A constant of 500 or 1000 is used in the formula. With a constant of 1000, air has a CT number of -1000, bone has a CT number of $+1000$, and soft tissues, with the exception of fat, have a range of CT numbers between 10 and 80. Fat, with its low density, has a CT number between -80 and -100.

Historical Perspective

The first clinical CT unit was developed by Godfrey Hounsfield, a physicist with EMI Ltd. in England. The machine examined the head exclusively. The unit used two sodium iodide crystal detectors for data gathering and produced an image based upon an 80×80 matrix after a scanning time of four and one-half minutes. It was put to clinical use in 1971.[4] Applying the same principles, Ledley in 1974 developed a CT unit that was capable of imaging the body.[5] All of the CT images illustrated in this chapter were produced by the CT unit developed by the American Science and Engineering Corporation. The A.S. & E. Scanner employs a fixed array of 600 bismuth germinate crystal detectors. After a 10-second scan period, the computer reconstructs an image based upon a 512×512 matrix. Since 600 separate calculations are required to compute the CT number for each pixel, the computer performs over 157 million ($512 \times 512 \times 600$) operations for each scan. With the large amount of data available, a very high fidelity reconstruction is delivered. This unit is capable of distinguishing objects that differ in linear attenuation coefficient by 1.0 percent; it also achieves a spatial resolution of 1.25 mm for high-contrast objects.

THE CLINICAL ROLE FOR COMPUTED TOMOGRAPHY

Computed tomography of the head was rapidly perceived as a revolutionary, valuable, noninvasive method for the evaluation of disorders of the brain.[6] In institutions where the equipment is available it is employed almost routinely for the evaluation and management of patients at risk for the full range of intracranial disorders: congenital abnormalities, hydrocephalus, tumors, infections, hemorrhage, infarction, edema, and the sequelae of trauma. The definitive role for CT of the body is yet to be established.[7] In November 1974 a body CT unit developed by the Ohio Nuclear Corporation was placed in clinical service at the Cleveland Clinic.[8] In October 1975 body CT units manufactured by EMI Ltd. were installed at the Mayo Clinic,[9] and the Mallinckrodt Institute of Radiology of the Washington University School of Medicine.[10] Subsequent reports from these institutions have indicated a promising role for CT in the evaluation of the pancreas, liver, and retroperitoneum.[11–16] Initial reports on the value of CT of the thorax were pessimistic.[9,10] Views of the transaxially sectioned thorax offered an additional perspective, but in all the early cases CT was done only after an abnormality was recognized on plain chest roentgenography. It was predicted that CT of the thorax would be far less effective as a clinical tool than CT of the head, or of the organs of the pelvis and abdomen. After further experience, however, subsequent reports have been more optimistic.[17–19] A number of clearly defined indications for CT of the thorax is emerging. There are few clinical situations that call for "routine" use of thoracic CT. The major role for the instrument in our view is to serve in a "problem-solving" capacity when other noninvasive techniques have failed to provide adequate information. In the recent past CT examinations of the thorax comprised 10 percent of the body examinations (i.e., non-head) at the Mallinckrodt Institute[18] and 6 percent of the body studies at the Cleveland Clinic.[19] At the Johns Hopkins Hospital, 210 of the first 1000 body CT examinations involved the thorax. Our current indications for CT of the thorax are outlined in Table 5-1.

INDICATIONS FOR CT EXAMINATIONS OF THE THORAX

Pulmonary Nodules

One of the primary current indications for CT of the thorax is to detect pulmonary parenchymal nodules that are not apparent on plain chest roentgenography or whole-lung tomography. What are the principles that determine our ability to detect nodules in the lung? The *size* of the nodule is of primary importance. Lesions smaller than 3 mm in diameter will not be seen on standard chest roentgenography.[20,21] Moody et al. reviewed 42 cases of metastatic lung disease and noted that all pulmonary metastases that were 15 mm or larger were detected on plain chest roentgenography.[22] In experiments in which lucite balls (to simulate pulmonary neoplasms) are incorporated into roentgenograms for test purposes, 10–12-mm nodules are seen with great regularity.[21] Four to ten millimeters appears to be the critical size range. The visibility of such nodules is markedly influenced by many factors.

The ability of a sophisticated observer to detect a lesion in the plain

Table 5-1
Indications for CT Examination of the Thorax

I. Pulmonary Parenchyma
   1. To search for pulmonary nodules.
      A. Prior to definitive therapy for a patient with bone, tumor, melanoma, soft tissue sarcoma.
      B. Prior to pulmonary resection for presumed localized metastatic disease.
      C. Sputum positive for cancer, chest x-ray negative.
   2. To detect parenchymal disease in the presence of pleural effusion.
   3. To determine if an abnormality is pulmonary or pleural.
   4. To distinguish granuloma from carcinoma.
   5. To detect suspected lesions hidden by the mediastinum.

II. Mediastinum
   1. To establish the cause for the widened mediastinum: fat versus vascular structure versus tumor.
   2. To locate anterior mediastinal tumors.
      A. Thymoma.
      B. Parathyroid adenoma.
   3. To evaluate paraspinal widening.
   4. To study the questionably abnormal hilum.
   5. To stage lung tumors.

III. Pleura
   1. Determination of extent of pleural tumors.
   2. To detect loculated pleural effusions.

IV. Chest Wall
   1. Evaluation of the sternum.
   2. Determination of extent of chest wall tumors.
   3. Planning for radiotherapy of chest wall masses.

V. Diaphragm
   1. To locate subphrenic abscess.
   2. To make a positive diagnosis of diaphragmatic herniation of fat.

VI. Trachea
   To map infiltrating submucosal masses.

VII. Heart
   1. To detect pericardial effusion.
   2. To distinguish between pericardial cysts and pericardial fat pads.

chest roentgenogram depends not only on the size and density of the lesion but also upon the nature of the surrounding structures. The density and the complexity of the anatomic structures in the area of the lesion have an important influence on its visibility.[23] When ribs or blood vessels are immediately adjacent, they tend to obscure the details of the outline of the lesion. Six-millimeter nodules are generally seen only when they are projected directly over rib interspaces.[21] Lesions most apt to be obscured on the basis of location are those at the lung apex, in the inferior recesses about the diaphragm, and in the subpleural area.

Another important factor is the coarse random fluctuations in density of a radiograph, which are called "radiographic mottle."[23,24] The intensity of background mottle is a function of the kilovoltage employed in the examination, the speed of the film, the chemical composition of the screens, and the temperature of the developer. Increased background mottle definitely results in reduced detectability of lesions. The effect of kilovoltage is an example of the complex interrelationships involved. Raising the energy of the x-ray beam from 100 to 150 kVp has a salutary effect on the detectability of 4–6-mm nodules in a chest phantom.[25] Increasing the energy produces a decreased prominence of the bones, and therefore, the ribs and clavicles are less likely to obscure the fine structure of the pulmonary parenchyma. Even though the contrast between the nodules and the surrounding lung is decreased at 150 kVp, the nodules are more readily detected because of the decreased interference from the overlying osseous structures. As kilovoltage increases beyond 200 kVp, lesions become more difficult to detect because bone–soft tissue contrast exhibits no further decrease, whereas contrast between the lesion and normal lung decreases and background mottle increases.[25]

Occasionally, if small nodules are present, the partial superimposition of one nodule upon another can result in a loss of smoothness in the outline and hence a loss of detectability. Heitzman has an excellent discussion on the interactions of multiple nodules.[20] Sufficient size of nodules will, of course, compensate for the distractions produced by overlying structures and film technique.

If one were to examine excellent quality P-A and lateral chest roentgenograms in a group of patients harboring pulmonary nodules, in what percentage would the nodules be detected? A reasonable answer to this question is that 50–60 percent of the patients with lesions would be detected. All lesions 3 mm and smaller would be missed. Many lesions in the 4–10-mm range would be missed as a function of size and location. Ten to twenty percent of clearly observable lesions would be overlooked because of observer error. Moody et al. found P-A and lateral chest roentgenograms positive in 33 of 50 examinations (66 percent) in patients with proven metastatic disease.[22] The investigators, however, were aware that they were examining chest films in patients with proven metastases and made efforts to locate the lesions. A somewhat lower percentage should be expected in most clinical situations.

Whole chest tomography is a more efficient manner of examining the pulmonary parenchyma for nodular lesions. Without listing, tabulated data, Miller et al. of the Mayo Clinic, have stated that in studying oncology patients with a high risk of pulmonary metastases whole lung tomography revealed nodular lesions that were not present on P-A and lateral chest roentgenograms in 12 percent of patients examined by both modalities.[26] The additional yield is attributable to elimination of the obscuration by overlying ribs, heart, diaphragm, or pulmonary vessels and hence the detection of smaller nodules. Tomography will frequently disclose lesions that are 3 to 4 mm in diameter.[27] The best recent data on the role of tomography in increasing the yield of pulmonary nodules comes from the Surgery Branch of the National Cancer Institute, where since 1969 all patients have had whole lung tomography as a routine part of their initial evaluation. Neifeld et al. reported that of 152 patients with extrathoracic malignant disease evaluated by whole lung tomography, 25 had lesions found on tomography that were not present on plain chest roentgenography. Nineteen of the 25 lesions proved to be metastases at thoracotomy. More important, of 64 patients with nodules on plain chest roentgenography, 14 (21.9 percent) also had contralateral lesions demonstrated on tomography.[27] Polga and Watnick noted that 8 of 28 patients with a solitary metastasis seen with conventional chest x-rays had additional lesions detected by tomography.[28] Based upon this experience, it is reasonable to estimate that in a survey of patients for metastatic nodules, whole lung tomography will detect 20 percent more cases of metastases than plain chest roentgenography. Despite the greater yield when contrasted to plain chest roentgenography, whole lung tomography fails to detect numerous lesions. From the NIH experience, 8 of 38 patients (21 percent) with extrathoracic malignancies in whom solitary nodules were found at whole lung tomography had multiple unilateral nodules at thoracotomy, and 35 of 48 patients with multiple nodules during whole lung tomography, had additional nodules detected at thoracotomy.[27]

Computed tomography is significantly more sensitive than whole chest tomography in detecting lung nodules. There is less scattered radiation with the CT examination, and the ability to achieve a spatial resolution of 2 mm is an easy task for CT equipment. With the gray scale adjustment of the CT examination, it is possible to display nodules as white against a dark background. The difference in density between the nodule and the surrounding tissue is greater than on either plain chest roentgenography or tomography (Fig. 5-2). Computed tomography will detect smaller lesions and will detect more subpleural lesions than will conventional tomography (Fig. 5-3). Muhm et al. at the Mayo Clinic, studied 29 patients with whole lung and CT tomography; CT showed more nodules in 10 of the 29 patients.[29] Most of the additional nodules detected by CT were 5 to 10 mm in size. Three of the 10 patients had no nodules shown by conventional tomography, and CT revealed one or more. Two of the 10 patients had unilateral nodules, and CT revealed bilateral nodules. Jost et al. also reported five patients with lung nodules on CT not seen on conventional tomography. Four of these patients had solitary nodules on whole lung tomography. The additional nodules found on CT markedly affected patient management.[18] Schaner et al. reported that there were twice as many nodules detected with CT as with conventional tomography.[30] Most of the additional nodules were between 3 and 6 mm in size. All of the aforementioned authors have noted that the additional nodules detected by CT tended to be located in the lung apices, the subpleural regions, or in the recesses of the lung near the diaphragm.

The matter of establishing precisely the existence of pulmonary nodules is of major importance in directing therapy for the patient with malignant disease. Recent experience at NIH indicates that if all metastatic pulmonary nodules are removed at surgery, the five-year survival is 50 percent for metastatic carcinoma and 32 percent for sarcoma.[27] These figures represent an improvement over those from an earlier Mayo Clinic series in 1965 which indicated a five-year survival of 32 percent for carcinoma and 23 percent for sarcoma.[31]

What are the roles for plain chest roentgenography (PCR) whole lung tomography (WLT) and CT of the thorax in the preoperative evaluation of the patient with known extrathoracic malignant disease? If a group of patients at risk for pulmonary metastases were examined by each modality, our current estimate, based upon the preceding discussion, is that CT is the most sensitive method and will detect nodules in 40 percent of patients with negative WLT. WLT, however, is more sensitive than PCR and will detect nodules in 20 percent of patients with negative PCR. Of 100 patients with nodules seen on CT, 72 would also have nodules on WLT, and only 60 would have nodules detected by PCR. If the overall incidence of lung metastases was very low in the group of patients being studied, as in patients with Stage I cancer of the cervix, the extra cost and effort to detect additional lesions by CT would not be justified. (If PCR shows lesions in 60 of 2000 patients, then 1940 CT examinations would be required to show an additional 40 patients with lung metastases). There are a number of populations in which the anticipated incidence of lung metastases is high. In such populations we can anticipate that PCR will fail to detect lesions in a significant percentage of the group, and hence, routine CT is indicated. Thus, a clear-cut role exists for routine CT of the thorax in patients with primary bone tumors, soft tissue sarcomas, and melanoma, despite the presence of normal PCR. Metastases from sarcomas are more frequent, and more apt than carcinomatous metastases to be overlooked on PCR.[27] In institutions where CT is not available, WLT should be performed on such patients prior to the determination of the primary mode of therapy. The role for WLT and CT is less clear in patients with primary carcinoma of the cervix, bladder, prostate, kidney, colon, and breast who have normal PCR. Muhm et al. advocate routine CT for all patients with primary tumors "who would benefit from additional treatment . . . for a pulmonary metastasis if it were detected."[29] This recommendation has been criticized on the grounds that the additional cost to implement such an uncritical approach would not be justified by the anticipated benefits to the population of cancer patients.[32] The management strategy for such patients is also complicated by the fact that not all pulmonary nodules are metastatic. Additional evaluation of this question is in order. The final resolution will probably be to employ CT in patients with normal PCR only if the patient fits into a well-defined category of high risk for metastatic disease.

Computed tomography to search for additional pulmonary parenchymal

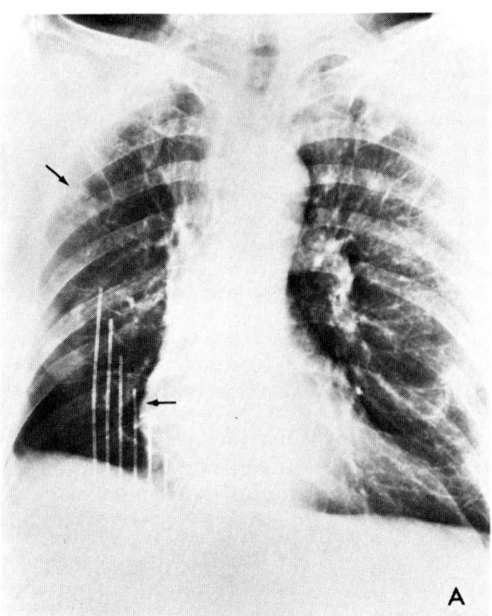

Fig. 5-2. Pulmonary nodule seen clearly by CT examination. 61-year-old man with abnormal sputum cytology. (A) Chest roentgenogram with catheter markers. A probable nodule was detected in the right upper lobe projected over the right fourth posterior interspace (oblique arrow). There was also a suspicion of scattered patchy areas of radiodensity in the left lower chest. The catheters placed on the posterior chest wall serve as a guide to the level of the CT images of the lower chest. The horizontal arrow indicates the section of the thorax corresponding to Figure 5-2B, (since cross-sections of four catheters appear in Figure 5-2B); (B) CT image of chest corresponding to the location indicated by horizontal arrow in Figure 5-2A. Four catheters are seen in cross-section on posterior chest wall. No abnormalities are present in the lung at this level; (C) CT image of the thorax at level of trachea and aortic arch. A subpleural parenchymal mass is present in the right lung (arrow). The lesion proved to be an epidermoid carcinoma of the lung.

nodules is also definitely indicated at this time in several other specific groups of patients with malignant disease. Since the likelihood of discovery of additional lesions is great, and since the knowledge of the total number of lesions is vital to treatment planning, CT should be performed on patients with proven malignancies who have either a single nodule or a series of nodules localized to one lung by PCR or WLT. Routine CT of the thorax should also be considered in selected research protocols which deal with new methods of cancer therapy whenever precise information on the existence of lung metastases is required. Computed tomography of the thorax is also in-

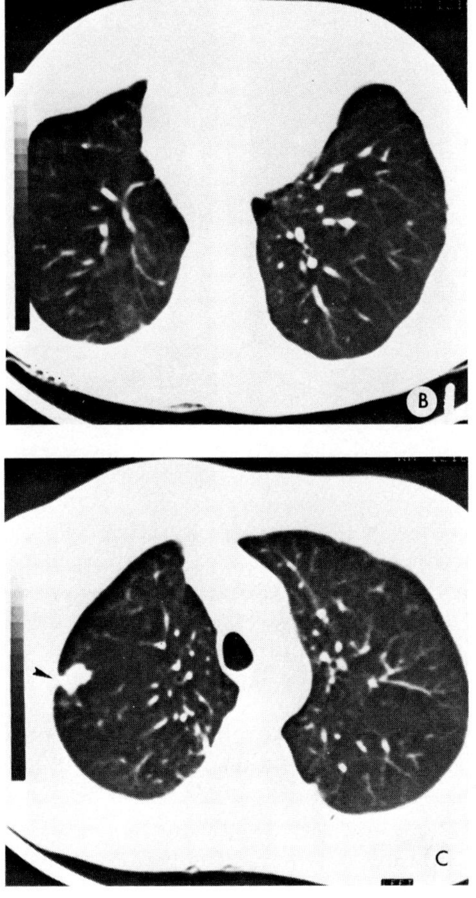

Figs. 5-2B and C.

dicated for patients with sputum cytology indicating cancer and normal PCR, although fiberoptic bronchoscopy and tantalum bronchography also play roles in evaluating such patients (see Chapters 2 and 8). Muhm et al. reported that CT detected lesions in two of six patients with malignant cells in sputum but negative PCR and WLT.[29]

As a diagnostic test for the presence of metastatic pulmonary nodules CT is definitely superior to PCR and WLT. There are limitations which should be recognized, however. The CT examination will not detect a nodule if the axial section of the lung containing the lesion is not imaged. The screening CT examination consists of a sequential series of 1-cm sections of the thorax. The patient rests on an examining table that is moved in 1-cm increments after each exposure. If the patient makes a significant undetected movement on the examining table, it is possible to exclude a section of the thorax from the examination. It is important to devise a strategy whereby the patient is examined with the same lung volume for each chest

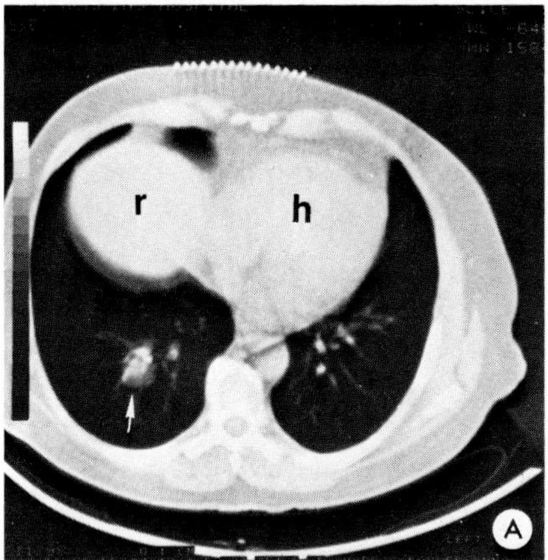

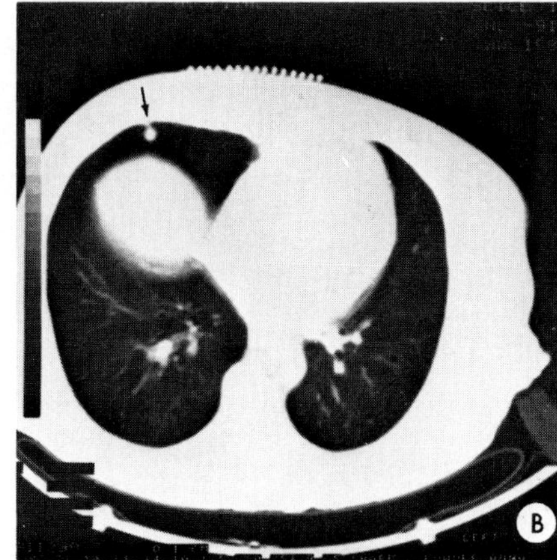

Fig. 5-3. Detection of nodule not seen on routine chest roentgenography. A 69-year-old female with carcinoma of the cervix had an apparent solitary lesion in the right lower lobe on routine chest roentgenography. (A) CT section obtained from the inferior portion of the thorax showing right hemidiaphragm (r) inferior portion of heart (h) and a 2-cm nodule in right lower lobe (arrow); (B) CT section at slightly higher level. A 6-mm subpleural nodule (arrow) is apparent in the anterior portion of the right lung. The 6-mm lesion was not detectable in the chest roentgenogram, even in retrospect. Both nodules proved to be granulomas.

section. With a cooperative patient, the best maneuver is to examine with breath-holding at maximum inspiration. However, if in the judgment of the supervising radiologist, the patient is unlikely to be capable of sustaining a series of held maximum inspirations, it is preferable to examine during resting lung volume (end tidal volume). The patient is instructed to inspire at this usual tidal volume and then to breathe out and to relax. In this situation the natural recoil forces of the lung create a reproducible state of lung volume, i.e., the resting lung volume. Muhm et al. reported four false-negative CT scans among 52 cases attributable to faulty positioning or patient movement.[29] This problem will not occur if a cooperative patient is given proper instructions prior to the examination.

Granuloma Versus Carcinoma

Not all nodules detected by PCR, WLT, or CT will represent metastatic disease. In the NIH study, 182 thoracotomies were performed to remove noncalcified nodules in a group of patients with known malignant disease.[27] Of these lesions, 9.3 percent represented a second primary cancer and 74.3 percent represented metastases, but 16.4 percent represented benign granulomatous disease. In one small series of 15 patients with sarcomas, CT examination of the thorax showed twice as many nodules as WLT, but the majority of the additional small nodules detected by the CT were found at thoracotomy to be due to benign disease.[33] Further evaluation is required to assess the capacity of CT to distinguish between granuloma and carcinoma. Theoretically, CT has the capacity for recognition of granulomas by means of CT number. If a scattering of calcium (too small to be detected by standard tomography) were present in the lesion, the CT number should increase since calcium has a high atomic number relative to lung tissue. Sagel et al. first illustrated this phenomenon.[34] They reported an asymptomatic 70-year-old woman who had two well-circumscribed nodules which had no detectable calcium when studied by conventional tomography. One of the nodules had a CT number identical to an adjacent blood vessel and proved to be a carcinoma. The CT number of the second nodule was 30 units higher than a comparable-sized artery and proved to be a granuloma. Jost et al. later reported that by means of this phenomenon (CT number within lesions significantly higher than CT number of blood vessel in the field of examination), 3 of 42 coin lesions were diagnosed as granulomas.[18] Kollins at the Cleveland Clinic has not shared the early success of the radiologists at the Mallinckrodt Institute. Kollins reports that he has been unable to use CT to detect calcium in lesions that did not appear calcified when studied by conventional tomography.[19] Raptopoulos et al. performed a retrospective study of the results of CT in 31 patients with solitary lung nodules—18 benign and 13 malignant.[35] In 16 of the 18 benign nodules there was evidence of either attenuation values in the range of calcium or distinctive high-density foci within the nodules. All 13 malignant nodules had low-density values and none exhibited high-density foci. All nodules seen to contain calcium with conventional techniques had calcium confirmed by CT. In addition, CT detected calcific foci in five benign nodules in which no calcium was apparent on conventional tomography. Muhm et al. have also found that high CT numbers with a lung lesion are a reliable indication of calcium, but these investigators believe that conventional tomography remains more accurate than CT in detecting small amounts of calcification.[29] This is an area of potentially great economic significance if CT could reliably diagnose benign disease in nodules without manifest calcium on conventional tomography.

There are at least two reasons for the current inadequacy of CT in this area: the partial-volume effect and the beam-hardening artifact. The partial volume effect (Fig. 5-4) refers to variation in CT numbers as a function of the volume of the lesion which occupies the area of examination. Although the picture matrix, the product of a single CT examination, is a two-dimensional display, the data summarized in the image are derived from a three-dimensional slice of tissue. The thickness of the tissue slice is an important variable. The final CT number calculated is derived from an average of multiple measurements of *all* of the tissue within the three-dimensional area. If a 5-mm lesion is imaged in a CT slice with a thickness of 13 mm, the CT number readings for the area of interest also receive an important contribution from the air in the lung inferior and superior to the lesion. The partial-vol-

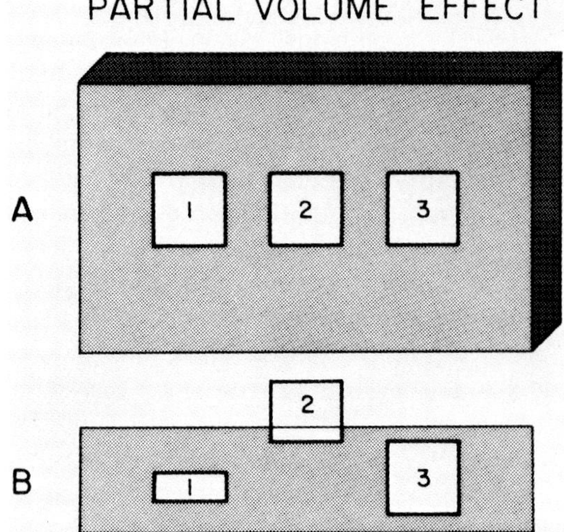

Figure 5-4. Diagrammatic illustration of partial volume effect. "A" represents a hypothetical CT image of a section of the lung. It appears as if the areas within Boxes 1, 2, and 3, are comparable. "B" represents the same lung section viewed on end. If Boxes 1, 2, and 3 contain identical materials, the CT number determined for Boxes 1 and 2 would be significantly lower than the CT number determined for Box 3, because Boxes 1 and 2 include a considerable volume of lung tissue. It should be apparent that as the width of the slices decreases, the partial volume effect is minimized.

ume effect may be minimized by using thinner sections. In the A.S. & E. scanner it is possible to obtain reliable images that are only 3-4 mm in thickness. An additional factor that prevents absolute reliance on the fidelity of CT numbers is the heterogeneity of the energies in the x-ray beam. The theory of image reconstruction assumes that the total attenuation of an x-ray beam along a fixed pathway is a function of the sum of the absorption coefficients of the tissues at regularly spaced intervals along the pathway. This basic assumption is true only if the x-ray beam has a single energy. In practice, the beam consists of x-rays with a spectrum of differing energies. As the beam traverses tissues containing heterogeneous absorbing materials, the energy of the beam changes.[36] The chief manifestation is a beam-hardening artifact. After passing through a dense object, such as bone, a disproportionate number of low-energy components of the beam will be attenuated. The effect is to create a beam with higher energy which sustains less attenuation than anticipated in a subsequent pathway. The result of this phenomenon is the perception of artificially low attenuation numbers in the vicinity of dense tissue. The converse of this phenomenon generally does not occur and hence, artificially high CT numbers are not a problem.

Thus if we get a high CT reading on a pulmonary nodule, we can presume that it is benign. If we fail to detect a high reading, we are uncertain of the significance of the findings. There are various means to monitor the transmitted beam and make appropriate adjustments, but more work is required to perfect the corrections for beam hardening.

OTHER USES

Pulmonary Parenchyma

CT examination offers an additional perspective in that it provides a cross-sectional view of the thoracic contents. Since the pulmonary parenchyma and pleura are always superimposed in frontal, oblique, or lateral roentgenograms, it is not unusual to encounter a case in which it is not possible to distinguish between loculated effusion and pulmonary consolidation. Computed tomography has been of value in distinguishing between the pulmonary and pleural contributions to a radiographic abnormality, as illustrated in Figure 5-5. Another frequent problem confronting the clinician is our inability by standard means to evaluate any area of the lung that is surrounded and being obscured by pleural effusion. Under most circumstances the fluid should be completely removed after appropriate diagnostic procedures and the underlying parenchyma evaluated by PCR. When a significant amount of fluid cannot be removed, the horizontal display by CT permits visualization of the parenchyma underlying the pleural effusion. Computed tomography will occasionally uncover parenchymal lesions which are otherwise hidden by the normal mediastinal contents.[18] Also, CT may be used to distinguish between segmental atelectasis and pleural fibrosis.[19]

The Mediastinum

Computed tomography has several distinctive features that make it suitable for examination of the mediastinum. Fat, with its characteristic range of CT numbers, can always be recognized and distinguished from other mediastinal structures. After standard radiographic contrast media are injected intravenously, the CT numbers of vascular structures are increased beyond the range of other pulmonary tissues; thus, the superior vena cava, aorta, and pulmonary vessels may be identified with regularity and confidence. Finally, the unique horizontal cross-sectional view offers an additional means of visualizing the mediastinal contents. A list of indications for CT of the mediastinum has been offered in the table. The indications listed represent typical situations in which CT may serve in a "problem-solving capacity" when conventional noninvasive radiographic techniques have failed to provide a solution to a clinical problem or to a question raised by an

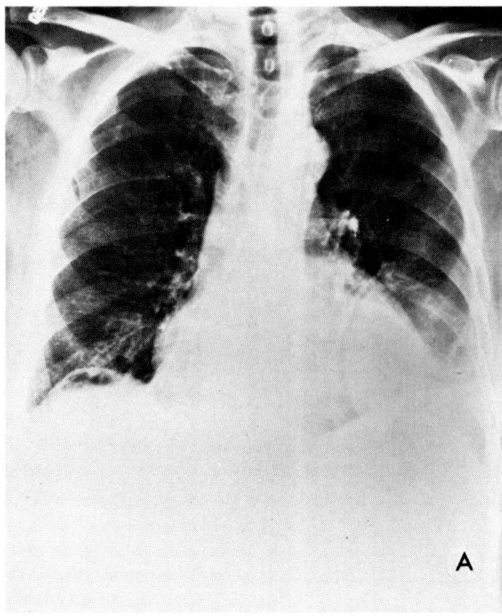

Fig. 5-5. The distinction between intrapulmonary and intrapleural abnormalities. (A) A 62-year-old man with cough and fever. A right pleural effusion has been drained with a tube. Figure 5-5A shows a rounded collection in the left lower chest. It was not possible to determine from studies including decubitus films whether this represented pleural fluid or pulmonary consolidation.

abnormal chest roentgenogram. At this point we cannot state whether CT should replace standard tomography in any of these situations. Efficacy studies of CT versus other modalities in diagnosis of mediastinal disease have not been completed.

Analysis of the widened mediastinum is a natural task for CT. It should enable us to determine with regularity whether the mediastinal enlargement is due to fat deposits, to dilated vascular structures, or to tumor.[37]

Computed tomography may be used to evaluate the anterior mediastinum, especially in patients in whom a mediastinal mass has not been detected by standard tomography despite a strong clinical suspicion of the existence of a lesion. Mink et al. studied five patients with myasthenia gravis and thymomas by chest radiography, conventional anterior mediastinal tomography, and CT.[38] In one of the five patients, plain chest roentgenograms were normal and repeated mediastinal tomography was equivocal, but CT clearly defined an anterior mediastinal tumor. These authors also found that CT visualized all of the thymomas. In addition CT provided useful additional information in two of the patients: the detection of unsuspected pleural metastases and the localization of a "possible lung mass" to the an-

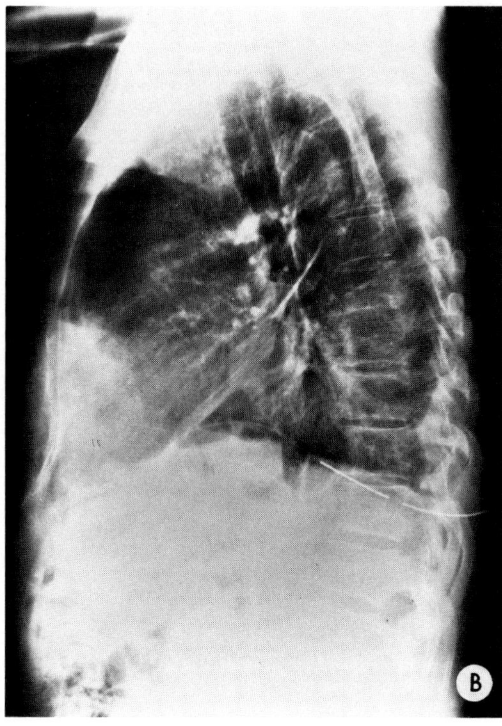

Fig. 5-5. (B) Lateral view of the chest. Right chest tube present posteriorly. Left chest abnormality is not well localized.

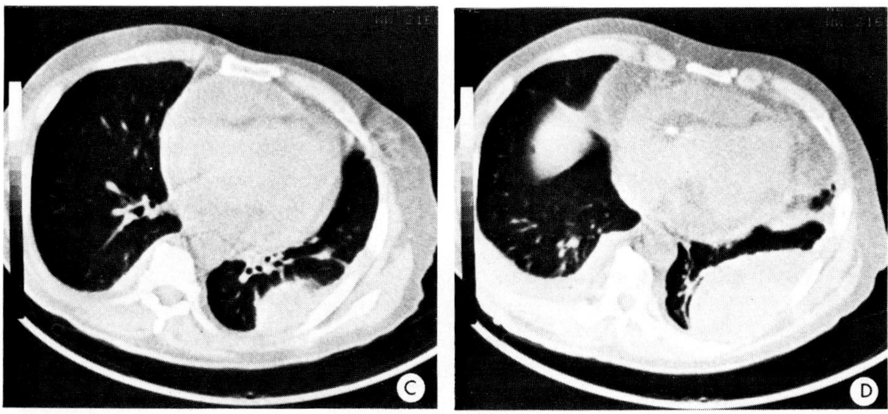

Fig. 5-5. (C) CT scans showing that the lesion is a loculated pleural fluid collection. A tube was inserted and the loculated effusion was drained. (D) It should also be noted that there is a small right pleural effusion in this figure.

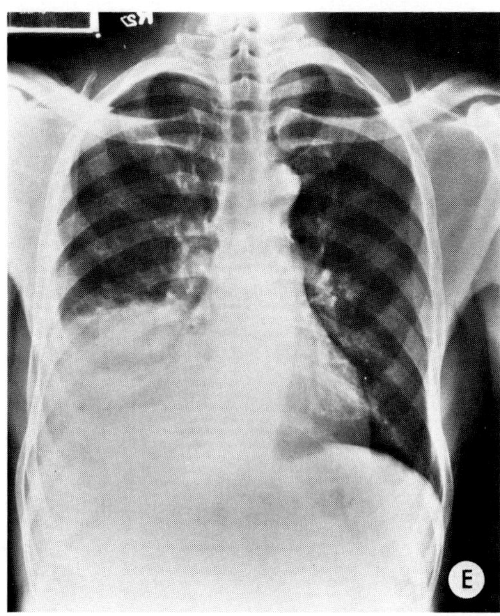

Fig. 5-5. (E) A 52-year-old man with two-month history of cough and fever. Chest x-ray shows right consolidation of the right lower chest. It could not be determined whether this represented a pulmonary or pleural abnormality.

terior mediastinum. Doppman et al., employing CT, localized four anterior mediastinal parathyroid adenomas in patients in whom chest roentgenography revealed no abnormality.[39]

In Figure 5-6, another useful role for CT is presented: evaluation of the patient with a posterior thoracic paraspinal widening that is not resolved by conventional radiographic techniques. In the case illustrated, the soft tissue prominence was attributable to a dilated aorta. When a paraspinal mass is due to adenopathy the enlarged nodes can generally be clearly identified.[18]

Heitzman et al., after experience with 150 cases of CT of the thorax, reported that CT has real merit in the evaluation of the abnormal or questionably abnormal hilum.[17] Since during standard roentgenography the mediastinal structures are seen en face in lateral or oblique projections, the profile view provided by CT may be of considerable assistance. After intravenous administration of contrast medium, an enlarged hilum can frequently be attributed to an innocent dilatation of the pulmonary artery. Standard tomography of the hilum in the oblique position is an excellent technique which has found increasing acceptance in recent years.[40–43] There are many groups who believe that there is little need for an additional means of hilar evaluation because of the excellent studies provided by oblique hilar tomography.

The final possible indication for CT of the mediastinum is to evaluate

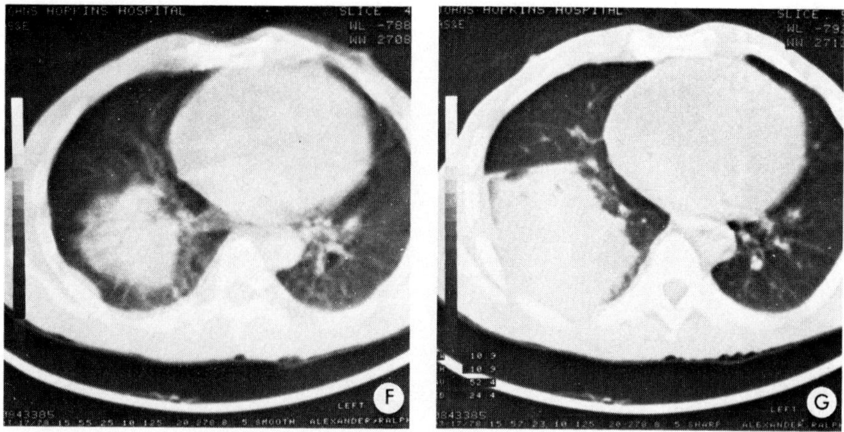

Fig. 5-5. (F) CT scan of the lower chest showing that the abnormality represents an area of parenchymal consolidation. (G) Slightly higher section shows the better advantage the area of pulmonary consolidation.

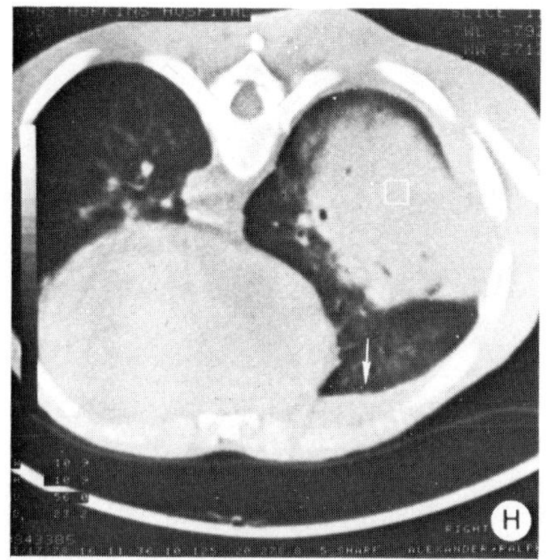

Fig. 5-5. (H) To ascertain this finding the patient was placed prone and a small amount of fluid is seen layering in the right pleural cavity (arrow). The dense area of pulmonary consolidation remains.

the extent of disease in order to stage tumors. The reader is referred to Chapter 10, "Mediastinoscopy," to underline the importance of knowing the extent of disease before planning definitive therapy for lung cancer. CT should provide excellent information on the existence of subcarinal, peritracheal, hilar, and mediastinal nodes. Whether CT is superior to conventional tomography in this regard is yet to be determined. Castellino et al. found that routine whole lung tomography in patients with lymphoma revealed information that was not suspected on plain chest films which resulted in a

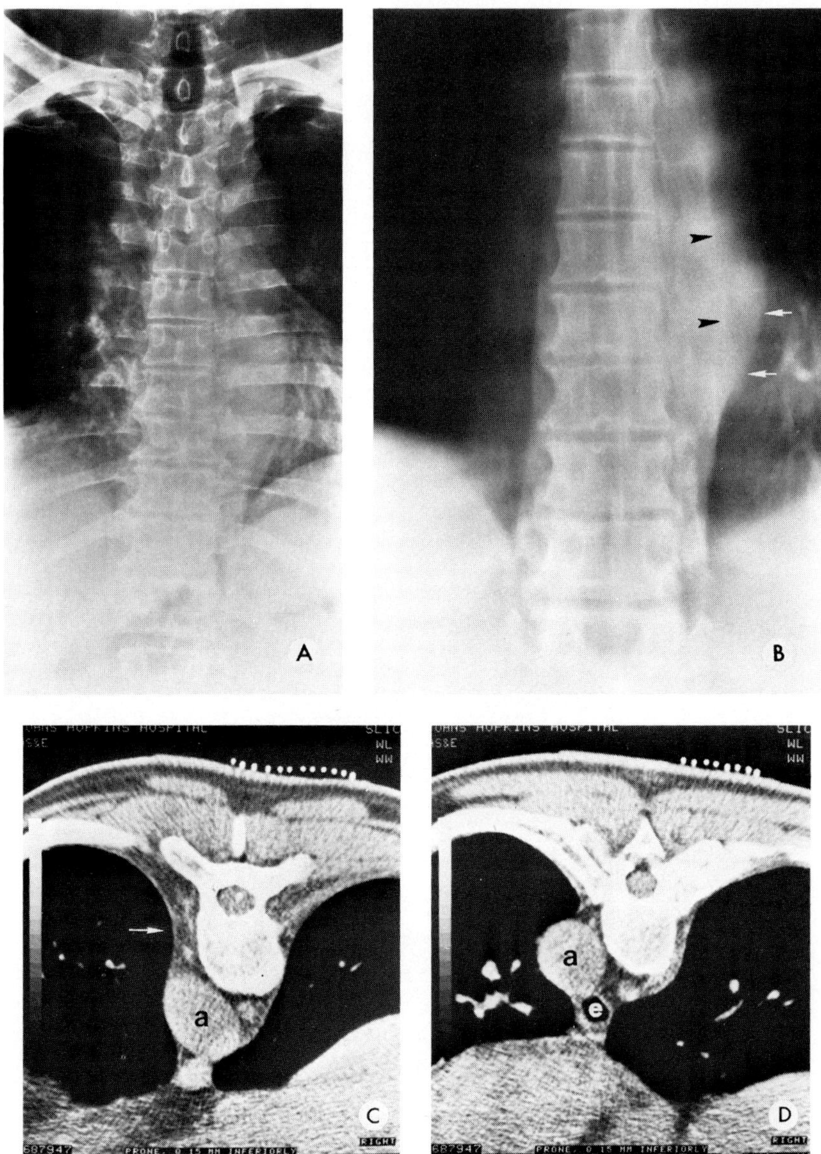

Fig. 5-6. A 52-year-old male with apparent paraspinal mass noted on routine chest roentgenogram. (A) AP view of thoracic spine shows excessive fullness of the soft tissue structures to the left of the spine; (B) AP tomogram shows widening of the left paraspinal soft tissue stripe (black arrows). A prominent aorta (white arrows) was also present; (C) CT scan obtained in prone position. No mass is present. The prominent paraspinal shadow (arrow) is due to a displacement of extrapulmonary soft tissue structures by a slightly dilated aorta (a); (D) CT scan at slightly higher level than Figure 5-6C. Normal aorta (a) and esophagus (e) are visualized.

change in the staging or treatment of the disease in only 11 of 243 patients.[44] Whether CT can alter this low percentage of useful examinations must await further study.

Pleura

The third general area in which CT of the thorax should prove useful is in the imaging of pleural disease. Pleural collections have a circumferential distribution which is usually more easily imaged by CT than by frontal or lateral radiography. The pleural and subpleural zones have less inherent contrast than other regions of the lung,and CT is superior to other imaging techniques in this area.[45] The rind-like growth of mesothelioma was illustrated by Sheedy et al.[9] In general the extent of pleural tumors can be demonstrated much more effectively by CT than by any other means. Loculated pleural effusions are easily distinguished from localized areas of pulmonary consolidation.

Chest Wall

CT is particularly suited to imaging the details of the bone, muscle, and subcutaneous tissues of the chest wall.[19,30] It can determine whether a lesion projected over the periphery of the chest is pulmonary, pleural, or extrapleural (Fig. 5-7). The extent of tumors of the chest wall and the degree of infiltration of the thoracic contents can best be mapped by CT for radiotherapy treatment planning. Computed tomography is probably the procedure of choice to image lesions of the sternum, which are notoriously difficult to visualize by other techniques.

The Diaphragm

The use of CT for problem solving when other imaging techniques have failed to establish a diagnosis is well illustrated with two recent Johns Hopkins Hospital patients with abnormalities related to the diaphragm. The first patient (Fig. 5-8) had a lobulated soft-tissue mass located at the base of the right lung which had not been present three years previously. The mass had a constant relationship to the diaphragm and seemed to be of suitable appearance for a diaphragmatic hernia, but an upper gastrointestinal series and a barium enema examination showed no bowel in the chest. The CT examination (Fig. 5-8D) shows that the lesion is a well-circumscribed soft-tissue mass. The CT number within the lesion was -119, indicating that the mass is composed of fat. The mass represents either herniation of omental fat or a benign lipoma. Surgery has not been performed on this patient. The value of CT in several very similar cases has been recognized by others, and histologic confirmation is not required in such cases.[18,34,46] The patient shown in Figure 5-9 had a prolonged history of recurrent episodes of pleuro-

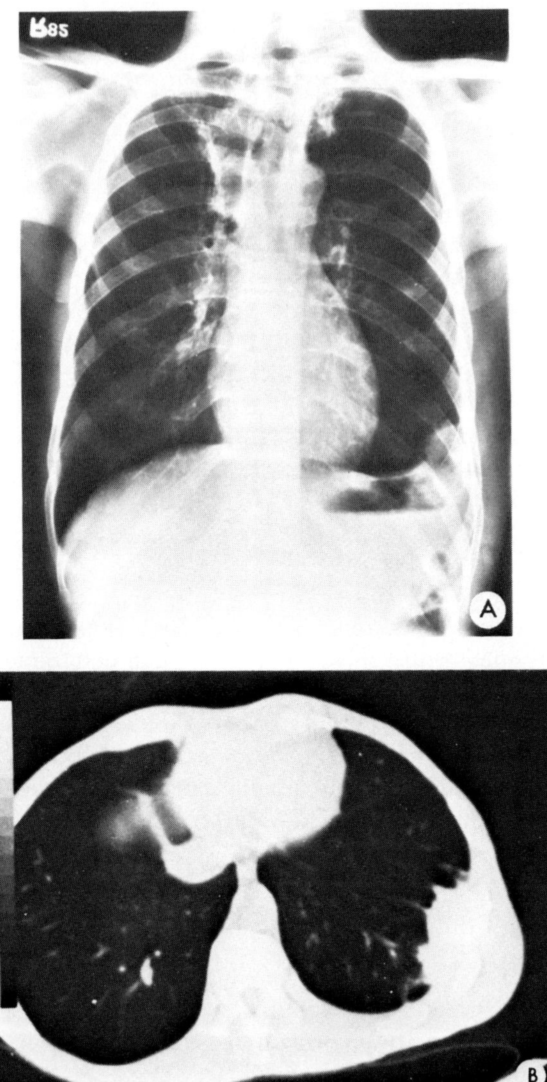

Fig. 5-7. Chest wall evaluation. A 50-year-old man with proven actinomycosis of the thorax. (A) A chest roentgenogram shows soft tissue swelling along the left lateral inferior portion of the chest wall. There is a localized bulge at the left costophrenic angle; (B) CT image shows a diffuse swelling of the chest wall and the involvement of the underlying pleura and pulmonary parenchyma.

pulmonary inflammation involving the right lower chest. The patient was hospitalized on several occasions over a period of years. An extensive work-up, including fiberoptic bronchoscopy and transtracheal lung biopsy, failed to reveal the cause for the patient's recurring pulmonary difficulties. Computed tomography scan of the diaphragm demonstrates a chronic subphrenic abscess. Although the reader may be surprised by the chronic history, the abscess in our patient was promptly drained. Rosenberg has emphasized that subphrenic abscesses may persist for months or years to serve as a source of recurring fever or anemia.[47]

Trachea

The trachea can usually be successfully examined by a variety of endoscopic and radiographic procedures. On occasion, however, additional useful information may be derived from the unique transaxial view afforded by CT. Such a case is illustrated in Figure 5-10, a patient with an adenocystic carcinoma of the trachea with submucosal infiltration. Computed tomography helped to determine the extent of disease and hence to establish a plan for appropriate therapy. This patient had the endobronchial component of the tumor removed by laser surgery. The use of CT provides a noninvasive way of following such lesions.

Heart and Pericardium

Experimental studies with isolated animal hearts have shown that it is possible by means of CT to localize acute myocardial infarction.[48,49] Infarcted myocardium has a lower attenuation number by virtue of an increase in intracellular water. Human hearts, when studied in vivo, have CT characteristics similar to animal hearts; an area of myocardial infarction has been identified by means of its low attenuation values.[50] It is anticipated that CT of the myocardium will be feasible if the CT unit can be gated to the electrocardiogram. This technology is being developed, and it is anticipated that CT scanning to evaluate for myocardial ischemia will be performed in the early 1980s. Pericardial effusions can be diagnosed by CT, but cardiac ultrasound is the procedure of choice for detecting and monitoring pericardial collections. Computed tomography can also be used to distinguish pericardial fat pads from pericardial cysts.[8]

COSTS

The installation of a computed tomography unit is an expensive undertaking. Initially the units were priced at $350,000–$400,000, but in 1978 the price was apt to be in the range of $500.000–$600,000. Most of the direct technical costs for the examination are fixed; i.e., they are expenses that

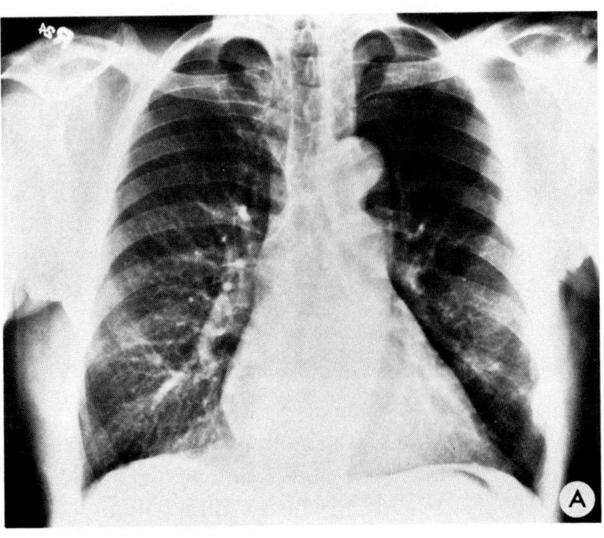

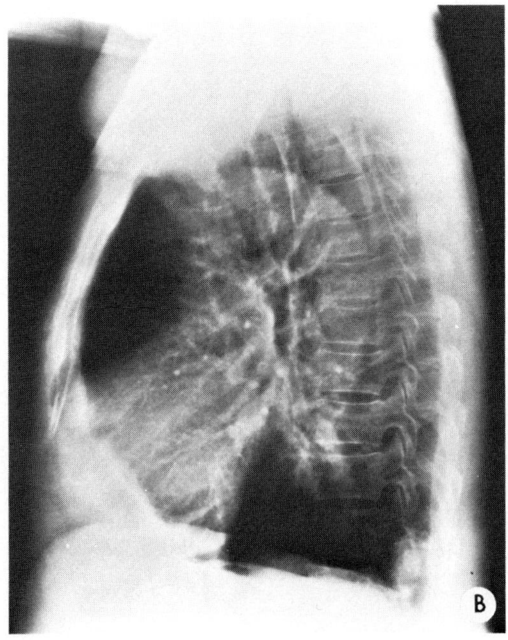

Fig. 5-8. Mass containing fat. A 67-year-old man hospitalized for severe arthritis. (A) Chest roentgenogram shows soft tissue fullness above the right hemidiaphragm; (B) Lateral chest roentgenogram. An abnormal density is present at the posterior cardiophrenic angle.

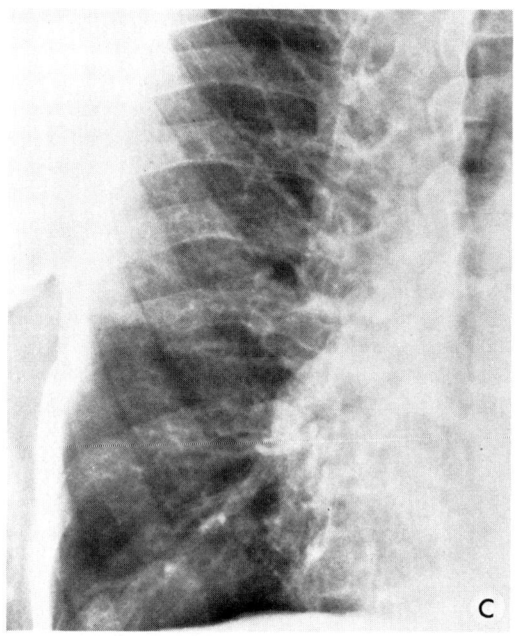

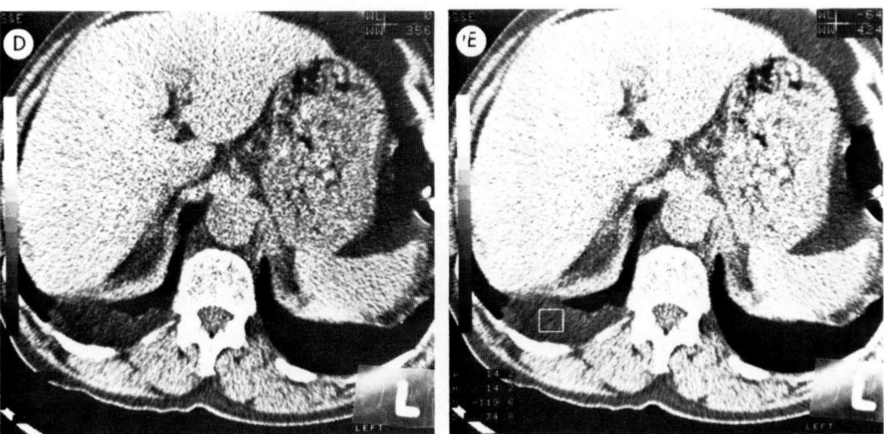

Fig. 5-8. (C) Oblique chest roentgenogram shows the lobulated density above the diaphragm. (D) CT Scan. A well-defined soft tissue mass is evident; (E) The white box (cursor) within the mass indicates that the average CT number within the lesion is being calculated. The readout at the bottom left of the figure shows the calculations which were obtained. The width of the cursor was 14.2 mm, the height of the cursor was 14.2 mm. The average attenuation number within the lesion is −119 and the standard deviation is 34.

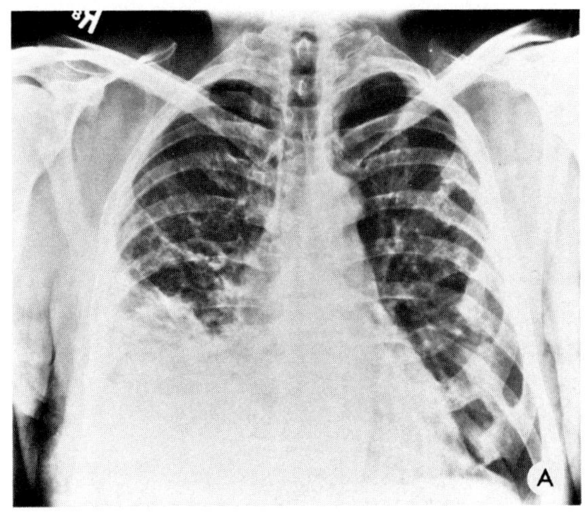

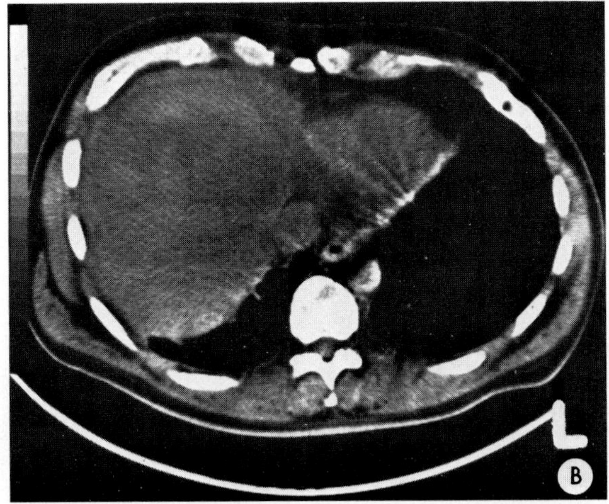

Fig. 5-9. A 54-year-old male with recurrent episodes of cough and fever. Bronchoscopy showed purulent material draining from the right lower lobe but no evidence of an endobronchial lesion. (A) Chest roentgenogram discloses pleural pulmonary inflammation in the right lower chest; (B) CT scan through the base of the right lung shows a circular area of reduced attenuation which was interpreted as a subdiaphragmatic abscess. An abscess in this location was indeed found at surgery and a drain was left in place.

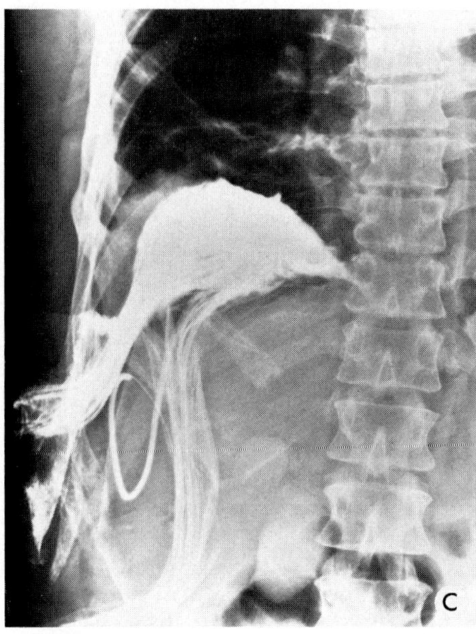

Fig. 5-9. (C) The abscessed cavity is outlined by injection of contrast material into the drain.

must be covered whether one is examining two patients or twenty patients per day. The high fixed costs include allocations for the cost of the equipment, room alterations, a maintenance contract, and full-time technical personnel. A survey in early 1976 of 98 operating units revealed that 83 percent of direct costs was fixed.[51] With further increases in the price of the equipment, the expenses for direct costs are approaching 90 percent. The upshot of this is that patient volume has very little effect on total cost, because only variable costs (for items such as contrast media and film) increase as the number of procedures increase. In order to keep total costs at a reasonable level, a hospital that plans to operate a CT unit must have the assurance of a reasonable patient load. At The Johns Hopkins Hospital, the CT unit is employed in examining 16 patients per day, and the total charge for each examination is $175. This is to be contrasted with a total charge of $120 for a whole lung tomography. If 8 instead of 16 patients a day were examined, the charge for the procedure would have to be doubled.

OVERVIEW

We believe that CT scanning of the thorax will play a significant role in the evaluation of selected patients with chest diseases. One item we have not emphasized sufficiently in the prior discussion is the value of a negative examination. In many areas CT is the single most sensitive imaging method

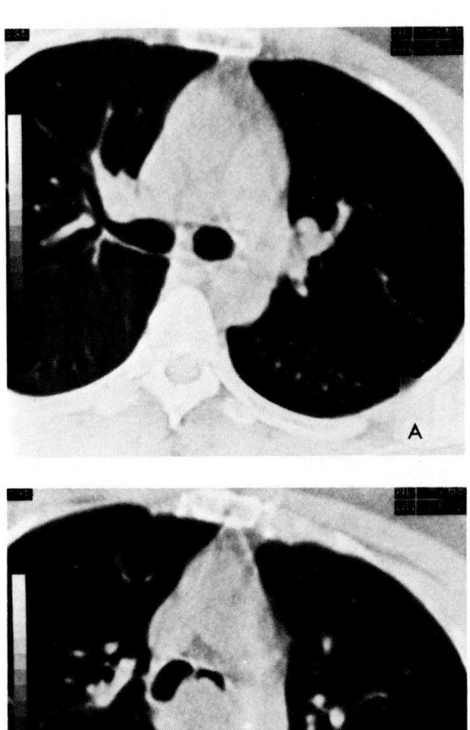

Fig. 5-10. A 47-year-old man with hemoptysis. Bronchoscopy showed a lesion of the lower trachea which proved to be an adenocystic carcinoma. The extent of the lesion could not be readily determined by conventional methods. (A) CT scan 2 cm below the tracheal bifurcation showing that both major bronchi are free of tumor at this point; (B) CT scan directly at the tracheal bifurcation showing that the tumor involves the bifurcation with narrowing of the posterior medial aspect of the right and left major bronchi.

for thoracic disease. Knowledge that a questionable mediastinum is normal or that a patient definitely does not have nodules in the lung is extremely useful and valuable information. Computed tomography provides a unique display of anatomy of the chest which provides very accurate localization. This accurate localization is useful for planning needle biopsy of the lung, surgical resections, and radiotherapy treatment. The main shortcoming of CT at this point seems to be a high cost, which can be offset in part by adequate use of the equipment.

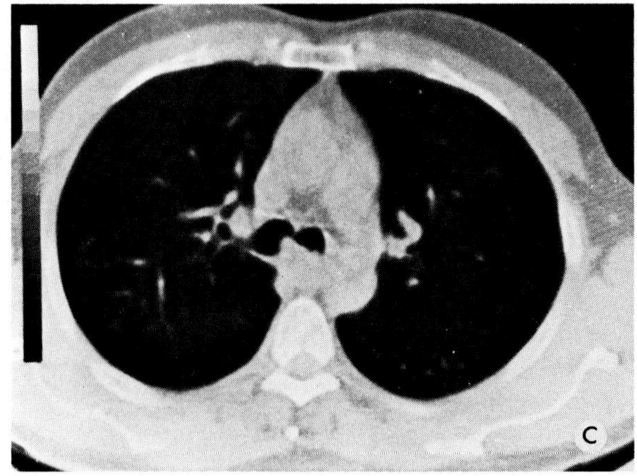

Fig. 5-10 (C) Post-op CT scan at the same level as Figure 5-10B following subtotal removal of the tumor by laser surgery.

REFERENCES

1. Radon J: On the determination of function from their integrals along certain manifolds. Berichte über die Verhandlungen der Königlich Sächsischen Gesellschaft der Wissenschaften zu Leipzig. Mathematisch-Physische Klasse 69:262–277, 1917
2. Gordon R, Herman GT, Johnson SA: Image reconstructions from projections. Scientific Am 233:56–68, 1975
3. Brooks RA, DiChiro G: Theory of image reconstruction in computed tomography. Radiology 117:561–572, 1975
4. Hounsfield GN: Computerized transverse axial scanning (tomography) Part 1. Description of system. Br J Radiol 46:1016–1022, 1973
5. Ledley RS, DiChiro G, Luessenhop AJ, Twigg HL: Computerized transaxial x-ray tomography of the human body. Science 186:207–212, 1974
6. Ambrose J: Computerized transverse axial scanning (tomography): Part 2. Clinical application. Br J Radiol 46:1023–1047, 1973
7. Abrams HL, McNeil BJ: Medical implications of computed tomography ("CAT scanning"). N Engl J Med 298:255–261; 310–318, 1978
8. Alfidi RJ, Haaga J, Meaney TF, et al: Computed tomography of the thorax and abdomen: A preliminary report. Radiology 117:257–264, 1975
9. Sheedy PF II, Stephens DH, Hattery RR, et al: Computed tomography of the body: Initial clinical trial with the EMI prototype. Am J Roentgenol Radium Ther Nucl Med 127:23–51, 1976
10. Stanley RJ, Sagel SS, Levitt RG: Computed tomography of the body. Early trends in application and accuracy of the method. Am J Roentgenol Radium Ther Nucl Med 127:53–67, 1976
11. Haaga JR, Alfidi RJ, Havrilla TR, et al: Definitive role of CT scanning of the pancreas: The second year's experience. Radiology 124:723–730, 1977
12. Havrilla TR, Haaga JR, Alfidi RJ, et al: Computed tomography and obstructive biliary disease. Am J Roentgenol Radium Ther Nucl Med 128:765–768, 1977

13. Levitt RG, Sagel SS, Stanley RJ, et al: Accuracy of computed tomography of the liver and biliary tract. Radiology 124:123–128, 1977
14. Sheedy PF II, Stephens DH, Hattery RR, et al: Computed tomography in the evaluation of patients with suspected carcinoma of the pancreas. Radiology 124:731–737, 1977
15. Stanley RJ, Sagel SS, Levitt RG: Computed tomographic evaluation of the pancreas. Radiology 124:715–722, 1977
16. Stephens DH, Sheedy PF II, Hattery RR, et al: Computed tomography of the liver. Am J Roentgenol, Radium Ther Nucl Med 128:579–590, 1977
17. Heitzman ER, Goldwin RL, Proto AV: Radiologic analysis of the mediastinum utilizing computed tomography. Radiol Clin North Am 15:309–329, 1977
18. Jost RG, Sagel SS, Stanley RJ, Levitt RG: Computed tomography of the thorax. Radiology 126:125–136, 1978
19. Kollins SA: Computed tomography of the pulmonary parenchyma and chest wall. Radiol Clin North Am 15:297–308, 1977
20. Heitzman ER: The Lung. Radiologic-Pathologic Correlations. St. Louis, C. V. Mosby, 1973, pp 64–70
21. Spratt JS Jr, TerPogossian M, Long RT: The detection and growth of intrathoracic neoplasms. Arch Surg 86:283–288, 1963
22. Moody DL, Edlich RF, Gedguadas E: The roentgenologic identification of pulmonary metastases: Evaluation of an operatively proved series. Dis Chest 51:306–310, 1967
23. Kundel HL, Peversz G: Lesion conspicuity, structured noise, and film reader error. Am J Roentgenol 126:1233–1238, 1976
24. Starr SJ, Metz CE, Lusted LB, Goodenough DJ: Visual detection and localization of radiographic images. Radiology 116:533–538, 1975
25. Christensen EE, Dietz GW, Murry RC, et al: Effect of Kilovoltage on detectability of pulmonary nodules in a chest phantom. Am J Roentgenol 128:789–793, 1977
26. Miller WE, Crowe JK, Muhm JR: The evaluation of pulmonary parenchymal abnormalities of tomography. Radiol Clin North Am 14:85–93, 1976
27. Neifeld JP, Michaelis LL, Doppman JL: Suspected pulmonary metastases—Correlation of chest x-ray, whole lung tomograms and operative findings. Cancer 39:383–387, 1977
28. Polga JP, Watnick M: Whole lung tomography in metastatic disease. Clin Radiol 27:53–56, 1976
29. Muhm JR, Brown LR, Crowe JK: Use of computed tomography in the detection of pulmonary nodules. Mayo Clin Proc 52:345–348, 1977
30. Schaner EG, Head GL, Kalman MA, et al: Whole-body computed tomography in the diagnosis of abnormal and thoracic malignancy: Review of 600 cases. Cancer Treat Rep 61:1537–1560, 1977
31. Thomford NR, Wolner LB, Clagett OT: The surgical treatment of metastatic tumors in the lungs. J Thorac Cardiovasc Surg 49:357–363, 1965
32. Savoca CJ, Gamsu G: Critical reviews. Invest Radiol 12:474–475, 1977
33. Schaner EG, Chang AE, Doppman JL, et al: Comparison of computed and conventional whole lung tomography in the detection of pulmonary metastases. J Comput Assist Tomogr 1:363, 1977
34. Sagel S, Stanley RJ, Evens RG: Early clinical experience with motionless whole body computed tomography. Radiology 119:321–330, 1976

35. Raptopoulos V, Schellinger D, Katz S: Computed tomography of solitary pulmonary nodules: Experience with scanning times longer than breath-holding. J Comput Assist Tomogr 2:55–60, 1978
36. Zatz LM, Alvarez, RE: An inaccuracy in computed tomography: The energy dependence of CT values. Radiology 124:91–97, 1977
37. Goldwin RL, Heitzman ER, Proto AV: Computed tomography of the mediastinum. Normal anatomy and indications for the use of CT. Radiology, 124:235–241, 1977
38. Mink JH, Bein ME, Siekow R, et al: Computed tomography of the anterior mediastinum in patients with myasthenia gravis and suspected thymoma. Am J Roentgenol 130:239–246, 1978
39. Doppman JL, Brennan MF, Koehler JO, et al: Computed tomography for parathryoid localization. J Comput Assist Tomogr 1:30–36, 1977
40. Brown LR, DeRemee RA: 55° Oblique hilar tomography. Mayo Clin Proc 51:89–95, 1976
41. Favez G, Willa C, Heinzer F: Posterior oblique tomography at an angle of 55° in chest roentgenography. Am J Roentgenol 120:907–915, 1974
42. McLeod RA, Brown LR, Miller WE, DeRemee RA: Evaluation of the pulmonary hila by tomography. Radiol Clin North Am 14:51–84, 1976
43. Pajewski M: The diagnostic value of the latero-oblique tomogram of the lungs. Br J Radiol 38:430–436, 1965
44. Castellino RA, Filly R, Blank N: Routine-Full-lung tomography in the initial staging and treatment planning of patients with Hodgkin's disease and non-Hodgkin's lymphoma. Cancer 38:1130–1136, 1976
45. Kreel L: Preliminary evaluation of the EMI whole body scanner. J Belge Radiol 59:267–280, 1976
46. Rohlfing BM, Korobkeu M, Hall AD: Computed tomography of intrathoracic omental herniation and other mediastinal fatty masses. J Comput Assist Tomogr 1:181–183, 1977
47. Rosenberg M: Chronic subphrenic abscess. Lancet 2:379, 1968
48. Adams DF, Hessel SJ, Judy PF, et al: Computed tomography of the normal and infarcted myocardium. J Roentgenol 126:786–791, 1976
49. Powell WP Jr, Wittenberg J, Maturi RA, et al: Detection of edema associated with myocardial ischemia by computerized tomography in isolated, arrested canine hearts. Circulation 55:99–108, 1977
50. White RI Jr, Leo EP, Kaufman SL, et al: In vitro computed tomography of the human heart. Radiology 123:777–778, 1977
51. Evens RG, Jost G: Economic analysis of computed tomography units. Am J Roentgenol 127:191–198, 1976

Yener S. Erozan, M.D.

6

Cytopathology in the Diagnosis of Pulmonary Disease

Microscopic examination is usually required to establish a definitive diagnosis of pulmonary neoplasms and certain nonneoplastic diseases of the lung so that proper treatment can be administered. During the last two decades, significant progress has been made in developing less aggressive but accurate techniques to provide cellular or tissue specimens for microscopic examination, and consequently the need for diagnostic thoracotomy has been decreased. It has also become evident that radiologically occult, early bronchogenic carcinomas can be diagnosed by cytopathologic examination of sputum and localized by new, sophisticated bronchographic and bronchoscopic techniques.[1–7] (See Chapters 2 and 8.)

These more sophisticated collection techniques have broadened the field of cytopathology as a reliable diagnostic tool in pulmonary diseases.

This chapter deals with the applicability and diagnostic yield of cytopathology in pulmonary diseases.

TECHNIQUES FOR COLLECTION AND PROCESSING OF CYTOPATHOLOGY MATERIAL

The efficacy of cytopathologic examination depends greatly upon the selection and application of proper techniques for collection of cellular specimens. Spontaneous or induced cough, tracheobronchial instrumentation, transthoracic needle aspiration, and thoracentesis are the most valuable and

This work was supported in part by National Cancer Institute Contract No. NIH-No. 1-CN-45037 commonly used techniques for collecting specimens for the diagnosis of pulmonary disease.

Sputum Collection

SPONTANEOUS COUGH SPUTUM

Sputum produced by spontaneous cough is the most frequently used and generally valuable pulmonary material for cytologic examination. Following proper instruction, the majority of symptomatic patients are able to produce satisfactory samples that contain material from all lung fields. A satisfactory specimen should contain carbon-bearing histiocytes. Optimum results are obtained when separate sputum samples are examined for five consecutive days.

The patient should be instructed how to produce a "deep sputum" sample with deep inhalation and forceful expiration using his diaphragm. Ideal receptacles for sputum are clear plastic containers or Petri dishes. The unfixed material should be sent to the laboratory as soon as possible, although a few hours at room temperature will not cause significant damage to the cells. We prefer to have fresh samples because (1) these preparations give better morphological detail, (2) areas can be selected which most likely contain diagnostic cells (i.e., blood-tinged, nonsaliva), and (3) the remaining material can be processed by one of the concentration techniques (i.e., Saccomanno).[8] However, if a long delay is expected between collection and processing, fixation is necessary. Saccomanno has described the best technique; that is, to use 50 percent ethyl alcohol with 2 percent Carbowax. Then homogenized and concentrated cellular samples are prepared from this fixed material by blending and centrifugation. Using this technique, when fresh procurement is not possible, early-morning sputum samples can be collected singly, or three to five morning specimens can be pooled.

POSTBRONCHOSCOPIC SPUTUM

Sputum samples collected during the few hours following bronchoscopy and early-morning sputum samples collected for the following three consecutive days provide valuable diagnostic material. We are uncertain of the cost effectiveness of postbronchoscopy sputum analysis, but we have encountered several dramatic cases in which bronchoscopy and prior sputum analysis were totally negative but subsequent sputum cytology showed definite evidence of malignancy.

INDUCED SPUTUM

Sputum induction is used for individuals who cannot produce deep pulmonary material by spontaneous cough. Various techniques[9–12] have been developed utilizing tap water, hypotonic or hypertonic saline, or additives such as propylene glycol, mucolytic agents, or SO_2.[13] We have found the following two techniques to be very effective:

1. A nonirritating aerosol lavage technique has been designed to screen high-risk, asymptomatic individuals for lung cancer at The Johns Hopkins Medical Institutions. A balanced salt solution (Hanks' BSS) is aerosolized by an ultrasonic nebulizer (DeVilbiss, Model 3583) to deliver a larger volume of mist. Twenty-five minutes of aerosolization during normal breathing has been found to produce the desired results.
2. For the heated hypertonic saline technique, a solution containing 15 percent sodium chloride and 20 percent propylene glycol is delivered either by a disposable jet nebulizer with a wraparound heater or by a nondisposable nebulizer with an immersion heater. The solution is heated to near body temperature before it is delivered.

The early-morning sputum specimen collected on the day following induction usually contains good pulmonary material.

OTHER SPUTUM TECHNIQUES

There are several techniques that may be used in association with those described above, or alone in certain conditions. Percussion or vibration of the chest wall, either manually or mechanically, can be used in conjunction with spontaneous cough or other techniques, such as aerosol induction[14] or postural drainage.[15] In certain cases, because of obstruction by inflammation, mucosal edema, or mucus, negative cytology results are obtained despite the presence of a large neoplasm. In these cases, a five-day course of broad-spectrum antibiotics, bronchodilators, and expectorants may reduce the bronchial obstruction and increase the flow of secretions from involved lung segments. A new sputum series is then started on the third day of therapy and is continued for five consecutive days.[16]

Tracheobronchial Instrumentation

BRONCHOSCOPY

Introduction of the fiberoptic bronchoscope significantly improved the yield of cytopathologic diagnosis.[17] With this instrument, material can be collected by lavage, brush, or curette. A detailed description of these techniques is given in Chapter 8. Two points, however, are important enough to be mentioned here. First, the combined results of multiple samples obtained by various techniques (brush, curette, lavage) always give a better yield than a single sample obtained by any one of these techniques alone; and second, material obtained for cytopathologic examination should be processed promptly. We prefer to collect the brush or curette material in a physiological solution such as Hanks' balanced salt solution. Membrane filters and cellular spreads are then prepared in the laboratory from this unfixed material. If a direct smear is to be done from the brush, fixation should be done promptly to avoid air-drying, which makes cytopathologic interpretation very difficult in Papanicolaou-stained slides.

BRUSHING UNDER FLUOROSCOPIC GUIDANCE

This procedure has been employed successfully for the diagnosis of peripheral lung lesions.[18–20] Cytologic material is collected by a brush inserted through a catheter which has been guided to the lesion under fluoroscopic control. The processing techniques are the same as those for bronchoscopic brush material.

Transthoracic Needle Aspirations

This technique is used generally to obtain a microscopic diagnosis for pulmonary lesions when other techniques fail or are not likely to succeed. Its effectiveness has been documented in the recent literature.[21–25] Using thin-walled needles, one can obtain satisfactory cytologic material from which to diagnose malignant neoplasms. For benign lesions the yield of specific diagnosis by lung aspiration techniques is somewhat lower. The latter can be improved by using a needle capable of obtaining tissue fragments in addition to cytologic material (Chapter 9). Cell spreads made directly from these samples should be fixed immediately in 95 percent ethyl alcohol for Papanicolaou staining. We prefer to collect the aspirated material by rinsing the syringe and needle in Hanks' balanced salt solution. The fresh, unfixed solution is then sent to the laboratory for filter preparations and direct smears.

Intrathoracic Fluid Aspiration

Primary and metastatic tumors of the lung, including pleural neoplasms and certain nonneoplastic lesions involving the pleura and pericardium, can be diagnosed by cytopathologic examination of effusions from these areas.[26–31] Proper collection and processing techniques affect the results significantly. Material should be collected into a bottle containing three units of heparin for each milliliter of fluid to be aspirated. The bottle is gently agitated as the specimen is added and is sent to the laboratory as soon as possible. If delay is unavoidable, the material can be kept in a refrigerator or can be fixed by adding an equal amount of 95 percent ethyl alcohol or Saccomanno fixative. A combination of cytologic preparations (i.e., smears, filters, cell blocks) allows optimal use of the cytologic material for routine and special stains.

Factors Affecting Specimen Quality

Several rules that apply to all types of techniques and that are essential for optimal results follow:

1. Cytologic samples, if they are unfixed, should be sent to the laboratory for processing without delay. This is especially important for broncho-

scopic and needle aspiration material. Keeping the material in a physiological solution (i.e., Hanks' balanced salt solution) helps to preserve the cells.

We prefer fresh (unfixed) cytologic material for all types of pulmonary cellular specimens (sputum, bronchoscopic samples, needle aspirations, and pleural tap). In our experience, fresh specimens give better morphological detail and flexibility to apply various preparation techniques.

2. If there will be an unavoidable delay before the specimen reaches the laboratory, the material should be fixed immediately after collection. The best fixative for all types of pulmonary material is a solution of 50 percent ethyl alcohol and 2 percent Carbowax (Saccomanno's fixative).
3. If smears are made from the material obtained, they should be fixed immediately in 95 percent ethyl alcohol. Any delay, even a matter of seconds, will cause drying of the cells, which hampers the microscopic interpretation of Papanicolaou-stained slides.
4. Concentration (i.e., Saccomanno) and filter techniques (in effusions, bronchoscopic material, and needle aspiration material) give optimal results with representative sampling of material and minimum loss of cells.

CYTOPATHOLOGIC DIAGNOSIS OF NONNEOPLASTIC PULMONARY DISEASES

Cytopathology can be of significant use in the diagnosis of certain nonneoplastic pulmonary diseases by revealing etiologic agents or specific patterns. The diagnostic yield varies depending upon the type of etiologic agent, the specificity or morphological changes, and the technique used to collect the cytologic material.

Infectious Diseases

BACTERIAL

Cytopathology has little to offer in the specific diagnosis of bacterial pulmonary infections. The identification of etiologic agents can be done more efficiently by bacteriological techniques. The cellular patterns, although sometimes significantly altered, are usually nonspecific; perhaps the only exception is tuberculous pleuritis. Predominance of lymphocytic cells and either absence of or a small number (less than 1 percent) of mesothelial cells in an exudative effusion suggest a tuberculous pleuritis.[29,32] These findings are by no means pathognomonic for tuberculosis; malignant effusions can show the same mixture of cellular components. In addition, on very rare occasions tuberculous effusions may have a high number of mesothelial cells.

VIRAL

Most viral infections involving the respiratory system cause specific bronchopulmonary epithelial changes that can be recognizable by cytologic techniques. Herpes simplex, parainfluenza, adenovirus, and cytomegalic viral infections are among those with characteristic morphological features.[33–36]

FUNGAL

Cytopathology is a valuable technique to diagnose fungal diseases. Pulmonary infections caused by *Cryptococcus neoformans, Blastomyces dermatitidis, Coccidioides immitis, Histoplasma capsulatum, Candida albicans,* and phycomyces can all be diagnosed in cytologic material by the identification of the etiologic agent.[33,34] Most of these fungi can be identified on routine cytologic preparations stained with Papanicolaou stain; however, for some (i.e., *H. capsulatum*) special stains such as Gomori's silver methenamine are needed. Special attention should be given to the screening of this material, since the organisms might be few in number or obscured by inflammatory cells.

PARASITIC

In this group of diseases, cytopathology is probably most valuable for the diagnosis of *Pneumocystis carinii* pneumonia (because of the importance of specific diagnosis for therapy). Transthoracic needle aspirations, bronchial brushings, and pulmonary lavages have been reported to give a better yield than sputum or other respiratory material.[34–36] Special stains (i.e., Gomori's silver methenamine, Gram-Weigart, Giemsa) are required because these organisms are difficult to identify on Papanicolaou-stained slides.[34–39]

On rare occasions, other parasites are diagnosed in cytologic material.[34,40] The filariform larval stage of *Strongyloides stercoralis* has been found in the sputum of patients with pulmonary involvement by this parasite. We have seen one such case, and three others have been reported in the literature.[34]

Benign, Noninfectious Diseases

The role of cytopathology in the diagnosis of benign noninfectious diseases of the lung is limited. Most of the disease processes in this category are identified by their tissue pattern rather than by individual cellular changes. There are, however, some exceptions. In certain conditions, a specific diagnosis, or valuable clues leading to a diagnosis, can be obtained by examination of proper cytologic material. For example, in *bronchial asthma* a large number of eosinophils, and Charcot-Leyden crystals, as well as fragments of hypersecretory respiratory mucosa (Creola bodies) can be found in sputum.[41,42] In some cases of *pneumoconiosis,* such as silicosis and asbestosis, silica and protein-iron coated asbestos fibers (ferruginous bodies) are seen in sputum or other material from the lung.[43] Specific changes for *alveolar proteinosis* can be observed in material obtained by transthoracic needle aspiration or pulmonary lavage. These changes include abundant amounts of granular eosinophilic material containing deep eosinophilic, lamellar, or homogeneous round bodies. The proteinaceous material and round bodies give positive staining reaction with periodic acid-Schiff but a negative reaction with alcian blue. Sputum samples from patients with *lipid pneumonia* may show a large number of "foamy" histiocytes in which fat droplets can be demonstrated with special stains.[44] The presence of Langhans-type giant cells, occasionally containing Schaumann bodies or asteroids and clusters of epithelioid histiocytes, has been described in pulmonary *sarcoidosis*.[45]

Specific changes can be found in pleural effusions of patients with *systemic lupus erythematosus* and *rheumatoid pleuritis*. The former may show the characteristic L.E. cells, which are identifiable by routine preparation and staining techniques, whereas the latter may demonstrate a background of eosinophilic, granular material, large elongated cells, and round or oval multinucleated giant cells.[46]

CYTOPATHOLOGIC DIAGNOSIS OF PULMONARY NEOPLASMS

Cytopathology is an effective technique for detection and diagnosis of malignant pulmonary neoplasms. Benign tumors of the lung are rare and are less likely to be diagnosed in routine cytologic specimens (i.e., sputum, bronchoscopic material). Certain benign tumors, for example, hamartomas, can be diagnosed by needle aspiration.[47,48] The efficacy of cytopathologic diagnosis in pulmonary tumors is largely dependent upon the location, type, and size of the neoplasm, and the proper selection and application of collection techniques.

Occult Lung Cancer

Cytopathology has a definite place in the detection of early lung cancer. Neoplasms arising from the surface of the bronchial mucosa, primarily epidermoid carcinomas, can be detected by cytopathologic examination of sputum before they can be seen on chest x-ray films[1–7]; however, tumors originating in distal bronchi or peripheral lung tissues are less likely to be detected by sputum cytology in their early stages. Certain other tumors, even centrally located ones, cannot be detected by cytologic examination in their early stages because they lie deep in the bronchial mucosa. Some adenocarcinomas, including the so-called bronchial adenomas and probably oat cell carcinomas, fall into this category. In addition, the extremely rapid growth of the oat cell carcinoma makes it very difficult to detect it in its early stage.

A combination of sputum cytology and chest x-ray examination has been frequently used in screening studies for the early detection of lung cancer.[5,49] Recently this type of screening program has been undertaken by the National Cancer Institute. Carefully designed and coordinated cytologic and x-ray screening studies of populations at high-risk for developing lung cancer (i.e., male, heavy smoker, over 45 years of age) are being carried out by The Johns Hopkins Medical Institutions, the Mayo Clinic, and the Memorial Sloan-Kettering Cancer Center, to determine if lung cancer can be detected at an early stage and if the early detection improves the cure rate in this disease. Preliminary findings from these[50–53] and earlier studies,[5,49] suggest that a combination of sputum cytology and chest x-ray can be more effective than either technique alone in the early detection of lung cancer. Initial results also suggest that early detection improves resectability of lung cancer, which should increase the cure rate.

Again, proper collection techniques are essential for optimum results. A series of early-morning samples is preferred. Those individuals who cannot produce spontaneous sputum should be induced; and utilizing the ultrasonic physiologic aerosol technique described earlier, we were able to obtain satisfactory specimens in 93.9 percent of the asymptomatic, high-risk screenees. When multiple specimens were examined (i.e., induced sample and a subsequent series of early morning specimens), the rate of satisfactory samples increased to 97.86 percent.[53,54]

Clinical Lung Cancer

In experienced hands, multiple, combined, proper techniques can diagnose 70–95 percent of lung cancers. The cell type of most can be accurately determined by cytopathologic examination alone.[23,54–57] Selection and proper application of collection and processing techniques, and the location, size, and type of neoplasm affect the diagnostic yield.

CENTRAL BRONCHOGENIC NEOPLASMS

Tumors of the main and lobar bronchi give higher diagnostic rates on sputum specimens than do peripheral lesions.[56,58,59] Deeply located tumors, such as carcinoid, and slow-growing adenocarcinomas of bronchial glands, which lack access to the bronchial lumen, cannot be detected on sputum examination. For these, bronchoscopic techniques such as biopsy, brushing, or curetting give best results.[60] On the other hand, epidermoid carcinomas, which arise from the surface epithelium, give the highest diagnostic yield (67–85 percent) in either sputum or bronchoscopic material.[52,55,56] Small-cell anaplastic carcinomas also give a high diagnostic yield on sputum examination (64–70 percent).

The size of centrally located neoplasms is related inversely to the incidence of definitive sputum cytology diagnosis.[53] Larger tumors give lower diagnostic rates because bronchial obstruction prevents the cells from appearing in the sputum. In addition, these larger neoplasms tend to be necrotic, and degenerative changes in the neoplastic cells make the cytopathologic diagnosis difficult. In these cases, microscopic diagnoses can be obtained by bronchoscopic techniques.

PERIPHERAL PULMONARY NEOPLASMS

In sputum samples, tumors of the smaller bronchi, bronchioles, and terminal airways produce a lower diagnostic yield than centrally located bronchogenic carcinomas. There is a parallelism between the diagnostic rate and the proximity of the tumor to the trachea. Small, peripheral lesions, especially scar carcinomas, are usually not detected by sputum examination; however, samples obtained by fiberoptic bronchoscopy or brushing under fluroscopic guidance can provide the diagnosis.[18–20,60–62] Best results for the most peripheral lesions are obtained by transthoracic needle aspirations.[22,25]

Large peripheral masses and diffuse neoplastic alveolar infiltrates are more likely to be diagnosed by sputum than the smaller peripheral lesions, but again fiberoptic bronchoscopy under fluoroscopic guidance and transthoracic needle aspirations provide better diagnostic yields.

Rarely neoplasms will involve only the alveolar septae. These can only be diagnosed by needle aspiration or transbronchial biopsy.

SECONDARY NEOPLASMS OF THE LUNG

About 50 percent of the tumors metastatic to the lung can be diagnosed on sputum examination.[63,64] Like primary tumors, the diagnostic yield is influenced by the location and extent of the tumor. Small peripheral lesions are less likely to be diagnosed by sputum examination. Metastatic peripheral lesions can be diagnosed more effectively by cytologic examination of the material obtained by aspiration of pleural fluid.[26–31] Multiple taps may be required before a diagnosis can be made. Although cytologic examination of pleural effusion gives a higher diagnostic yield than pleural biopsy, optimum results are obtained by a combination of these techniques.[30] Pleural biopsies should be attempted when cytologic examination fails to diagnose a suspected neoplasm.

ACCURACY OF CYTOPATHOLOGIC DIAGNOSIS

The diagnostic accuracy is affected by (1) the techniques used to collect and process the specimen, (2) the number of specimens examined, (3) the type and location of the lesion, and (4) proper interpretation of the findings.

Role of Collection and Processing Techniques

SELECTION OF TECHNIQUE

Since the efficacy of cytopathologic techniques for collecting representative pulmonary material varies according to the location and nature of the lesion, selection of proper techniques for various conditions is important to the final diagnostic outcome. Obviously, certain clinical factors influence this decision in each case. Familiarity with the diagnostic potentials of the various techniques will enable the physician to choose the technique to fit the requirements of any given clinical condition.

Sputum. Sputum is the easiest material to collect and provides representative sampling of large areas of the lung as well as the upper respiratory tract. Cells from cancer of the oral cavity, pharynx, and in some instances esophagus, may be found in sputum samples. Cytopathologic examination of sputum is especially valuable for screening of populations at high risk of respiratory cancer, for differential diagnoses of pulmonary lesions, and for microscopic confirmation of clinically evident lung cancer. Definitive cytologic diagnosis of lung cancer can be made in 60–75 percent of the cases by sputum examination alone.[54–59,65]

For the diagnosis of nonneoplastic diseases, cytopathologic examination of sputum may provide valuable information by identifying special agents (i.e., fungi, parasites) or specific cellular patterns (i.e., viral infections, asthma), but it is of little value in bacterial infections or peripheral lesions involving mainly alveolar septae.

Bronchoscopy. Cellular samples obtained by washing or aspiration during conventional rigid bronchoscopy yield 70–90 percent cytologic detection in clinically suspicious, centrally located lesions.[56,65–67] The diagnostic yield of rigid bronchoscopy for cancers in all areas of the lung, however, is lower than that obtained by examination of a series of five sputum specimens.[58,59,68]

Diagnosis of lesions outside the central region can be established more effectively by fiberoptic bronchoscopy.[60,61,69–71] This technique allows direct sampling of segmental and subsegmental lesions which cannot be reached by a rigid bronchoscope; and with fluoroscopic guidance, more peripheral lesions may also be sampled by brush, curette, or microbiopsy forceps. Occult, x-ray negative/sputum positive carcinomas have been successfully localized by fiberoptic bronchoscopy in the vast majority of cases (see Chapter 8).

Transthoracic Needle Aspirations. Peripheral neoplasms not diagnosed by other techniques can be diagnosed by this one; a definitive cytologic diagnosis can be made in 80–90 percent of the cancer cases.[21–24] Thin needles usually provide satisfactory cellular samples for the diagnosis of malignant neoplasms. In addition, certain benign neoplasms such as hamartomas have been diagnosed accurately using this technique.[47,48] It should be noted that, although certain nonneoplastic diseases (i.e., fungal infections, *Pneumocystis carinii,* alveolar proteinosis) can be diagnosed by examining cytologic material obtained by thin needles, tissue provides a more specific diagnosis in most of the benign lesions. In these cases, better results are obtained by using larger needles (i.e., Turner needle) with which one can obtain tissue in addition to cytologic material (see Chapter 9).

Thoracentesis. Cytopathologic examination of pleural effusions provides valuable information for the differential diagnosis of benign diseases and a definitive diagnosis in the majority of the malignant tumors.[26–31] In two separate series studied at The Johns Hopkins Hospital, of 43 and 95 cases of malignant neoplasms involving pleura, 77 percent and 72 percent, respectively, were cytologically diagnosed.[29,30] Combining cytopathology with pleural biopsies increased the diagnostic yield up to 90 percent.[30] Several taps may be required to establish a diagnosis in certain cases.[29,30] Biopsy should be attempted when repeated pleural taps fail to provide the diagnosis.

COLLECTION AND PROCESSING

Proper collection and processing of the cytologic specimens is critical for optimal diagnostic results. Because the cytopathologic diagnosis is based essentially on individual cellular changes and one does not have the benefit of the tissue pattern, preservation of cellular structures is more crucial than for biopsies. Degeneration and artifactual changes in the cells resulting from improper collection or preparation of the material can cause misinterpretation of the findings and serious consequences. Various cytopathologic collection techniques for pulmonary material and factors affecting specimen quality have been discussed earlier.

NUMBER OF SPECIMENS

The value of multiple specimens in the cytopathologic diagnosis of lung cancer has been well established.[58,59,65,71,72] In a group of 197 patients with primary bronchogenic carcinoma seen at The Johns Hopkins Hospital and the University of Maryland between 1956 and 1959, the detection rate increased from 45 percent on the first sputum samples, to 86 percent on three sputum samples, and to 95 percent when five sputum samples were examined. In this group, a definitive cytopathologic diagnosis was established in 20 percent, 40 percent and 56 percent of the cases when one, three, and five sputum samples respectively, were evaluated.[16]

In another group of 141 cases of histologically proven lung cancer with a definitive cytopathologic diagnosis by sputum or bronchoscopic cytology, only 42 percent were diagnosed on the first sample. This rate increased to 73 percent with three samples, and to 84 percent with five. When eight samples were examined, 97 percent of the cases were diagnosed.[68]

Lesion

The influence of the location, type, and size of the lesion on the diagnostic yield has been discussed earlier with collection techniques.

Interpretation

Reporting of cytopathologic findings should be handled in the same fashion as reporting of histopathologic findings. Numerical or other types of classification lack clarity and uniformity. Although cytopathology has limitations, a definitive diagnosis can be ascertained in the majority of malignant tumors and in certain benign lung diseases.

ACCURACY OF CANCER DIAGNOSIS

Cytopathologic diagnosis, in experienced hands, is highly accurate. In the literature, if the "positive" category is used strictly to indicate definitive cytologic diagnosis of cancer,[73] "false positive" diagnoses do not exceed 1 percent.[16,21,23,55,58,74] Most false cancer reports are the result of misinterpretation of atypical squamous metaplasia, reactive alveolar epithelium or histiocytes, and mesothelial proliferation. Chronic bronchitis, bronchiectasis, lung abscess, tuberculosis, and viral infections can cause atypical metaplasia mimicking cancer cells; and alveolar cell proliferation and histiocytes in healing pneumonia or infarct can resemble adenocarcinoma. Experience with the various atypical changes associated with benign conditions and use of very strict criteria for establishing cytologic diagnosis[73] will prevent the majority of false cancer diagnoses. It is also very important for the pathologist to have all pertinent clinical information available to avoid misinterpretation of certain cytologic changes.

ACCURACY OF CELL TYPING OF TUMORS

The tissue type of the tumor can be determined accurately from adequate cytologic samples.[75–78] Approximately 80 percent of the neoplasms diagnosed cytologically in sputum can be properly typed. Well-differentiated carcinomas (epidermoid or adeno) and small cell anaplastic carcinomas give the highest accuracy (epidermoid carcinoma, 89–91 percent; adenocarcinoma, 72–100 percent; small cell anaplastic carcinoma, 76–86 percent). On the other hand, poorly differentiated carcinomas and large cell undifferentiated carcinomas are difficult to type.

In sputum samples from 241 patients and bronchoscopic material from 223 patients with primary lung carcinoma at the Johns Hopkins Medical Institutions, 98 percent of the well-differentiated or moderately well-differentiated epidermoid carcinomas in sputum and all of the same type carcinomas in bronchoscopic material were diagnosed accurately. Eighty-five percent of patients with cytopathologic diagnosis of small cell carcinoma in sputum and 100 percent of the same type in bronchoscopic material had the same tissue diagnosis. Poorly differentiated carcinomas and large cell undifferentiated carcinomas showed a lower degree of correlation (poorly differentiated epidermoid carcinomas, 48 percent in sputum and 71 percent in bronchoscopy; poorly differentiated adenocarcinomas, 65 percent in sputum and 47 percent in bronchoscopic material; and large cell undifferentiated carcinomas, two of four in sputum and only one of six in bronchoscopic material).[54] The type of tumor can also be accurately determined in pleural effusions.[79,80] The primary site of the tumor, however, may be difficult to ascertain on a morphologic basis alone.[81] Adequate clinical information often helps to establish the diagnosis.[80,81] In some cases, examination of other types of material (i.e., sputum, bronchoscopic material, needle aspiration material) is necessary to reach a specific diagnosis.

CONCLUSIONS

Cytopathology has been proved a valuable, highly accurate technique in the diagnosis of malignant pulmonary neoplasms and certain benign pulmonary diseases. Its diagnostic yield in sputum and bronchoscopic samples is high for centrally located malignant neoplasms and low for peripherally located lesions. The peripheral lesions can be diagnosed, however, by transthoracic needle aspirations or fluoroscopically guided bronchoscopic brushings or curettings. As a screening technique, sputum cytology, along with radiologic examination, is an effective means of detecting early neoplasms of the lung. Many lesions may be detected by sputum cytology before they are evident on chest roentgenography.

Cytopathologic techniques for the diagnosis of nonneoplastic diseases are successful only in those diseases with identifiable specific etiologic agents (i.e., fungal, parasitic) or in those with specific cellular changes. Examination of multiple specimens and proper application of techniques increase the efficacy of cytology.

An accurate cytopathologic diagnosis depends upon careful screening and interpretation of material in the light of the clinical findings. It is a team effort involving the cytotechnologist, the cytopathologist, and the clinician who supplies the necessary, pertinent clinical data. Optimum results can only be obtained through the cooperation and experience of each member of this team.

REFERENCES

1. Melamed MR, Koss LG, Cliffton EE: Roentgenologically occult lung cancer diagnosed by cytology: Report of 12 cases. Cancer 16:1537–1551, 1963
2. Pearson FG, Thompson DW, Delarue NC: Experience with the cytologic detection, localization, and treatment of radiographically undemonstrable bronchial carcinoma. J Thorac Cardiovasc Surg 54:371–382, 1967

3. Meyer JA, Bechtold E, Jones DB: Positive sputum cytologic tests for five years before specific detection of bronchial carcinoma. J Thorac Cardiovasc Surg 57:318–324, 1969
4. Woolner LB, David E, Fontana RS, et al: In situ and early invasive bronchogenic carcinoma. Report of 28 cases with postoperative survival data. J Thorac Cardiovasc Surg 60:275–290, 1970
5. Grzybowski S, Coy P: Early diagnosis of carcinoma of the lung. Simultaneous screening with chest X-ray and sputum cytology. Cancer 25:113–120, 1970
6. Marsh BR, Frost JK, Erozan YS, et al: Occult bronchogenic carcinoma. Endoscopic localization and television documentation. Cancer 30:1348–1352, 1972
7. Martini N, Bains MS, Beattie EJ: Radiologically occult lung cancer. NY State J Med 75:1699–1701, 1975
8. Saccomanno G, Saunders RP, Ellis H, et al: Concentration of carcinoma or atypical cells in sputum. Acta Cytol 7:305–310, 1963
9. Barach AL, Beck GJ, Bickerman HA, et al: Physical methods simulating mechanisms of the human cough. J Appl Physiol 5:85–91, 1952
10. Bickerman HA, Sproul EE, Barach AL: An aerosol method of producing bronchial secretions in human subjects: A clinical technic for the detection of lung cancer. Dis Chest 33:347–362, 1958
11. Barach AL, Bickerman HA, Beck GJ, et al: Induced sputum as a diagnostic technique for cancer of the lungs and for mobilization of retained secretions. Arch Intern Med 106:230–236, 1960
12. Roberts TW, Pollak A, Howard R, et al: Tracheo-bronchial cytology utilizing an improved tussilator (cough machine). Acta Cytol 7:174–179, 1963
13. Allan WB, Whittlesey P, Haroutunian LM, et al: The use of sulfur dioxide as a diagnostic aid in pulmonary cancer; preliminary report. Cancer 11:938, 1958
14. Masin F, Masin M: Sputum cytology (Letter to the Editor). Acta Cytol 10:391, 1966
15. Tweeddale DN, Harbord RP, Nuzum CT, et al: A new technique to obtain sputum for cytologic study: external percussion and vibration of the chest wall. Acta Cytol 10:214–219, 1966
16. Frost JK: Manual of Second Postgraduate Institute for Pathologists in Clinical Cytopathology. Baltimore, Johns Hopkins, 1961, Section 3
17. Ikeda S, Yanai N, Ishikawa S: Flexible bronchofiberscope. Keio J Med 17:1–16, 1968
18. Fennessy JJ: Bronchial brushing. Ann Otol Rhinol Laryngol 79:924–932, 1970
19. Hattori S, Matsuda M, Nishihara H, et al: Early diagnosis of small peripheral lung cancer—cytologic diagnosis of very fresh cancer cells obtained by the TV-brushing technique. Acta Cytol 15:460–467, 1971
20. Bibbo M, Fennessy JJ, Lu CT, et al: Bronchial brushing technique for the cytologic diagnosis of peripheral lung lesions. A preview of 693 cases. Acta Cytol 17:245–251, 1973
21. Dahlgren S, Nordenstrom B: Transthoracic Needle Biopsy. Stockholm, Alqvist and Wiksell/Gebers Förlag AB, and Chicago, Year Book Medical Publishers, 1966
22. Dahlgren SE: Aspiration biopsy of intrathoracic tumors. Acta Pathol Microbiol Scand 70:566–576, 1967

23. Dahlgren SE, Lind B: Comparison between diagnostic results obtained by transthoracic needle biopsy and by sputum cytology. Acta Cytol 16:53–58, 1972
24. Zelch JV, Lalli AF, McCormack LJ, et al: Aspiration biopsy in diagnosis of pulmonary nodule. Chest 63:149–152, 1973
25. Landman S, Burgener FA, Lim GH: Comparison of bronchial brushing and percutaneous needle aspiration biopsy in the diagnosis of malignant lung lesions. Radiology 115:275–278, 1975
26. Cardozo PL: A critical evaluation of 3,000 cytologic analyses of pleural fluid, ascitic fluid and pericardial fluid. Acta Cytol 10:455–460, 1966
27. Johnson WD: The cytological diagnosis of cancer in serous effusions. Acta Cytol 10:161–172, 1966
28. Jarvi OH, Kunnas RJ, Laitio MT, et al: The accuracy and significance of cytologic cancer diagnosis of pleural effusions (a follow-up study of 338 patients). Acta Cytol 16:152–158, 1972
29. Light RW, Erozan YS, Ball WC Jr: Cells in pleural fluid: Their value in differential diagnosis. Arch Intern Med 132:854–860, 1973
30. Salyer WR, Eggleston JC, Erozan YS: Efficacy of pleural needle biopsy and pleural fluid cytopathology in the diagnosis of malignant neoplasm involving the pleura. Chest 67:536–539, 1975
31. Grunze H: The comparative diagnostic accuracy, efficiency and specificity of cytologic technics used in the diagnosis of malignant neoplasm in serous effusions of pleural and pericardial cavities. Acta Cytol 8:150–163, 1964
32. Spriggs AI, Boddington MM: Absence of mesothelial cells from tuberculous pleural effusions. Thorax 15:169–171, 1960
33. Naib ZM: Exfoliative Cytopathology, ed 2. Boston, Little, Brown and Company, 1976, p 237
34. Johnston WW, Frable WJ: The cytopathology of the respiratory tract. Am J Pathol 84:372–414, 1976
35. Frable WJ, Frable MA, Seney FD: Virus infections of the respiratory tract. Cytopathologic and clinical analysis. Acta Cytol 21:32–36, 1977
36. Jordan SW, McLaren LC, Crosby JH: Herpetic tracheobronchitis. Arch Intern Med 135:784–788, 1975
37. Drew WL, Finley TN, Mintz L, et al: Diagnosis of Pneumocystis carinii pneumonia by bronchopulmonary lavage. JAMA 230:713–715, 1974
38. Hogkins JE, Anderson HA, Rosenow EC: Diagnosis of Pneumocystis carinii pneumonia by transbronchoscopic lung biopsy. Chest 64:551–554, 1973
39. Kim H, Hughes WT: Comparison of methods for identification of Pneumocystis carinii in pulmonary aspirates. Am J Clin Pathol 60:462–466, 1973
40. Willie SM, Snyder RN: The identification of Paragonimus Westermanii in bronchial washings. Acta Cytol 21:101–102, 1977
41. Naylor B, Railey C: A pitfall in the cytodiagnosis of sputum of asthmatics. J Clin Pathol 17:84–89, 1964
42. Sanerkin NG, Evans DMD: The sputum in bronchial asthma: Pathognomonic patterns. J Pathol Bacteriol 89:535–541, 1965
43. Greenberg SD, Hurst GA, Matlage WT, et al: Sputum cytopathological findings in former asbestos workers. Texas Med 72:39–43, 1976
44. Losner S, Volk BW, Slade WR, et al: Diagnosis of lipid pneumonia by examination of sputum. Am J Clin Pathol 20:539–545, 1950

45. Aisner SC, Gupta PK, Frost JK: Sputum cytology in sarcoidosis. Acta Cytol 21:394–398, 1977
46. Nosanchuk JS, Naylor B: A unique cytologic picture in pleural fluid from patients with rheumatoid arthritis. Am J Clin Pathol 50:330–335, 1968
47. Dahlgren S: Needle biopsy of intrapulmonary hamartoma. Scand J Respir Dis 47:187–194, 1966
48. Ramzy I: Pulmonary hamartomas: cytologic appearances of fine needle aspiration biopsy. Acta Cytol 20:15–19, 1976
49. Lilienfeld A, et al: An evaluation of radiologic and cytologic screening for the early detection of lung cancer: a cooperative pilot study of the American Cancer Society and the Veterans Administration. Cancer Res 26:2083–2121, 1966
50. Baker RR, Marsh BR, Frost JK, et al: The detection and treatment of early lung cancer, in Murray GF (ed): Cancer of the Lung. New York, Stratton Intercontinental Medical Book Corp, 1976
51. Fontana RS, Sanderson DR, Miller WE, et al: The Mayo Lung Project: preliminary report of "early cancer detection" phase. Cancer 30:1373–1382, 1972
52. Fontana RS, Sanderson DR, Woolner LB, et al: The Mayo Lung Project for early detection and localization of bronchogenic cacinoma. A status report. Chest 67:511–522, 1975
53. Melamed M, Flehinger B, Miller D, et al: Preliminary report of the lung cancer detection program in New York. Cancer 39:369–382, 1977
54. Erozan YS, Frost JK: Cytopathologic diagnosis of lung cancer, in Straus MJ (ed): Lung Cancer: Clinical Diagnosis and Treatment. New York, Grune & Stratton, 1977, Chapter 7
55. Grunze H: A critical review and evaluation of cytodiagnosis in chest diseases. Acta Cytol 4:175–198, 1960
56. Umiker W: The current role of exfoliative cytopathology in the routine diagnosis of bronchogenic carcinoma. A five-year study of 152 consecutive, unselected cases. Dis Chest 40:154–159, 1961
57. Grunze H: Cytologic diagnosis of tumors of the chest. Acta Cytol 17:148–159, 1973
58. Koss LG, Melamed MR, Goodner JT: Pulmonary cytology—a brief survey of diagnostic results from July 1st 1952 until December 31st, 1960. Acta Cytol 8:104–113, 1964
59. Rosa UW, Prolla JC, Gastal ES: Cytology in diagnosis of cancer affecting the lung. Results in 1,000 consecutive patients. Chest 63:203–207, 1973
60. Marsh BR, Frost JK, Erozan YS, et al: Role of fiberoptic bronchoscopy in lung cancer. Semin Oncol 1:199–203, 1974
61. Zavala DC: Diagnostic fiberoptic bronchoscopy: techniques and results of biopsy in 600 patients. Chest 68:12–19, 1975
62. Kownat DM, Rath GS, Anderson WM, et al: Bronchial brushing through the flexible fiberoptic bronchoscope in the diagnosis of peripheral pulmonary lesions. Chest 67:179–184, 1975
63. Koss LG: Diagnostic Cytology and Its Histopathologic Bases. Philadelphia, J. B. Lippincott, 1968
64. Kern WH, Schweizer CW: Sputum cytology of metastatic carcinoma of the lung. Acta Cytol 20:514–520, 1976
65. William S: The cytologic diagnosis of lung cancer. Med J Aust 48:233–236, 1961

66. McKay DG, Ware PF, Atwood DA, et al: Diagnosis of bronchogenic carcinoma by smears of bronchoscopic aspirations. Cancer 1:208–222, 1948
67. Herbut PA, Clerf LH: Bronchogenic carcinoma; diagnosis by cytologic study of bronchoscopically removed secretions. JAMA 130:1006–1012, 1946
68. Erozan YS, Frost JK: Cytopathologic diagnosis of cancer in pulmonary material: a critical histopathologic correlation. Acta Cytol 14:560–565, 1970
69. Zavala DC, Richardson RH, Mukerjee PK, et al: Use of the bronchofiberscope for bronchial brush biopsy. Diagnostic results and comparison with other brushing techniques. Chest 63:889–892, 1973
70. Ikeda S: Flexible bronchofiberscope. Ann Otol Rhinol Laryngol 79:916–923, 1970
71. Farber SM, Benioff MA, Frost JK, et al: Cytologic studies of sputum and bronchial secretions in primary carcinoma of the lung. Dis Chest 14:633–664, 1948
72. Russell WO, Neidhardt HW, Mountain CF, et al: Cytodiagnosis of lung cancer. A report of a four-year laboratory, clinical, and statistical study with a review of the literature on lung cancer and pulmonary cytology. Acta Cytol 7:1–44, 1963
73. Frost JK: The Cell in Health and Disease. Basel, Karger AG, and Baltimore, Williams & Wilkins, 1969
74. Umiker W: False positive reports in the cytologic diagnosis of lung cancer. Br J Cancer 11:391–397, 1957
75. Lukeman JM: Reliability of cytologic diagnosis in cancer of the lung. Cancer Chemother Rep (Part 3) Suppl 4:79–93, 1973
76. Foot NC: The identification of types of pulmonary cancer in cytologic smears. Am J Pathol 28:963–983, 1952
77. Lange E, Høeg K: Cytologic typing of lung cancer. Acta Cytol 16:327–330, 1972
78. Kanhouwa SB, Mathews MJ: Reliability of cytologic typing of lung cancer. Acta Cytol 20:229–232, 1976
79. Luse SA, Reagan JW: A histocytological study of effusions. II. Effusions associated with malignant tumors. Cancer 7:1167–1181, 1954
80. Murphy WM, Na ABP: Determination of primary site by examination of cancer cells in body fluids. Am J Clin Pathol 58:479–488, 1972
81. Foot NC: Identification of types and primary sites of metastatic tumors from exfoliated cells in serous fluids. Am J Pathol 30:661–677, 1954

Darryl Carter, M.D.

7

Biopsies of the Lung

INTRODUCTION

The choice of procedure employed to retrieve an adequate sample of a pulmonary lesion for the histopathologist is in large part dependent upon the anatomic site of the lesion and an educated guess as to its nature. For the purpose of this discussion, pulmonary lesions are classified into three categories: central endobronchial lesions, midzonal endobronchial lesions, and peripheral or parenchymal lesions.

Central Endobronchial Lesions

The vast majority of lesions found in the trachea, mainstem bronchi, and lobar bronchi are benign or malignant neoplasms of the lung. Rarely inflammatory diseases such as sarcoidosis and tuberculosis appear as central endobronchial lesions. Central lobar mucus impaction associated with *Aspergillus fumigatus* has also been observed in patients with asthma and cystic fibrosis. All central lesions may be visualized with a rigid bronchoscope and sampled with the large forceps that can be passed through that instrument. This provides a maximum amount of tissue for preoperative histologic diagnosis. Other instruments such as a brush or a curette may be passed through the open-tubed bronchoscope to a visible lesion in order to obtain a sample of involved tissue. However, biopsy techniques retrieve more satisfactory material for histological examination. Any abnormality visualized in the central bronchial tree should be biopsied to provide a tissue diagnosis of the lesion. In addition, a proximal biopsy should be obtained to determine the adequacy of a proposed surgical margin for an otherwise resectable central lesion that is located more distally in the bronchial tree. The fiberoptic broncoscope with its 2-mm forceps may be used to obtain small biopsies of central lesions as well as brushed or curetted specimens. It can be used to obtain an adequate mucosal sample from a proximal bronchus to help delineate a proposed surgical margin.

Midzonal Endobronchial Lesions

Almost all lesions found in segmental or subsegmental bronchi are also either benign or malignant neoplasms of the lung. This area cannot be visualized with the rigid bronchoscope, and therefore samples of endobronchial lesions in these areas cannot be obtained with the large (5-mm cup) forceps that fit within that instrument. The midzonal bronchi are, however, accessible to the flexible fiberoptic bronchoscope. Satisfactory specimens may be obtained from the bronchial epithelium through that instrument, but the outside dimensions of the forceps which are usually used are limited to about 2 mm. The small samples require somewhat more careful processing techniques. Several specimens should be obtained to increase the yield of diagnostic material and ensure against the possibility that the small pieces are not lost in laboratory processing. The brush and curette techniques are more frequently used to remove cells and tissue from the surface epithelium of small bronchi than the larger bronchi.

Peripheral or Parenchymal Lesions

Peripheral or parenchymal lesions are associated with only small bronchi, bronchioles, or alveoli. They cannot be visualized through the flexible fiberoptic bronchoscope. Peripheral lesions may be either localized, or multiple and diffuse. Although endobronchial lesions are virtually all primary neoplasms, the peripheral lesions represent the full range of pulmonary pathology including primary or secondary neoplasms and inflammatory, infectious, and congenital diseases. Specimens can be obtained from this large area by three techniques: transbronchial biopsy with either the rigid or flexible bronchoscope, needle biopsy (aspiration, cutting, or trephine), or open biopsy. The efficacy of the diagnostic technique employed is dependent upon the anatomic site and the nature and configuration of the lesion.

HISTOPATHOLOGICAL APPROACH

Central Endobronchial Lesions

As noted earlier, virtually all of these lesions are neoplasms of the bronchi—either benign or malignant. The literature on bronchoscopy prior to 1969 refers only to lesions in this zone since examination was limited to the

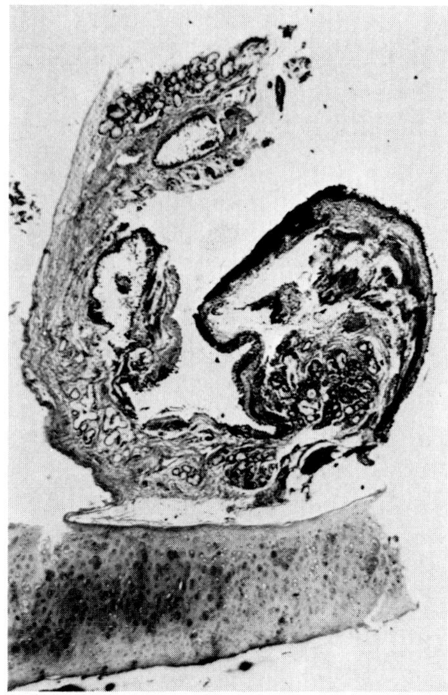

Fig. 7-1. Endobronchial biopsy obtained through a rigid bronchoscope. The tissue removed includes mucosa, submucosa, submucosal glands, and a full thickness of bronchial cartilage. The only pathologic abnormality present is squamous metaplasia. Hematoxylin and eosin stain. (H & E, from 6×)

area visualized with the rigid bronchoscope.[1] Biopsies obtained with large forceps from this area may yield good specimens that show mucosa; the full extent of the submucosa, including the blood and lymphatic vessels in the submucosa as well as the submucosal glands; and, frequently, cartilage (Fig. 7-1). The identification of a piece of tissue 5 mm in diameter is not difficult. The orientation of such a piece of tissue may pose a minor problem. Visualization of the tissue with either a hand lens or a dissecting microscope will enable the histologist to identify the mucosa and to orient the tissue in such a way as to produce sections that are cut at right angles to the surface. A properly oriented, thin-cut section enables the pathologist to identify and determine whether lesions: (1) are confined to the mucosa, (2) have invaded the submucosa, or (3) have spread from another site via the submucosal vessels as with adenocarcinomas or oat cell carcinomas (Fig. 7-2).

Although excellent biopsy material may be obtained from this area, fewer than 15 percent of bronchogenic carcinomas have a central endobronchial component. A definite limitation of central biopsy is the possibility of

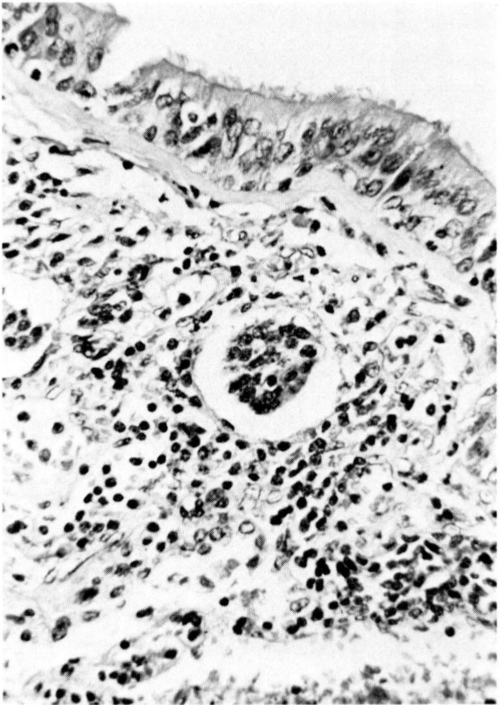

Fig. 7-2. Bronchial biopsy obtained through a rigid bronchoscope. Bronchial mucosa shows slight reserve cell or basilar hyperplasia and submucosa shows chronic inflammation. A submucosal lymphatic is dilated and filled with a group of cells which have spread from a carcinoma located more distally in the tracheobronchial tree. (H & E, from 250×)

producing a hemorrhage—particularly when biopsy of a carcinoid tumor is carried out. Figure 7-3 shows a resected lobe after emergency surgery following biopsy of a polypoid endobronchial carcinoid with consequent extensive hemorrhage. Zavala has noted that he diagnoses carcinoid tumors grossly rather than risking biospy even with microforceps.[2]

Midzonal Endobronchial Lesions

As noted earlier, the majority of primary endobronchial neoplasms are located in the midzone, which can be visualized with the flexible fiberoptic bronchoscope.[2–5] Whenever the lesion can be visualized, a biopsy should be attempted. In the majority of cases the tumor usually originates from a segmental or subsegmental spur. These areas are easily accessible to the microbiopsy of the fiberoptic bronchoscope. Material may be obtained

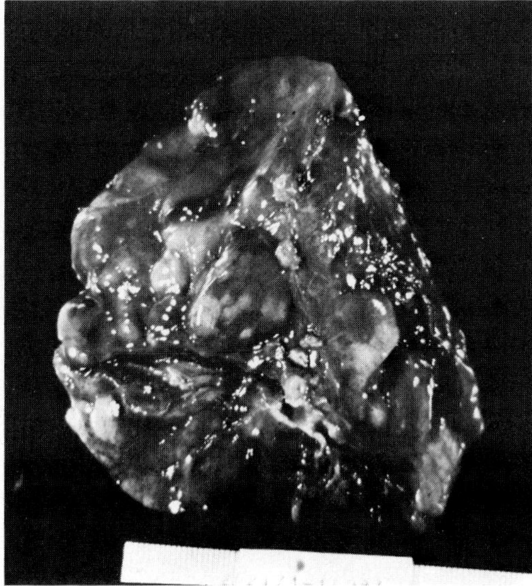

Fig. 7-3. Gross photograph of lobectomy specimen which is filled with fresh hemorrhage resulting from endobronchial biopsy of a carcinoid.

from the surface of these lesions by either brush or curette, and diagnostic results with this technique are good. In general, material obtained by brushing and curetting is better examined by cytologic techniques. Therefore, a discussion of the examination of these specimens is found in Chapter 6 (cytology). The brush and curette specimens have the distinct advantage to the endoscopist that they may be obtained from a broad surface area such as that involved by a squamous cell carcinoma. The diagnostic rate is high for these lesions. The brush and curette techniques are especially valuable for diagnosis of carcinoma in situ. The value in localization with this material is not as great as when the lesion is directly biopsied, however, since it is difficult to guarantee that individual cells and small fragments of tissue scraped from a surface have not spilled into the area or been picked up by the brush or curette from some other site. Hence, if there is no radiographic evidence of a lesion, some other verification for localization, such as a second positive brush or curette specimen or a microbiopsy, is needed. The microbiopsy forceps may be used to obtain a small fragment of tissue. The small size of the specimen obtained presents several problems. The first problem is finding the tissue, particularly at the time that it is to be imbedded in paraffin. This difficulty may be alleviated by staining the specimen with eosin, which colors it a pale pink that may be seen against the white background provided by the paraffin. Orientation is a problem that has not been solved since essentially all of the specimen is mucosa and the luminal side cannot be discriminated even with a dissecting microscope. Random imbedding and sec-

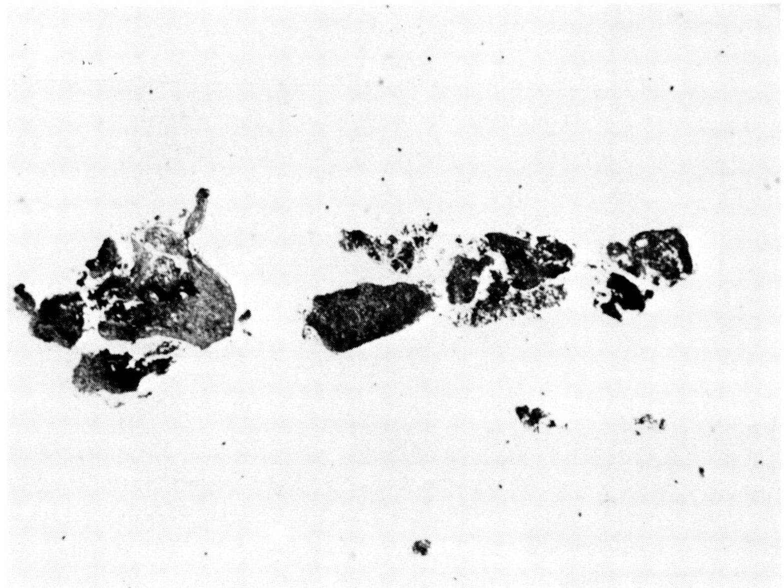

Fig. 7-4. Multiple microbiopsies obtained with a flexible fiberoptic bronchoscope from an x-ray negative squamous carcinoma of the lung. The specimens are all fragments of mucosa showing in situ squamous carcinoma. (H & E, from 6×)

tioning are all that can be anticipated. This problem may be alleviated if multiple biopsies are taken, and the possibility of achieving good orientation is improved by chance alone. The small size of the specimen also limits the ability to determine whether invasion of the submucosa has occurred (Fig. 7-4). This problem may also be overcome by the examination of multiple specimens. One disadvantage of the technique which cannot be alleviated is the mechanical arrangement of the forceps, which makes it difficult to obtain a biopsy from other than an exophytic lesion. Since exophytic lesions are uncommon and spurs may not be involved, it is not surprising that the brush and curette techniques have a higher diagnostic rate than the forcep biopsy. The one great advantage of the biopsy is the positive localization of the lesion to the area biopsied. Figure 7-4 shows a small specimen taken with the microforceps from an endobronchial lesion in a segmental bronchus (see Table 7-1).

Peripheral Parenchymal Lesions

These lesions are associated with very small bronchi and are beyond the range of endobronchial visualization of even the flexible fiberoptic bronchoscope. The etiology of many of these lesions can be suspected from the history, physical examination, and radiographic studies as well as a variety of noninvasive techniques, including examination of the sputum for microor-

Table 7-1
Problems with Microbiopsy Specimens from Midzone Endobronchial Lesions

Problem	Solution
Identification of small specimen	Eosin staining
Orientation of bronchial mucosa	Obtain and examine multiple specimens
Inadequate depth in some samples	Multiple specimens
Biopsies restricted to spurs and exophytic lesions	Supplement with multiple brush and curetted specimens

ganisms and malignant cells. On occasion, appropriate serological and skin tests may add helpful information. A significant number of these lesions defy attempts at diagnosis by noninvasive means, however. These lesions represent a full spectrum of disease, including primary and secondary tumors and toxic, infectious, circulatory, and idiopathic conditions. They may be separated into localized and diffuse lesions, which may alter the differential diagnosis but often do not negate the need for a tissue diagnosis. All of these lesions may be biopsied by one of three techniques: transbronchial biopsy with microforceps, directed needle biopsy, or open-lung biopsy.

TRANSBRONCHIAL BIOPSY (See also Chapter 8)

Transbronchial biopsy is perhaps the least invasive of the techniques, but it suffers from some limitations in producing a diagnostic specimen. It is a relatively blind procedure in that the endoscopist cannot visualize the area that is being biopsied, although he may be directed to the area of radiographic abnormality. The specimen produced is small by virtue of the limitation imposed by the size of the microforceps, and multiple biopsies are recommended (Fig. 7-5). Finding the specimen represents the same problem as it does for endobronchial microbiopsies, and the solution is the same. Orientation is not a problem, since there is no mucosal surface to be oriented. In spite of these limitations, reports from the literature indicate a diagnostic rate of 70–80 percent for primary malignant tumors.[2,6] The diagnostic rate is lower for nonneoplastic lesions. In infections, especially those in the immunologically compromised host, the reported experience is relatively small, but selected biopsies have been diagnostic for lesions such as *Pneumocystis carinii* infections. Zavala[2] reports a successfully diagnostic biopsy in all four patients in which it was attempted. One limitation of the transbronchial biopsy technique that is unavoidable is the sampling problem due to the small specimen size. Figures 7-6 to 7-11 show the pulmonary parenchymal lesions observed in a young boy with leukemia and a pulmonary infiltrate. The pulmonary lesions present at autopsy included a diffuse inter-

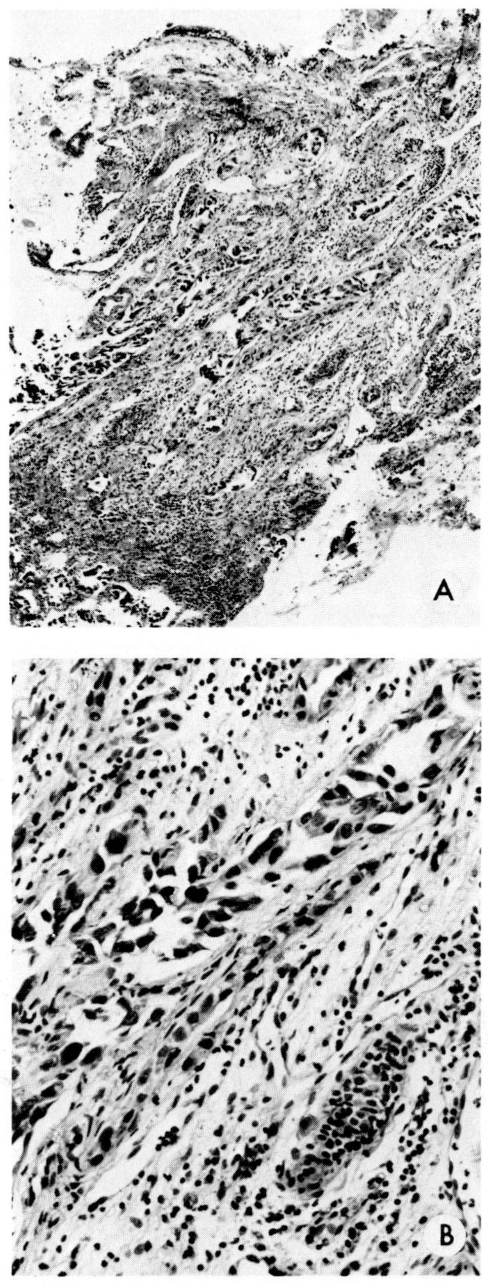

Fig. 7-5. Transbronchial biopsy of peripheral adenocarcinoma. (A) This figure shows the specimen with a small amount of respiratory epithelium at the top. The tumor lies in the lung surrounding the small bronchus (H & E, ×75); (B) This is a higher magnification of the tumor showing the malignant cells forming a small acinus. (H & E, ×275)

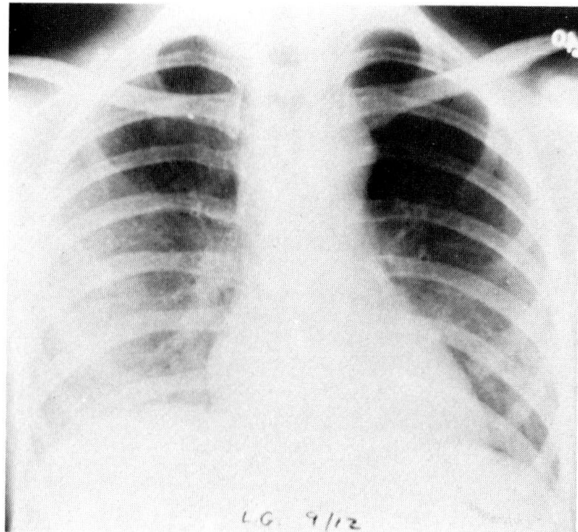

Fig. 7-6. 12-year-old boy with leukemia under therapy and in bone marrow remission when he developed respiratory insufficiency. Chest film shows diffuse pulmonary infiltrates.

stitial fibrosis, cytomegalovirus infection, aspergillus infection, and *Pneumocystis carinii* pneumonia. Any one of these diagnoses might have been established by transbronchial microbiopsy, but it is unlikely that all of them would have been established antemortem by such a limited technique. The immunologically compromised host is likely to have more than one lesion present. Therefore, the final determination of the full nature of a radio-

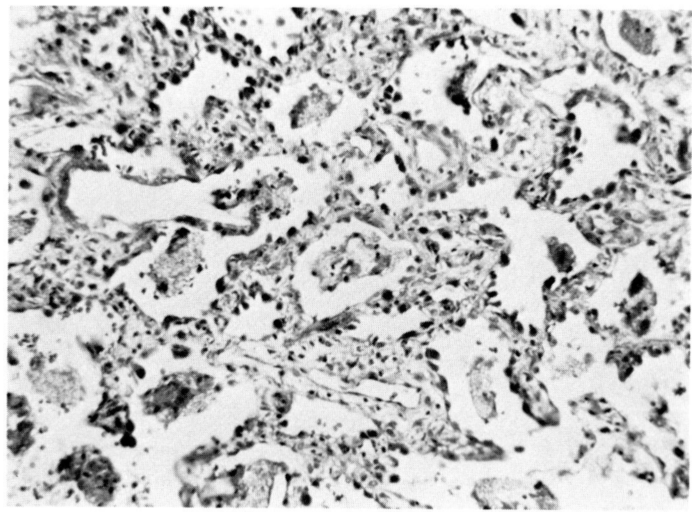

Fig. 7-7. Open lung biopsy from case above. The field shows a diffuse interstitial fibrosis of moderate severity and of indeterminate etiology. Cytotoxic agents may be associated with changes of this type. (H & E from 250×)

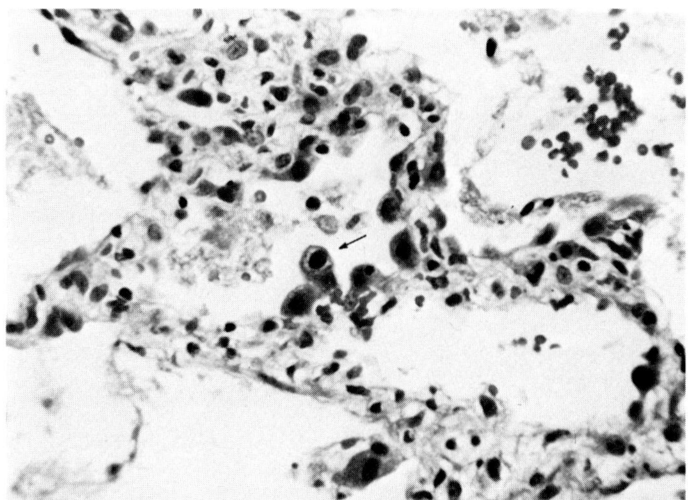

Fig. 7-8. From same open biopsy as that shown in Figure 7-6. Field shows marked prominence of alveolar cells one of which (arrow) shows the prominent eosinophilic nuclear inclusion with surrounding halo in an enlarged cell. The changes are characteristic of cytomegalic inclusion disease. (H & E, from 250×)

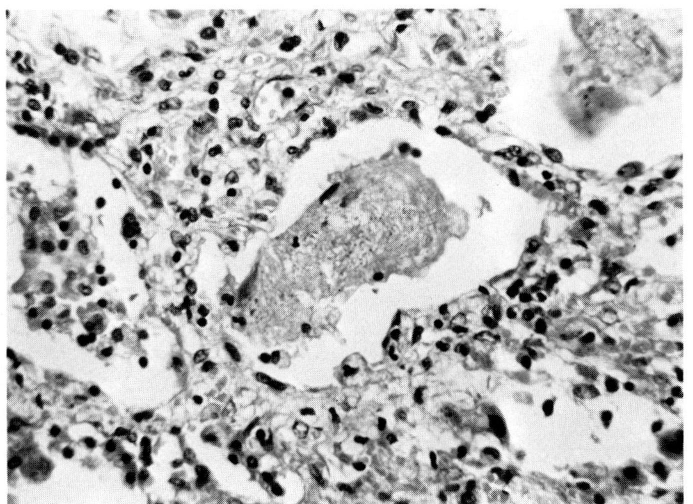

Fig. 7-9. From same open biopsy as that shown in Figure 7-6. Field shows interstitial infiltrate and eosiniophilic alveolar exudate that contains granular basophilic material. (H & E, from 350×)

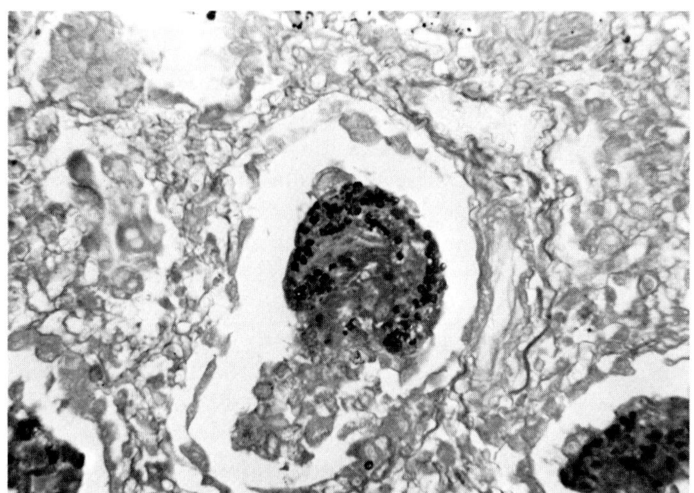

Fig. 7-10. Same area as in Figure 7-8. The methenamine silver stain outlines the capsules of the *Pneumocystis carinii* organisms which are present in the alveolar exudate. (From 350×)

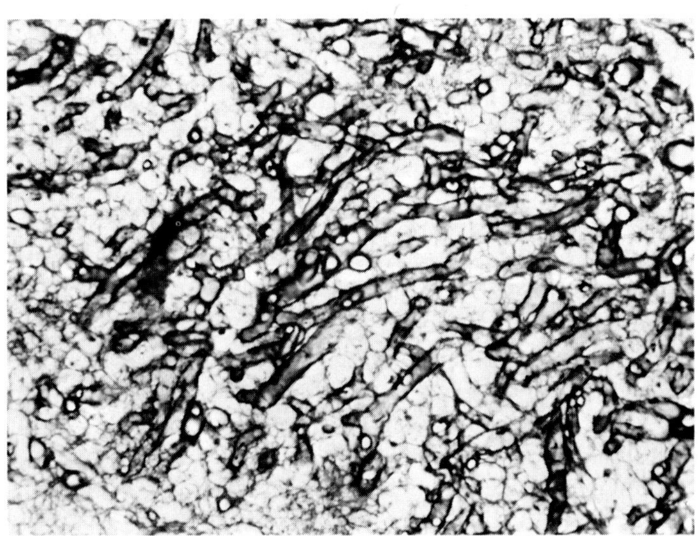

Fig. 7-11. The patient whose biopsy findings are illustrated in Figures 7-6 to 7-9 died shortly after the lung biopsy. In addition to the interstitial fibrosis, cytomegalovirus and *Pneumocystis carinii* infections which are evident in the biopsy, he was found at autopsy to have a significant infection with a fungus with the morphologic characteristics of aspergillus. The periodic acid Schiff stain shows the thin septate hyphae which branch at a relatively acute angle. (From 400×)

graphic abnormality may not be entirely certain even after examination of multiple microbiopsy specimens. Careful follow-up of cases in which a diagnosis is established by transbronchial microbiopsy is essential, especially in those cases in which a diagnosis of other than neoplasm is established, since the certainty of a tissue diagnosis in these circumstances is dependent to some extent on the amount of tissue available for diagnosis. Frozen sections may be carried out on a transbronchial biopsy if the situation is clearly an emergency. This technique is less than optimal, but in the interest of time it may give some helpful information. The frozen section requires about 30 minutes to process, whereas paraffin sections cannot be obtained in less than 5 hours with the best available techniques. Special stains for *Pneumocystis carinii* may be carried out on touch preps from the biopsy specimen, but frequently they are not as reliable as special stains on the tissue itself. Special stains employed include the Giemsa stain, methenamine silver stain, and a Bowling stain. These stains are also useful for the delineation of various fungus forms which may be present. Viruses are made evident only by the presence of specific inclusion bodies, and it is difficult to pick these up in a small biopsy.

NEEDLE BIOPSY (See also Chapter 9)

Several percutaneous biopsy techniques have been used with considerable success for removing a diagnostic core of tissue from lesions in the periphery of the lung.[6,7] These include various needle biopsy techniques. Although the process is somewhat more invasive than fiberoptic microbiopsy, the amount of tissue removed is greater. Needle aspiration techniques have been more successful in the resolution of the patient with a solitary pulmonary nodule or nodules than for the diagnosis of patients with diffuse pulmonary infiltrates. Although a variety of lesions may appear to be solitary pulmonary nodules, the most important differential diagnosis of this type of lesion is between a malignant tumor and a granuloma (or, less commonly, a benign neoplasm).

Sampling of a localized lesion of the lung by needle biopsy may produce material of two types, a core biopsy and a spread of cells. Examination of the cell spread by cytologic techniques is invaluable in establishing the diagnosis of carcinoma and may be more valuable in that respect than the core biopsy. A detailed discussion of the examination of the cell spread may be found in Chapter 6. Although the cytologic diagnosis is very helpful in establishing a carcinoma diagnosis, it is not very helpful in establishing a diagnosis of a benign lesion. The absence of cancer cells cannot be taken as conclusive evidence that a benign lesion is present; it only means that, for one reason or another, cancer cells are not present in the specimen examined. For these reasons, it is important that specimens be examined by both histologic and cytologic techniques. Fortunately, in our experience, cytolo-

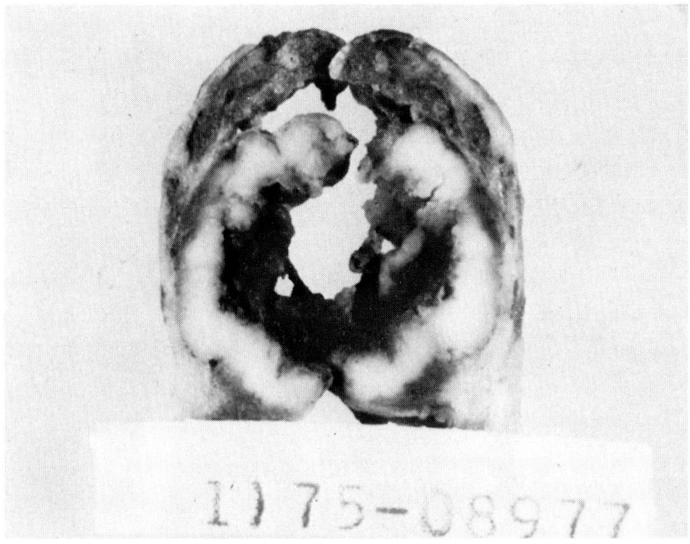

Fig. 7-12. Gross photograph of resected cariitary squamous carcinoma of lung. Needle biopsy from the center of the lesion yielded only necrotic material which was not diagnostic when examined both histologically and cytologically. The periphery of the lesion, represented by the white areas, is the viable squamous carcinoma. (6×)

gic and histologic examination of needle biopsy specimens results in a definite diagnosis of 90 percent of patients who are eventually proved to have primary or secondary localized malignant disease. Cavitary lesions are a special problem with this technique. Biopsy of the central portion of a cavitary lesion—either benign or malignant—may yield necrotic material that is of no value for an anatomic diagnosis. Biopsy of the periphery of the lesion is much more representative and diagnostic. Figure 7-12 shows a squamous carcinoma with a central cavity. Biopsy of the center of this lesion yielded no diagnosis. Biopsy of the periphery yielded a core of poorly differentiated squamous carcinoma. Figure 7-13 shows specimens of a lesion that were obtained with the needle biopsy technique.

OPEN BIOPSY

At present open biopsy is most frequently undertaken when other means of establishing a tissue diagnosis have been unsuccessful. Recently, we reviewed our experience with open-lung biopsy at this institution between 1952 and 1971.[8] One significant point in the procedure is that frozen section is performed on the tissue specimen as soon as it is obtained. Although the final diagnosis made from paraffin sections of the lung biopsy

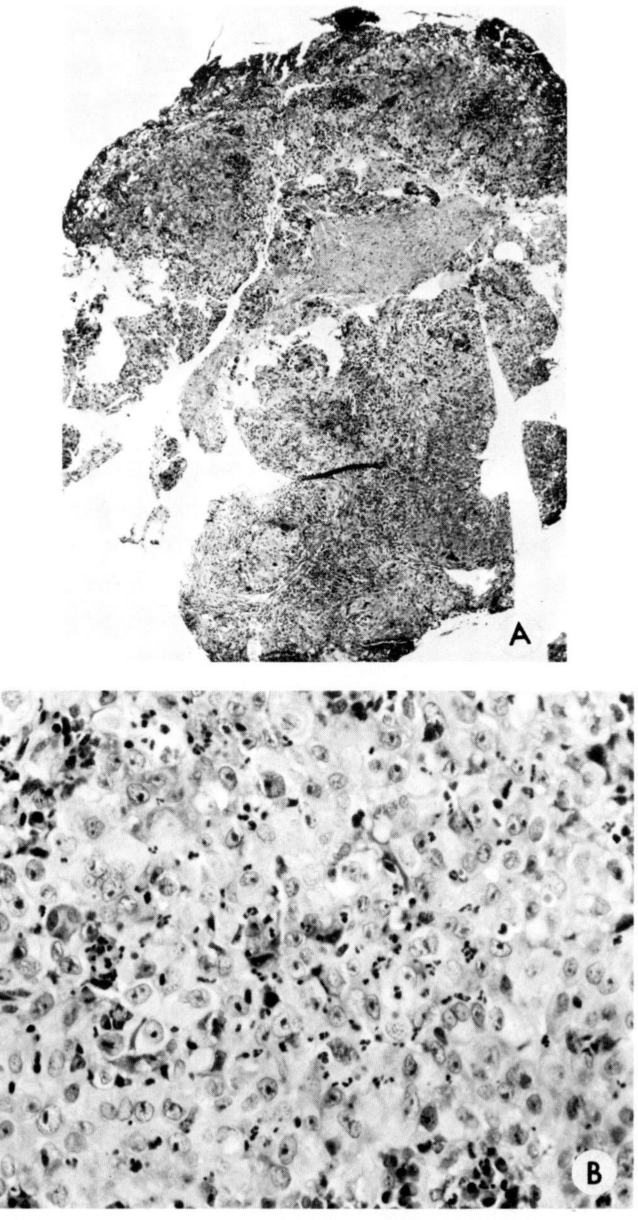

Figure 7-13. Percutaneous needle biopsy of peripheral large cell undifferentiated carcinoma of the lung. (A) This figure shows the mass of tissue obtained by several passes with the needle. (H & E × 50); (B) This shows the sheet of tumor cells in the center of the biopsy. The cells are large, polygonal in shape and have prominent vesicular nuclei with granular eosinophilic cytoplasm. (H & E, ×375)

may differ slightly from the frozen section diagnosis, the pathologist can ascertain whether there is an abnormality in the lung tissue, can make an estimate of whether the histologic abnormality can explain the radiographic abnormality, and frequently can provide information of immediate therapeutic significance, particularly in the immunosuppressed host. The frozen section can prevent the unfortunate situation in which the patient undergoes a thoracotomy for removal of an essentially normal piece of pulmonary tissue.

Another advantage of open biopsy is the relatively large amount of tissue that may be cultured on various media, examined histologically with a number of sections using various stains, and examined physically and chemically for crystalline foreign material that may be responsible for pneumoconioses. The bulk of the tissue obtained obviates sampling problems to some extent—especially in the patient with pneumoconioses and the immunosuppressed host. The wise surgeon should supply the pathologist with a generous sample of tissue which appears representative of the entire process. Occasionally more than one biopsy sample must be obtained to ensure that this is achieved.

If benign and malignant neoplasms, specific infectious agents, exudative and proliferative changes associated with cytotoxic drugs, and various inflammatory but noninfectious conditions can be excluded by histologic examination, the patients will frequently be left with a rather nonspecific diagnosis of interstitial pulmonary fibrosis. Ruttner et al. have recently suggested the steps required for identification of inhaled toxic agents which might be responsible for seemingly nonspecific pathologic alternations.[9] Transmission electron microscopy may reveal intracytoplasmic particles, but these are difficult to identify morphologically. Electron diffraction studies may be helpful in characterizing them, but frequently mineralogic analysis is required. It is particularly helpful to have the bulk of tissue obtained in an open biopsy when this type of analysis must be undertaken. An open biopsy is usually 1–2 cm in each of three dimensions and generates sufficient tissue to permit this type of study. No special handling is required at the time of biopsy.

Determination of the agents present in and presumably responsible for interstitial disease is of epidemiologic and diagnostic importance, but it may have relatively limited therapeutic implications. In our series of 41 patients with open-lung biopsy, the patients were divided into two groups on the basis of the type and severity of the histologic changes present. Patients with the degree and extent of interstitial fibrosis and alteration of the pulmonary parenchyma shown in Figure 7-14 had little chance of reversal of the process with steroid therapy regardless of the etiology. It is significant, however, that patients with an essentially inflammatory interstitial process such as the one shown in Figure 7-15 and the pulmonary alveolar proteinosis shown in Figure 7-16 frequently showed an almost complete return to normal pulmonary function following appropriate therapy.

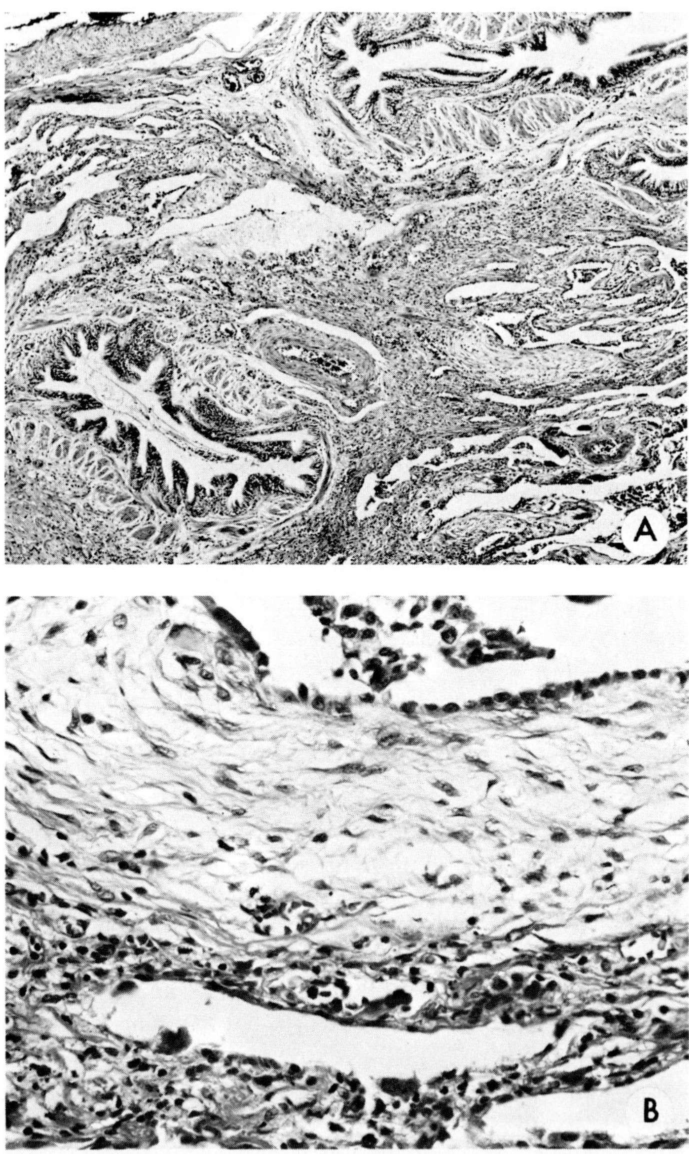

Fig. 7-14. (A) Open lung biopsy from a patient with diffuse pulmonary changes on chest x-ray. Histology of an irreversible case of interstitial fibrosis. The pulmonary architecture is markedly distorted. The alveolar spaces are virtually obliterated by fibrous tissue in which smooth muscle has proliferated. Pulmonary vessels show mild hypertensive changes. Along the few remaining air spaces there is proliferation of the alveolar lining cells. A small amount of lymphocytic infiltration is present (H & E, ×80); (B) Fibrosis of alveolar wall in irreversible case. The alveolar wall thickening is due to the proliferation of fibroblasts and the presence of collagen. Inflammatory cells are few in number and confined to the area around the air spaces. (H & E ×310). Reprinted from The Johns Hopkins Medical Journal, 132:103, 1973 (Baker RR, Lee JM, and Carter D: An evaluation of open lung biopsy. Figures 4A and 4B p. 109).

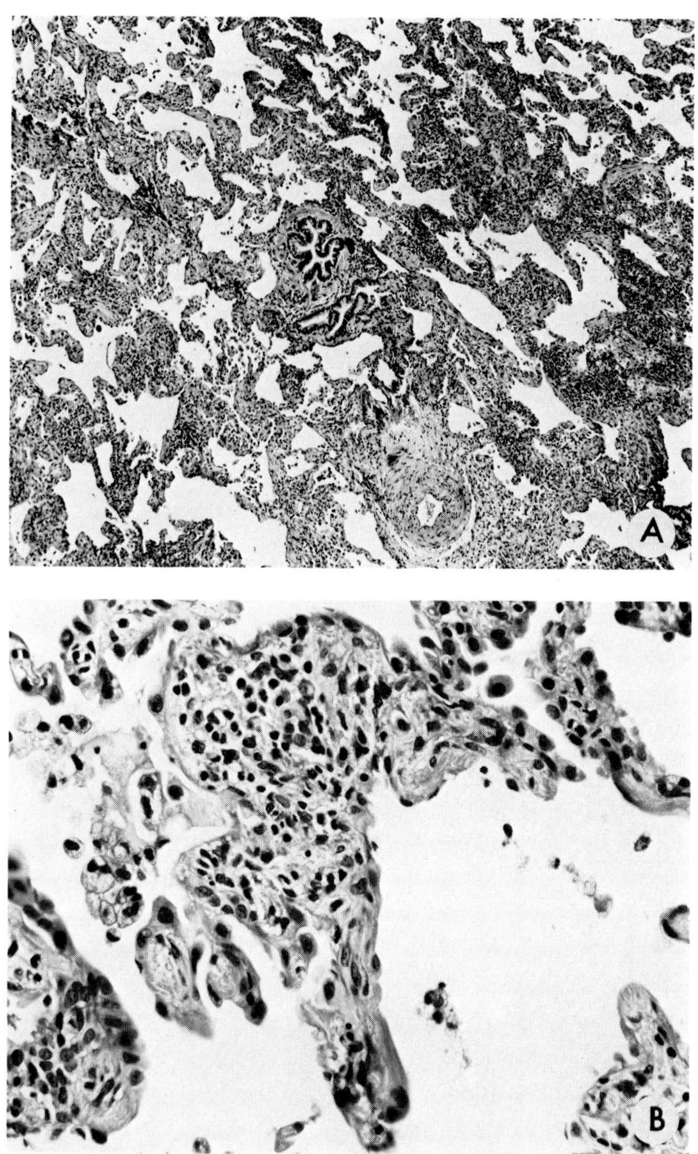

Fig. 7-15. Open lung biopsy of patient with diffuse pulmonary infiltrate on chest x-ray. Reversible changes evident on biopsy. (A) Histology of a potentially reversible case. The pulmonary architecture is essentially preserved. The abnormality present is a diffuse interstitial pneumonitis (H & E, ×50); (B) Marked interstitial thickening due to round cell infiltration in a potentially reversible case. Fibrosis is not present. Comparison with Figure 7-14B shows the essential difference between the two categories. (H & E, ×310). Reprinted from The Johns Hopkins Medical Journal, 132:103, 1973 (Baker RR, Lee JM, and Carter D: An evaluation of open lung biopsy Figures 5A and 5B, p. 110).

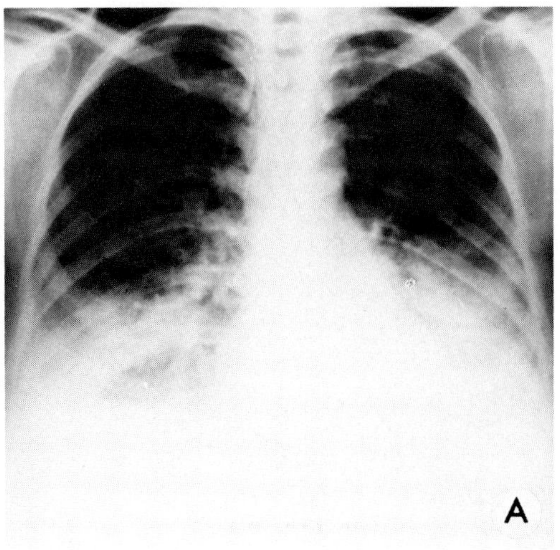

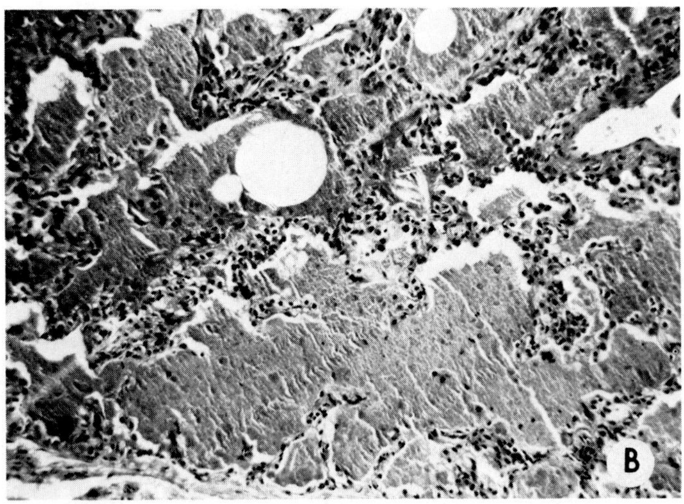

Fig. 7-16. (A) Chest x-ray of adult male with myeloproliferative disorder and pulmonary infiltrate. Open biopsy revealed pulmonary alveolar proteinosis. (B) Photomicrograph shows alveoli filled with granular eosinophilic material. Cholesterol crystals are evident to the right of center. (H & E, ×200); (C) Higher power photomicrograph shows alveolar wall essentially intact and lined by pneumocytes with a granular cytoplasm. The cytoplasmic material has been shown to be the same as that filling and distending the alveolar space. (H & E, ×325)

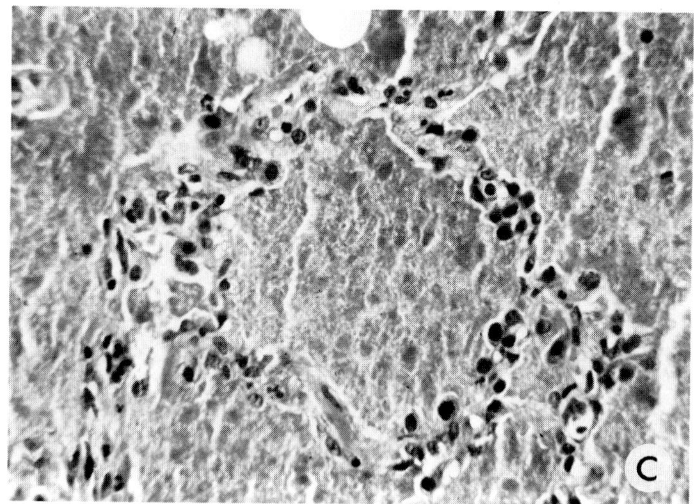

Fig. 7-16C.

REFERENCES

1. Bernstein L: Two thousand bronchoscopies in search of cancer. Ann Otol Rhinol Laryngol 76:242–249, 1967
2. Zavala DC: Diagnostic fiberoptic bronchoscopy: Techniques and results of biopsy in 600 patients. Chest 68:12–19, 1972
3. Marsh BR, Frost JK, Erozan YS, et al: Occult bronchogenic carcinoma. Endoscopic localization and television documentation. Cancer 30:1348–1352, 1972
4. March BR, Frost JK, Erozan, YS, et al: Flexible fiberoptic bronchoscope—Its place in search for lung cancer. Trans Am Broncho-esophologol Assoc 53:101–110, 1973
5. March BR, Frost JK, Erozan YS, et al: The role of fiberoptic bronchoscopy in lung cancer. Semin Oncol 1:199–203, 1974
6. Andersen HA, Miller WE, Bernatz PE: Lung biopsy: Transbronchoscopic, percutaneous, open. Surg Clin North Am 52:785–793, 1973
7. King EG, Bachynski JE, Mielke B: Percutaneous trephine lung biopsy. Chest 70:212–216, 1976
8. Baker RR, Lee JM, Carter D: An evaluation of open lung biopsy. Johns Hopkins Med J 132:102–116, 1973
9. Ruttner JR, Spycher MA, Sticher H: The detection of etiologic agents in interstitial fibrosis. Hum Pathol 4:497–512, 1973

Bernard R. Marsh, M.D.
Ko Pen Wang, M.D.

8

Bronchoscopy in the Diagnosis of Pulmonary Disease

In recent years the importance of bronchoscopy in evaluating pulmonary disease has been increasingly recognized and better understood. The advent of flexible instruments not only opened to our view larger areas of the bronchial tree but also provided a relatively simple means for obtaining specimens from areas beyond our view in nearly all parts of the lung. Not surprisingly this development has resulted in a surge of new interest in bronchoscopy as a means for evaluating a variety of pulmonary problems.

This chapter is devoted to some of the indications and applications of modern bronchoscopy in the study of patients with focal and diffuse pulmonary disorders. No attempt has been made to present an exhaustive treatise on the subject but rather its more practical aspects in representative clinical problems are discussed.

In the hands of a competent endoscopist modern bronchoscopy is a relatively safe procedure with minimal morbidity and a high diagnostic yield.[1–3] It should therefore be considered in any patient with an inadequately understood pulmonary problem. Whether in the study of conditions affecting the visible airways with more striking features such as foreign body, atelectasis, or hemoptysis or in diseases affecting principally the pulmonary parenchyma (e.g., granulomatous diseases, peripheral tumors, lung abscess) bronchoscopic techniques usually provide important information about the pathologic process. The value of these techniques depends upon a number of factors listed in Table 8-1.

The discussion that follows deals principally with the flexible fiberoptic bronchoscope (FOB) because of its increasingly widespread application in

Supported, in part, by National Cancer Institute, Contract No. 1-CM-45037.

Table 8-1
Factors Affecting Success in Bronchoscopy

1. The specific pathologic entity and its specific location
2. The skill and experience of the endoscopist
3. The availability of all necessary endoscopic equipment in proper working order
4. The adequacy of preoperative evaluation
5. The competence and interested cooperation of all laboratory and other support personnel
6. The cooperation of the patient
7. Availability of fluoroscopic guidance for localized lesions

the management of patients with pulmonary disorders. It should be emphasized, however, that even though the FOB is used in more than 95 percent of our bronchoscopic procedures the open-tube bronchoscope is by no means obsolete. There are circumstances in which the well-trained and experienced endoscopist still finds such instruments of great value. These circumstances are outlined in Table 8-2. Although each of the specific situations indicated in Table 8-2 may sometimes be managed satisfactorily with flexible instruments, a broad choice of instrumentation in the hands of a competent endoscopist will provide the most efficient and effective means of management.

NATURE OF THE FIBEROPTIC BRONCHOSCOPE

The commonly used fiberoptic bronchoscope consists of a flexible shaft 5–6 mm in diameter and about 60 cm long. At one end is the eyepiece and control handle; at the other, a directionally controllable tip and objective lens. Through the shaft runs an image bundle of coherent glass fibers, a pair of illumination bundles, a pair of control cables, and a lumen 1.8–2.6 mm in diameter. The lumen provides not only for insertion of various biopsy devices but also serves as a means for instilling anesthesia and other solutions as well as aspiration of secretions.

Table 8-2
Indications for Open Tube Bronchoscopy

1. Tracheal tumor or stricture
2. Massive hemoptysis
3. Foreign bodies
4. Need for suctioning of large amounts of inspissated or aspirated material
5. Tumors of the major bronchi
6. Biopsies of the carina and major spurs
7. Small children
8. Transtracheal or transbronchial needle aspiration of mediastinal or hilar tumors

The fiberoptic bronchoscope may be introduced via the nose or mouth. Although the nasal route may suffice for some examinations, we prefer to insert the fiberoptic bronchoscope through a previously placed endotracheal tube for most diagnostic procedures where brush and biopsy specimens are required.[4] The reasons for our particular preference include the following:

1. Airway control. The orotracheal tube provides an excellent means for delivering supplemental oxygen or for assisted or controlled ventilation when necessary even for prolonged procedures.
2. Ease of cleaning. The facility with which the bronchoscope may be removed for lens cleaning, clearing an occluded channel, or the retrieval of large and multiple specimens. If brush and curette are pulled through the instrument lumen, the specimen may be stripped off. Some of the larger biopsies may likewise be damaged or partially avulsed.
3. Management of hemorrhage. A larger catheter may be used to aspirate. The endotracheal tube may be directed into the non-bleeding lung to maintain ventilation. If necessary, the open-tube bronchoscope can be passed through a bloodless field and into the larynx before removal of the tube and application of more direct control measures.
4. Adaptability for general anesthesia. Immediate provision for proceeding, when necessary, to general anesthesia in technically demanding cases.
5. Patient acceptance. Excellent patient acceptance with either local or general anesthesia techniques.
6. Complications nil.

BIOPSY INSTRUMENTS

There are three principal instruments of value in retrieving pathologic specimens by means of the fiberoptic bronchoscope: the brush, the curette and the biopsy forceps (Fig. 8-1, by permission).[5] Some of the circumstances in which each has special value are discussed later in this chapter. A feature common to all, however, is the small specimen size. For best results in avoiding a sampling error, one should obtain multiple specimens, with a combination of brush, curette, and biopsy forceps. It is important that the specimen be dislodged from the brush or curette before it is extracted from the bronchoscope. This will increase the amount of material obtained for laboratory studies (Figs. 8-2, 8-3, 8-4, by permission).[5]

The importance of prompt and proper handling of cytologic materials cannot be overemphasized. An agreement should be reached with surgical and cytopathology laboratories regarding the desired techniques for handling this material. Understanding and cooperation in these areas frequently spell the difference between success and failure.

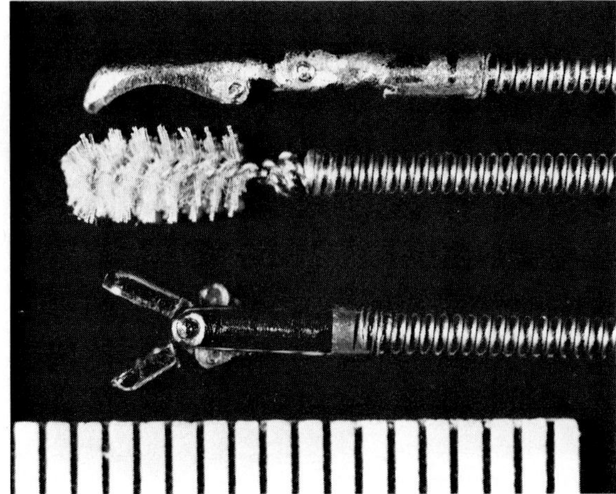

Fig. 8-1. Curette, brush and biopsy forceps. (Reprinted by permission, Marsh BR: Advances in bronchoscopy. Otolaryngol Clin North Am 11, 1978.)

INDICATIONS FOR BRONCHOSCOPY

Hilar Lesions

Tumors of the major bronchi can usually be diagnosed by endoscopic techniques. The principal exception to this rule is tumors that cause bronchial compression but have no endobronchial component. These are difficult to diagnose since the tumor tissue per se is inaccessible. This situation

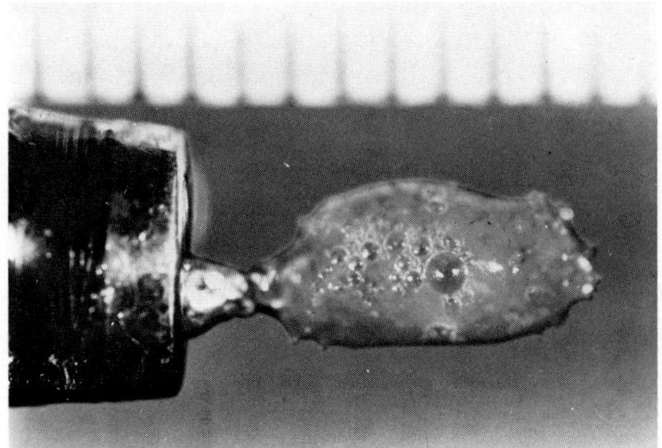

Fig. 8-2. Brush with specimen. (Reprinted by permission, Marsh BR: Advances in bronchoscopy. Otolaryngol Clin North Am 11, 1978.)

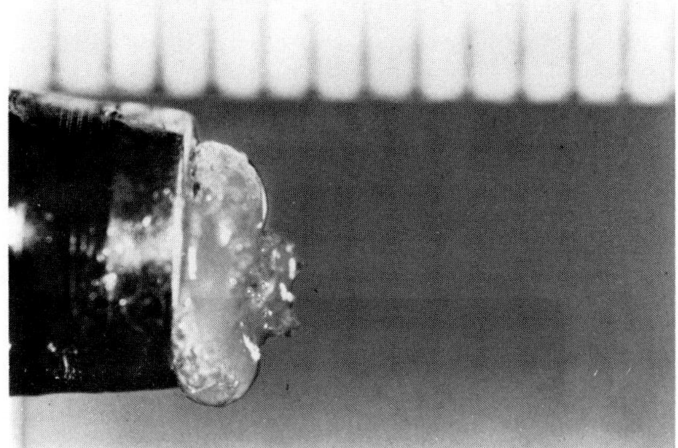

Fig. 8-3. Brush being drawn into bronchoscope. (Reprinted by permission, Marsh BR: Advances in bronchoscopy. Otolaryngol Clin North Am 11, 1978.)

is seen most commonly with oat cell carcinoma and in some cases of advanced squamous cell carcinoma. In contrast to the transbronchoscopic biopsy techniques used in the lung periphery, a biopsy through the intact wall of a major bronchus is quite hazardous and should not be attempted.

TECHNIQUE

On the evening before the procedure the patient should be told what to expect, why the procedure is being done, and what significant risks are involved. Appropriate sedation is ordered and the patient is made NPO after midnight. In the operating room (or similarly equipped and staffed area) an

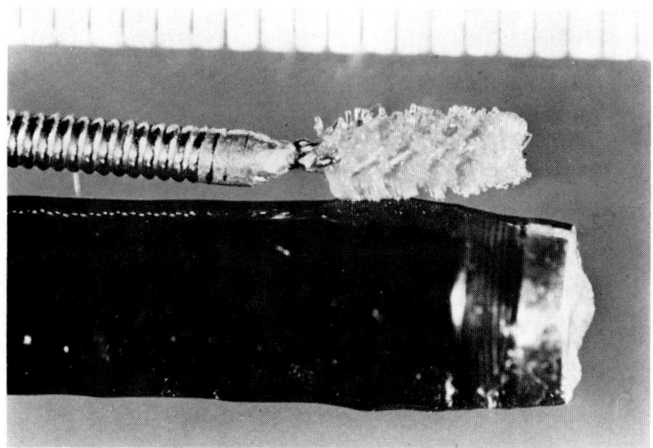

Fig. 8-4. Brush after being drawn through bronchoscope Note: Much of the specimen has been stripped off. (Reprinted by permission, Marsh BR: Advances in bronchoscopy. Otolaryngol Clin North Am 11, 1978.)

intravenous infusion is started, and the mouth, oropharynx, and larynx are examined. Routine examination of these structures is often rewarded by discovery of unsuspected pathology or additional useful information. Vocal cord paralysis and primary laryngeal carcinoma have been incidentally detected. The pharynx is then anesthetized with 4 percent lidocaine spray. A 3-cc syringe with a cannula allows increments of 2 percent lidocaine to be instilled under direct vision into the larynx and trachea. Care is taken not to exceed a safe dose. Seldom should more than 200–400 mg (10–20 cc of 2 percent lidocaine) be necessary. When adequate anesthesia has been obtained, a 9-mm (i.d.) endotracheal tube is lubricated with lidocaine jelly and fitted with a stylet to form a "J." Under guidance of a laryngeal mirror, the tube is gently passed through the mouth and larynx into the trachea. The stylet is removed, a bite block is secured over the tube, and both are secured with adhesive tape.

Alternatively the endotracheal tube may be slipped over the distal end of the FOB; the tip is then passed to just above the carina. The endotracheal tube is slipped over the bronchoscope and into the trachea.[6] The patient is then placed in a semi-recumbent position and the head draped by the nurse while the endoscopist is gowned and gloved. Oxygen is connected to the endotracheal tube via a "T" adapter (Fig. 8-5). The FOB is checked and lubricated with water-soluble jelly or silicone and passed through the endotracheal tube. Additional aliquots of 1 percent or 2 percent lidocaine may be added as necessary during the procedure. An examination of the bronchi in the involved lung is followed by a brief study of the uninvolved lung before any specimens are obtained. Special care is taken to note the appearance of the carina, major bronchi, and lobar spurs. These observations are often important for planning a surgical resection or radiotherapy.

If the tumor appears as a friable endobronchial mass, a biopsy should be obtained by passing the microforceps through the instrument channel and directing the tip of the tumor site where the specimen is taken from the most accessible area. If the specimen is larger than the forceps cup, the bronchoscope and forceps are removed together, and the specimen is dislodged into formalin. The forceps are then rinsed in saline to remove the formalin and are withdrawn from the bronchoscope. The bronchoscope is then replaced, and any bleeding or clots are aspirated. When bleeding has stopped, saline is aspirated through the instrument channel to remove blood and secretions. The brush is then placed in the instrument lumen and the bronchoscope is returned to the tumor site. The brush is extruded and passed well into the involved bronchus. After to-and-fro brushing for several seconds the brush is brought back to the tip of the bronchoscope and again both are removed. The brush is passed further out of the bronchoscope to facilitate removal of the specimen by one of two techniques: (1) the brush material may be smeared directly onto a slide and immediately placed into fixative or (2) the specimen may be dislodged into a balanced salt solution for prompt processing in the cytopathology laboratory. (We prefer the latter tech-

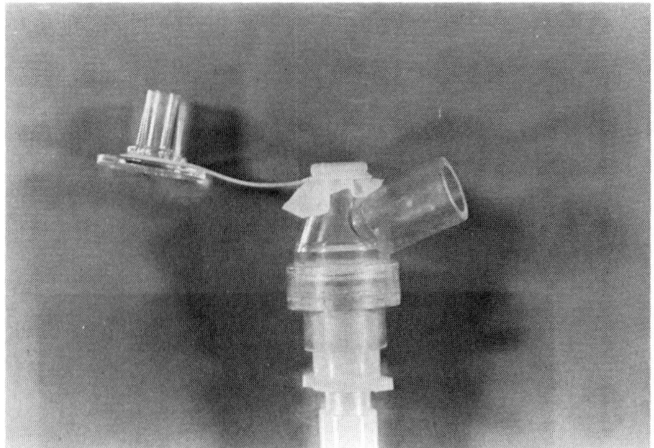

Fig. 8-5. "T" adapter with rubber diaphragm.

nique.) One should repeat the procedure by obtaining several more brushings and biopsies if possible. Finally a biosy is obtained from the next most proximal lobar spur and the carina. Specimens from these proximal sites must be carefully labeled to assist the surgeon in determining resectability and planning adequate bronchial margins. Microforceps obtain only a very superficial specimen, but it may be sufficient to detect inapparent carcinoma in situ.

If the tumor appears as a bronchial stenosis with no endobronchial mass, the curette should also be used. It should be passed 3–4 cm beyond the stenosis before the tip is bent and raked across the intervening bronchus wall. The tip is straightened and the procedure is repeated several times. With experience one learns to apply sufficient bend to the tip of the curette to obtain a positive scraping effect but to avoid an abrupt angulation which may cause injury. Both instruments are removed together and the specimen is dislodged in balanced salt solution for cytologic study. Alternatively the specimen may be smeared between two glass slides and immediately fixed in 95 percent alcohol. The curette should be manipulated into as many subsegmental bronchi in the tumor area as possible. Since tumors manifest as bronchial stenosis are more difficult to diagnose, a greater effort is required to reach a small subsegmental bronchus where the tumor may be exposed to biopsy instruments. In some resected carcinomas the pathologist may be unable to demonstrate *any* tumor within the bronchus lumen.

Finally, the bronchus involved is lavaged with several instillations of balanced salt solution and the patient is asked to cough. The aspirated material is retrieved in a trap and divided for cytologic examination and for bacteriologic analysis if indicated. These samples should be promptly delivered to the appropriate laboratories. The endotracheal tube is removed, and the patient is placed in a suitable area for observation until recovery from the anethesia and sedation.

RESULTS

In our most recent 50 patients with hilar tumors the lesion could be directly seen at bronchoscopy in 39 but was invisible in 11. A diagnosis, however, was established in 44 patients, indicating that some hilar tumors can be diagnosed by this technique even though they are not directly visible at bronchoscopy.

CASE REPORTS

Case #1. A 63-year-old white male cigarette smoker has an old history of tuberculosis. On his annual chest x-ray a left hilar mass was observed, and he was referred for bronchoscopy (Fig. 8-6). A friable lesion nearly filled the upper division bronchus of the left upper lobe and was proved on biopsy to be a squamous carcinoma (Fig. 8-7).[7] Unfortunately, a simultaneous but less extensive second primary carcinoma was also discovered in the apical segment of the right upper lobe (Fig. 8-8).[7] Because of limited pulmonary reserve he was treated with radiotherapy and succumbed to his disease 14 months later.

Bronchial Adenomas

Bronchial adenomas are usually found in the major airways and may be pedunculated. The glistening, smooth, nonulcerated surface with varying degrees of bossing distinguishes it from most other lesions. When such a mass occurs in a characteristic clinical setting, some surgeons proceed with thoracotomy without histologic diagnosis. Whenever there is any doubt, however, a biopsy should be obtained, even though excessive bleeding may result. We prefer an open-tube instrument in these patients not only because of the better aspirating capability but also to obtain a deeper biopsy. Microforceps are not always adequate to penetrate the overlying epithelium and obtain diagnostic tissue. For these reasons the inexperienced endoscopist may choose to leave such lesions alone.

Peripheral Lesions

Bronchogenic carcinomas, granulomas, metastatic tumors, and other lesions occurring beyond the directly visible bronchial tree may often be diagnosed by means of fiberoptic techniques with the aid of fluoroscopic guidance.

Lesions involving the mid-lung field and well seen on fluoroscopy can frequently be diagnosed by brushing, curetting, and microbiopsy. The brush and curette cover a large surface area and are therefore useful in detecting endobronchial disease. The biopsy forcep, however, provides a localized but somewhat deeper source of material necessary for diagnosis in some cases.

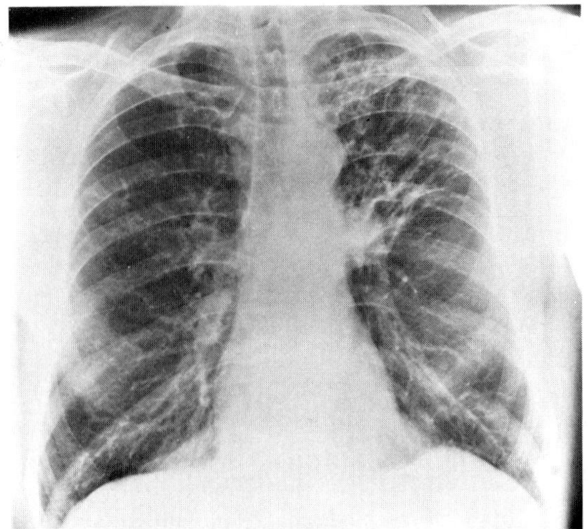

Fig. 8-6. Chest radiograph showing left hilar mass.

TECHNIQUE

Following induction of satisfactory anesthesia and intubation, the patient is placed on the fluoroscopy table. Biplane capability either with two tubes or a rotating cradle simplifies patient positioning.[8] First a brief view of all lobes and segments is carried out, followed by a detailed study of the involved lobe or segment. It is our standard routine to examine all areas of the bronchial tree even in the patient with an obvious roentgenographic lesion. Unsuspected additional focal primary neoplasms are not a rare occurrence. If no evidence of disease is found, the suspected segment is entered with the closed biopsy forcep, and under fluoroscopic control the instrument is passed into the involved area. When the correct position has been achieved in the P-A view, a check is made in the lateral view (or as near to that as possible). If the correct position is confirmed, the forceps is opened and withdrawn about 5 mm to assure full opening before advancing again the same distance and closing the jaws. The forceps is then withdrawn under

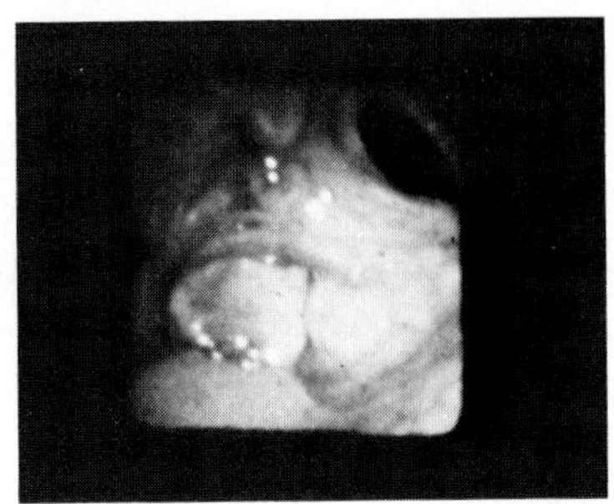

Fig. 8-7. Upper division bronchus, left upper lobe occluded by tumor. (Reprinted by permission, Marsh BR, et al: New horizons in lung cancer diagnosis. Cancer 37:437–439, 1976.)

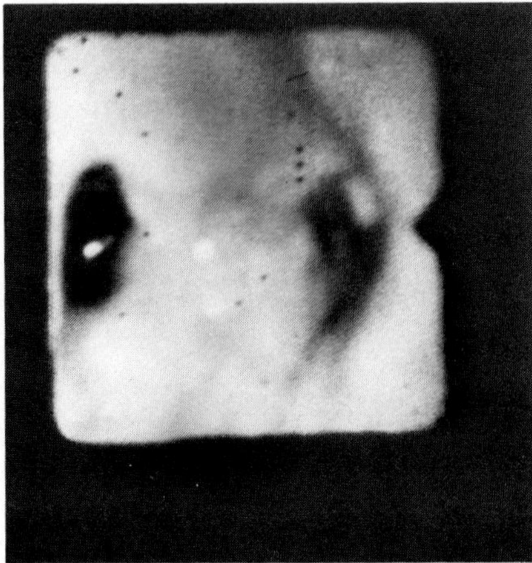

Fig. 8-8. Right upper lobe apical segment carcinoma. (Reprinted by permission, Marsh, BR, et al: New horizons in lung cancer diagnosis. Cancer 37:437–439, 1976.)

observation through the bronchoscope to see how much bleeding occurs. Normally bleeding is not a serious problem, but at times it may be troublesome for a few minutes. After the specimen is removed, the brush is reinserted. This procedure is repeated several times. For best results we also use the curette in these cases. Ultimately we should have four or five biopsies plus brushings, curettings, and lavage. Every effort is made to reach more than one bronchus in the area of the lesion. Some times this is fortuitous since the currette may take a different course than the brush or the biopsy forcep. Occasionally only one instrument can be successfully guided into the lesion. When it is impossible to reach the lesion with any instrument, specimens are obtained from the closest accessible area, since these may yield a diagnosis.

A postoperative chest x-ray is obtained later in the day unless acute shortness of breath, chest pain, or a change in vital signs warrants an earlier study.

RESULTS

Adequate tissue for diagnosis can be obtained in approximately 60 percent of cases of primary bronchogenic carcinomas greater than 2.5 cm in diameter and well seen on fluoroscopy (Case Report #2). Tumors less than 2 cm in diameter and especially those immediately subpleural frequently cannot be diagnosed from bronchoscopic specimens. In only 11 of our most recent 50 patients with these small tumors were we able to establish a diagnosis by this technique. Lack of directional control at the tip of the biopsy instrument often precludes precise entry into the smaller, peripheral lesions.

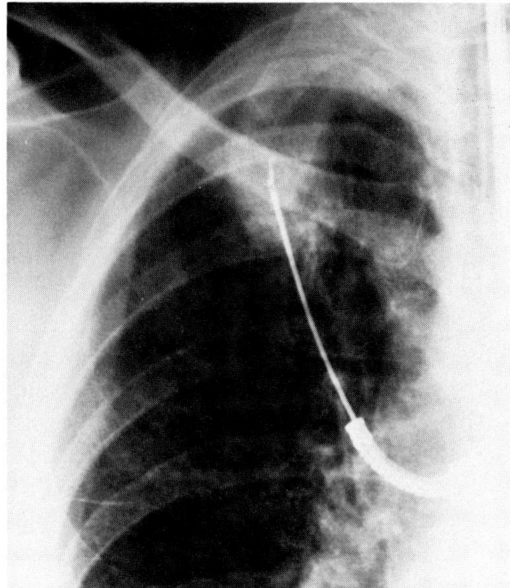

Fig. 8-9. Chest radiograph demonstrating 3 cm right upper lobe mass. Spot film during bronchoscopy shows curette located within the lesion.

Metastatic lesions may be located entirely outside of the bronchus and are more difficult to diagnose. Tumors arising in a "T" bronchus may prove completely inaccessible to biopsy instruments. When satisfactory directional control is developed for the tip of the biopsy instruments, we can expect improved results in cases in which we now have difficulty because of the geometry of bronchial bifurcation.

In benign tumors such as the hamartoma, the small biopsy specimen is inadequate for diagnosis. Granulomas on the other hand are frequently diagnosed from these specimens. In addition, a stained smear for organisms from the brush or curette has often allowed a rapid diagnosis of tuberculosis.

CASE REPORTS

Case #2. A 55-year-old white female cigarette smoker was admitted with a five-week history of right anterior chest and shoulder pain. She denied cough, dyspnea, fever, and chills but had sustained a ten-pound weight loss over the preceding six months. A chest x-ray revealed an ill-defined, 3-cm, right upper lobe mass (Fig. 8-9). Fiberoptic bronchoscopy under fluoroscopic control demonstrated on biopsy an undifferentiated large cell carcinoma which was subsequently proven unresectable and was treated by radiotherapy.

Pulmonary Infiltrates

In this group are patients with acute or chronic nonsuppurative pulmonary diseases, either diffuse or localized, alveolar, interstitial, or mixed in type. A visual examination by bronchoscopy may not allow definitive diagnosis, and thus pathologic material from the parenchyma must be obtained. Transbronchoscopic lung biopsy developed and evaluated by Andersen and Fontana with the rigid bronchoscope is now commonly performed with the fiberbronchoscope.[9–12] The technique using the FOB is similar, although it probably carries a somewhat lower risk of hemorrhage and pneumothorax since the biopsy forceps are smaller. When properly performed on selected patients, serious complications are rare, and pneumothorax should occur in less than 10 percent. In the immunosuppressed host, significant hemoptysis appears somewhat more frequently. The bronchoscopist must always be prepared to manage the unexpected or sudden complications associated with these techniques. A preoperative evaluation of the patient's prothrombin time, platelet count, and hematocrit should also be obtained. Relative contraindications are a prothrombin time less than 60 percent and a platelet count below 50,000 to 100,000 per cubic mm.

TECHNIQUE

The patient is premedicated and anesthetized as for routine bronchoscopy. In addition he is instructed to indicate any pain in the chest or back by means of a hand signal. The FOB is then introduced through the endotracheal tube, and the tracheobronchial tree is examined for any diagnostic clues. In the event of a segmental involvement, the appropriate segment is entered with the bronchoscope. If the disease is bilaterally diffuse, the basilar segments of the right lower lobe are most easily biopsied. Reaching these segments requires minimal angulation of the bronchoscope, thus providing a relatively friction-free system allowing a delicate sense of touch for determining how far to insert the biopsy forceps.

The middle lobe and lingula are usually avoided, since a pneumothorax may easily be created without warning by transversing the visceral pleura without causing pain at the chest wall.

The biopsy forceps should pass several centimeters into the basal segment in order to avoid taking a specimen from the midzone of the lung, where vessels remain large and bleeding complications are more severe. When a slight increase in resistance is felt, the jaws of the biopsy forcep are opened and it is withdrawn approximately 5 mm and then advanced 5 mm to ensure that the jaws have fully opened. With exhalation, the jaws are closed and the specimen is removed from the bronchus. It should not require significant force to avulse the specimen, and if it does, cartilage may have been grasped, an indication of too proximal a location. When considerable resistance is encountered, the forcep should be released and another more peripheral site chosen. After each specimen is removed a momentary observation is made for significant bleeding before the bronchoscope is removed. If necessary the instrument may be quickly wedged into a bleeding segment to tamponade or aspirate as required. So long as no untoward effects are noted, four to six acceptable specimens should be obtained from various subsegmental bronchi. Although these need not all be obtained from a single lobe, they should certainly be restricted to one lung because of the potential risk of bilateral pneumothorax.

Fluroscopy is usually used to aid in assessing the proper location for biopsy and should certainly be used by endoscopists who are gaining experience with the technique. Some recommend fluoroscopic use routinely. We find it especially important in the upper lobes where the sense of touch is compromised by friction resulting from angulation of the instrument. We do not, however, always use fluoroscopy in the performance of transbronchoscopic biopsy from the basal segments. Unless care is take to obtain several views, fluoroscopy may provide a false sense of security, encouraging the endoscopist to force the instrument too far, thus contributing to the risk of pneumothorax.

RESULTS

Transbronchoscopic biopsy in diffuse disease has proved its value in a high percentage of patients. In sarcoid the diagnostic yield with adequate specimens approaches 100 percent. In 29 of our most recent 31 cases noncaseating granulomata were discovered. In two patients there was no lung parenchyma present in the specimen.

CASE REPORTS

Case #3. Sarcoidosis. A 19-year-old black female complained of redness and pain in her left eye. Physical examination revealed mild conjunctival injection in the left eye and fine râles at the lung bases. A chest roentgenogram revealed diffuse nodular pulmonary infiltrates (Fig. 8-10). A transbronchial lung biopsy was performed, and the lung tissue showed noncaseating granulomata. Stains for AFB and fungi were negative (Fig. 8-11).

Even in Stage I disease a diagnosis can be expected in about 60 percent of cases.[13]

In various types of interstitial pneumonitis the histologic findings are, of course, nonspecific, but the diagnosis is frequently inferred from the absence of a more specific lesion.

Case #4. Interstitial Pneumonitis. A 20-year-old male had received a bone marrow transplant for aplastic anemia. While receiving therapy for graft-versus-host disease, he complained of dyspnea and a nonproductive cough. A chest roentgenogram revealed a diffuse interstitial infiltrate in the right lower lung field (Fig. 8-12). Transbronchial lung biopsy was performed. Histologic examination showed alveolar cells with intranuclear inclusion bodies (Fig. 8-13). Cultures of lung tissue grew cytomegalovirus.

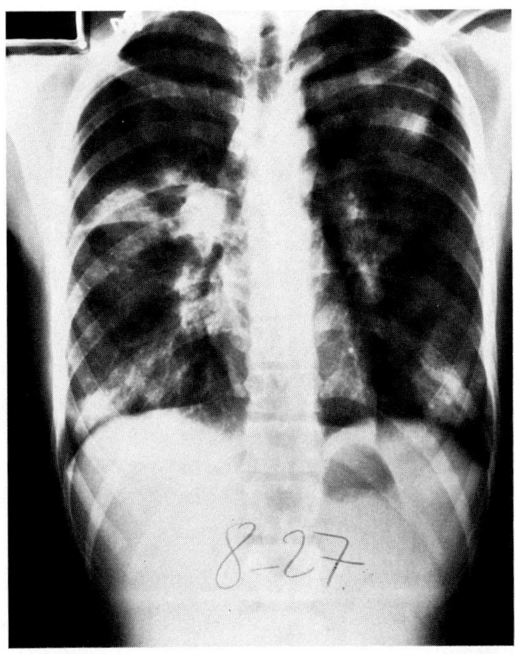

Fig. 8-10. Chest radiograph showing diffuse nodular infiltrates.

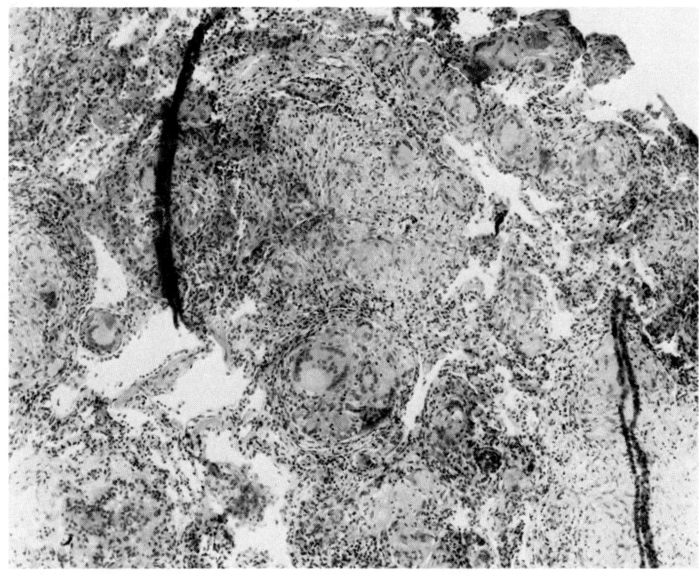

Fig. 8-11. Transbronchoscopic lung biopsy showing non-caseating granulomata. Strains for AFB and fungi were negative.

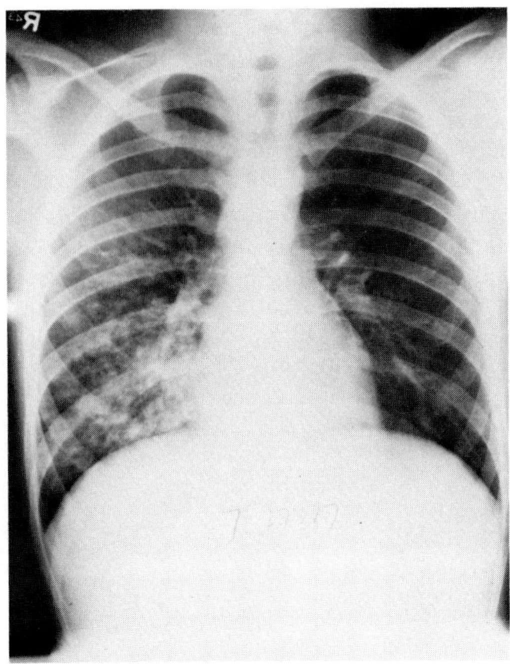

Fig. 8-12. Chest radiograph with diffuse interstitial infiltrate right lower lung field.

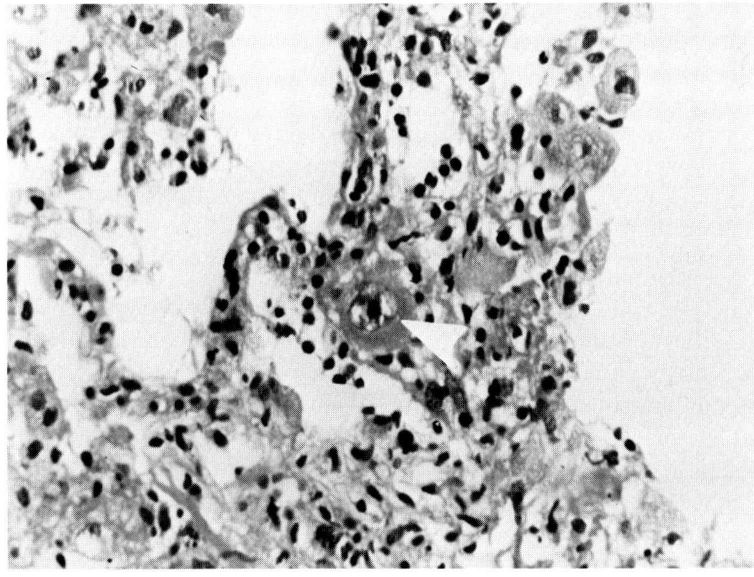

Fig. 8-13. Transbronchoscopic lung biopsy showing alveolar cells with intranuclear inclusion bodies. Cultures of lung tissue grew out Cytomegalovirus.

In *Pneumocystis carinii* the diagnosis is made in most cases where multiple specimens are obtained.[14] It is thus often the procedure of choice when these diagnoses are suspected.

In the immunosuppressed patient, one frequently discovers pulmonary infiltrates of a nonspecific or viral etiology where transbronchoscopic specimens provide no definitive diagnosis. These nonspecific results are, however, usually reliable in excluding such treatable conditions as *Pneumocystis,* fungus infection, bacterial pneumonia, and tuberculosis.

Metastatic cancer with lymphangitic spread can be readily diagnosed by fiberoptic bronchoscopy. In view of the infrequent complications and low morbidity associated with this technique it should be the procedure of choice in establishing the diagnosis unless other obvious peripheral sites are available for surgical excision.

Occult Bronchogenic Carcinoma

Localizing the source of malignant cells appearing in the sputum of a patient whose chest x-ray fails to demonstrate any evidence of tumor requires a careful and detailed study.[15,16]

TECHNIQUE

The upper respiratory tract should be examined for any evidence of malignancy in the oral cavity, pharynx, nasopharynx, and larynx. If these areas appear to be clear, a bronchoscopic study should then be undertaken.

In this situation we prefer general anesthesia for three principle reasons:

1. The procedure may require an hour or more in some difficult cases.
2. It is important to maintain a quiet tracheobronchial tree for ''uncontaminated'' brush specimens.
3. General anesthesia seems to provide a degree of bronchial dilatation improving exposure of the segments. This is probably due in part to the use of positive pressure ventilation and perhaps to a reduction in bronchial tone.

Once the endotracheal tube has been introduced, a bite block is placed over the tube and a ''T'' adapter is attached. This allows simultaneous general anesthesia and freedom to conduct an unhurried and as detailed a study as necessary. A segment-by-segment study is made with care to identify any area of roughening, friability, or thickening of a segmental spur. Normally the subsegmental spurs can be identified in most segments. All lobes and segments should be searched, even though a tumor is quickly identified. Sometimes a second primary tumor is also present and may be a more significant lesion than the first to be discovered (Figs. 8-14 and 8-15). If a tumor is found, both brushing and biopsy should be obtained in addition to a biopsy of the next most proximal lobar spur and the carina.

If no tumor is found, a series of differential brushings is required. Fol-

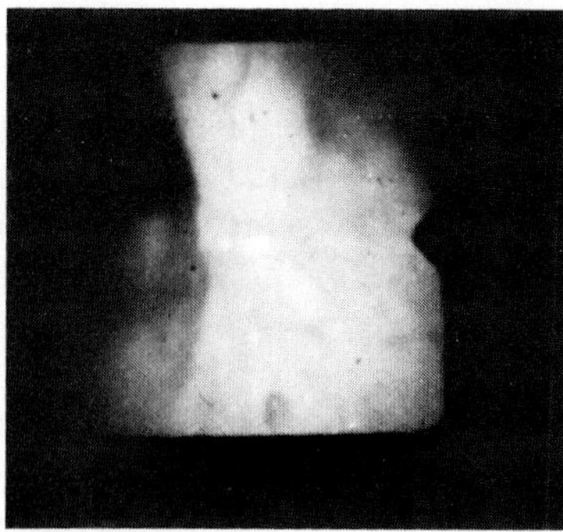

Fig. 8-14. Right upper lobe spur with discrete 3-mm carcinoma in situ.

lowing the complete visual search and aspiration of secretions, the bronchoscope channel is flushed with balanced salt solution and a clean brush is inserted within the channel. The bronchoscope is then carefully positioned at the right upper lobe orifice where the brush is extruded into one of the segments. The bronchoscope is then moved into the lobe. Each of the segments and as many of the subsegments as possible are brushed before the brush is drawn back to the tip of the bronchoscope. The bronchoscope is then removed, the brush extruded, and the specimen removed. Finally the brush is withdrawn from the channel, the channel is flushed with salt solution, and a new brush is placed within the lumen. This procedure is repeated for each lobe, and each specimen is identified as to its source. Ultimately several microbiopsies may be taken from representative areas at the segmental level. As soon as the cough reflex has returned, the entire tracheobronchial tree is lavaged for a cytologic specimen. As the endotra-

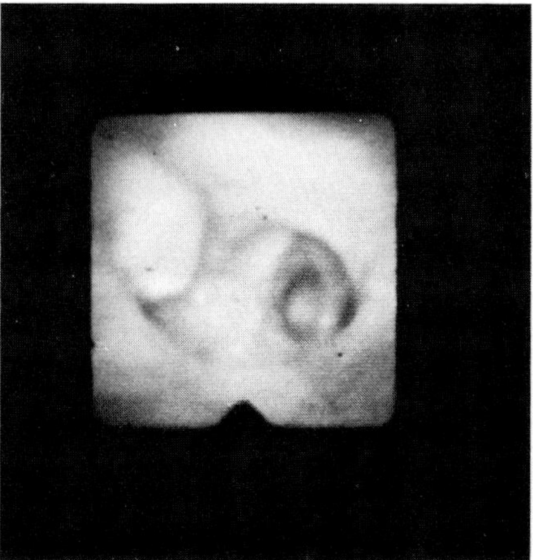

Fig. 8-15. Left upper lobe upper division bronchus of the same patient as in Figure 8-14 showing carcinoma in situ discovered later in the procedure.

cheal tube is withdrawn, the trachea is viewed through the bronchoscope to rule out a lesion that might have been overlooked.

Some have questioned the value of a postbronchoscopic sputum in patients with clinical tumors.[17] Although results with the brush and biopsy forcep are extremely good, we still obtain three morning sputum specimens following bronchoscopy when no endobronchial tumor is seen. In the event that all bronchoscopic material shows no evidence of cancer but the postbronchoscopic sputum demonstrates malignant cells, a strong case can be made for the existence of a tumor somewhere in the upper respiratory tract requiring additional search techniques.

RESULTS

In our experience with 28 patients with malignant cells in the sputum but no localizing information by chest x-ray, 4 were shown to be harboring cancer of the upper respiratory tract. Twenty-two of twenty-four of the remaining cases have been successfully localized. In 17 the lesion appeared to arise from a segmental bronchus and in 5 its origin was in a lobar or main bronchus. In 5 the disease was multifocal.

BRONCHOSCOPY LEAST VALUABLE

Having emphasized the importance and value of modern bronchoscopy in pulmonary problems, we have found that there are some situations in which it less often yields the correct diagnosis.

1. Small (less than 2.5 cm) subpleural lesions. These can sometimes be reached, but even with the aid of fluoroscopy, the diagnostic yield is probably less than 25 percent. Frequently they are difficult to see fluoroscopically and usually are visible in only one plane. In only 11 of our most recent 50 such patients were we able to establish a diagnosis by bronchoscopy.
2. Small metastatic nodules. Since these are usually extrabronchial in location they are more difficult to diagnose by bronchoscopy. The diagnostic yield is substantially less than in primary carcinomas.
3. Pancoast tumors. Inadequate control in the apex frequently makes these tumors difficult to reach.
4. Superior segment tumors. Small lesions occurring high in the apical subsegment of the superior segment of the lower lobe are notoriously difficult to reach by bronchoscopic techniques. The short, right-angled segmental bronchus coupled with a small subsegment requiring a sharp bending angle makes bronchoscopic diagnosis of these lesions rare.
5. Peripheral lesions visible by x-ray in only one plane. Localization may be accomplished by use of tomography, but such cases are seldom diagnosed by bronchoscopy unless they are 2.5 cm or larger in diameter.

6. Benign tumors in the peripheral bronchus. Microbiopsy forceps rarely prove adequate to obtain sufficient tissue for diagnosis. As improved forceps are developed, we can expect better results.
7. Mediastinal or hilar tumors adjacent to the trachea or major bronchus but without endobronchial involvement. These may sometimes be diagnosed by bronchoscopic needle aspiration but fiberoptic techniques currently available often prove inadequate.[18]
8. Diffuse pulmonary infiltrates in small children with respiratory failure (such as may occur in the immune-suppressed host). Maintenance of adequate ventilation in these circumstances is difficult at best, and transbronchoscopic lung biopsy is unwise.

CONCLUSION

Modern bronchoscopy is now a highly developed and essential service in the evaluation and treatment of patients with a broad range of pulmonary problems. For optimal value, however, a team approach is needed. Because the technique is associated with not only minimal morbidity but also a high diagnostic yield, it becomes an essential consideration in the work-up of most patients with focal or diffuse pulmonary disorders.

REFERENCES

1. Suratt PM, et al: Deaths and complications associated with fiberoptic bronchoscopy. Chest 69:747–751, 1976
2. Ikeda S: Flexible bronchofiberscope. Ann Otol Rhinol Laryngol 79:916–923, 1970
3. Zavala D: Diagnostic fiberoptic bronchoscopy: Techniques and results of biopsy in 600 patients. Chest 68:12–19, 1975
4. Smiddy JF: Transnasal fiberoptic bronchoscopy. RI Med J 55:351–352, 1972
5. Marsh BR: Advances in bronchoscopy. Otolaryngol Clin North Am 11:371–388, 1978
6. Hodgkin JE, Rosenow EC, Stubbs SE: Oral introduction of the flexible bronchoscope. Chest 68:88–90, 1975
7. Marsh BR, et al: New horizons in lung cancer diagnosis. Cancer 37:437–439, 1976
8. Schoenbaum SW, et al: Transbronchial biopsy of peripheral lesions with fluoroscopic guidance: Use of the fiberoptic bronchoscope. J Can Assoc Radiol 25:39–43, 1974
9. Andersen HA, Fontana RS: Transbronchoscopic lung biopsy for diffuse pulmonary diseases: Technique and results in 450 cases. Chest 62:125–128, 1972
10. Hanson RR, et al: Transbronchial biopsy via flexible fiberoptic bronchoscope: Results in 164 patients. Am Rev Respir Dis 114:67–72, 1976

11. Levin D, Wicks A, et al: Transbronchial lung biopsy via the fiberoptic bronchoscope. Am Rev Respir Dis 110:4–12, 1974
12. Joyner LR, Scheinhorn D: Transbronchial forceps lung biopsy through the fiberoptic bronchoscope. Chest 67:532–535, 1975
13. Koerner S, et al: Transbronchial lung biopsy for the diagnosis of sarcoidosis. N Engl J Med 293:268–270, 1975
14. Scheinhorn DJ, Joyner LR: Transbronchial forceps lung biopsy through the fiberoptic bronchoscope in pneumocystis carinii pneumonia. Chest 66:294, 1974
15. Marsh BR, et al: Flexible fiberoptic bronchoscopy, its place in the search for lung cancer. Ann Otol Rhinol Laryngol 82:757–764, 1973
16. Sanderson DR, et al: Bronchoscopic localization of radiographically occult lung cancer. Chest 65:609–612, 1974
17. Kvale PA, Bode F, Kini S: Diagnostic accuracy in lung cancer: Comparison of techniques used in association with flexible fiberoptic bronchoscopy. Chest 69:752–757, 1976
18. Wang, KP; Terry, PB, Marsh, BR: Bronchoscopic needle aspiration biopsy of paratracheal tumors. Amer Rev Respir Dis 118:17–21, 1978

Frederick P. Stitik, M.D.

9

Percutaneous Lung Biopsy

INTRODUCTION

Obtaining diagnostic material directly through the thoracic wall was done before the advent of radiology. In 1883 Leyden[1] performed the first needle aspiration biopsy to obtain microorganisms from a patient with pneumonia. Three years later, Ménétrier is credited with being the first to establish the diagnosis of carcinoma by transthoracic needle techniques.[2]

In the 1930s and 1940s needle biopsy was attempted by a number of investigators. At that time, large needles usually were used; often without the aid of a fluoroscope. The procedure gradually fell into disfavor due to a moderate morbidity, a few isolated case reports of deaths attributed to the procedure,[3–8] and some concern over local tumor spread to the pleura and chest wall following the biopsy.[9–11]

In 1966 Dahlgren and Nordenstrom reawakened the world's interest in needle biopsy of pulmonary lesions.[12] The technological advances that helped revitalize this procedure included (1) improved image-intensified fluoroscopy, (2) development of narrow-gauge, thin-walled needles, and (3) refinement of cytologic techniques in the diagnosis of pulmonary lesions.

The following discussion is based on experience with more than 300 patients undergoing needle biopsy at The Johns Hopkins Hospital. This procedure is a valuable addition to the diagnostic armamentarium. The physician performing needle aspiration biopsy has a wide variety of instruments from which he may choose. (Fig. 9-1) The selection of the needle should be tailored to the individual patient. In this chapter, there will be a discussion of the type of patient in whom needle aspiration biopsy is beneficial, the optimum time in the course of the work-up that biopsy is indicated, and the proper needle to be used.

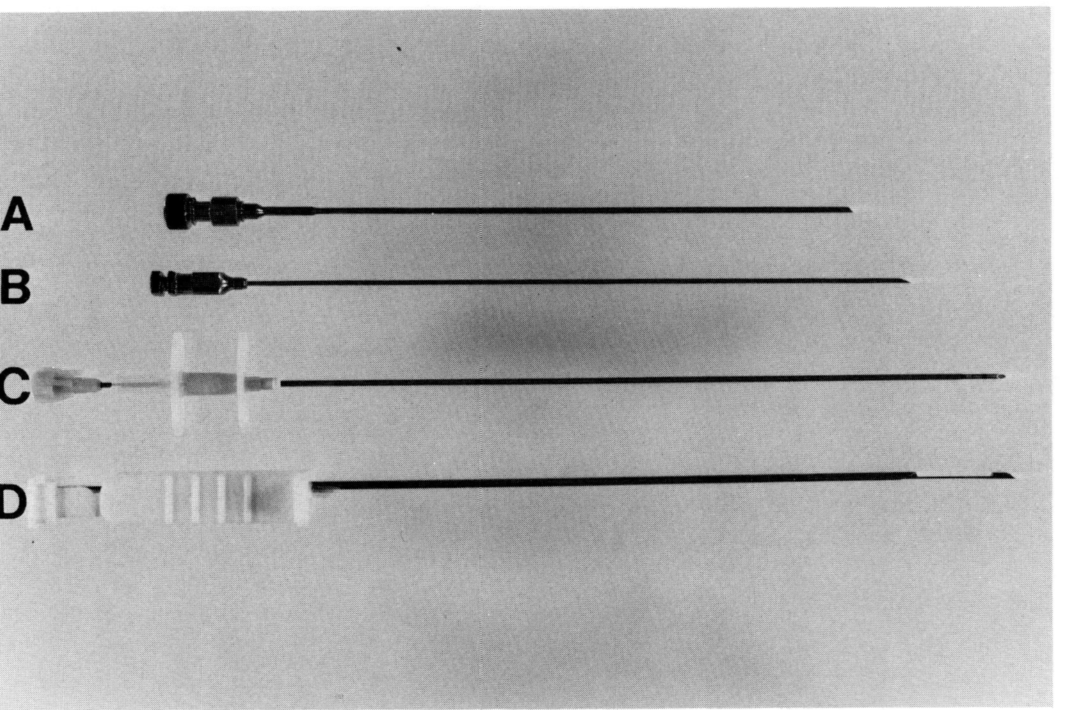

Fig. 9-1. *Needles:* (A) Turner Needle (Cook Incorporated, Bloomington, Indiana); (B) Spinal Needle; (C) Lee Needle (Becton-Dickinson Corporation, Rutherford, New Jersey); (D) Tru-Cut Needle (Travenol Laboratories, Inc. Morton Grove, Illinois).

INDICATIONS

Our indications for needle aspiration biopsy are listed in Table 9-1. Each is discussed briefly in the sections that follow.

Inoperable Patient with Suspected Bronchogenic Carcinoma

A tissue diagnosis is clearly indicated in patients with probable bronchogenic carcinoma who are considered inoperable due to poor cardiopulmonary reserve. Establishment of a tissue diagnosis for these patients is mandatory so that the radiotherapist and/or the chemotherapist will have a cytologic or tissue diagnosis from which to plan appropriate palliative therapy. Thoracotomy just to establish the diagnosis is to be discouraged. In patients with nonresectable cancer, the operative mortality rate may be as high as 9.3 percent.[13] We, however, disagree with other authors[9,14,15] who conclude that the diagnosis of inoperable bronchogenic carcinoma is the only indication for needle aspiration biopsy. Rarely, the pulmonary abnormality, although suggestive of bronchogenic carcinoma, may be due to benign disease.

Before needle aspiration biopsy is attempted, these patients should have sputum cytologic examinations for three days and bronchoscopy. These two techniques take precedence, as they are safer and are highly accurate, especially if the lesion is central and can be visualized and biopsied (see Chapters 6 and 8).

The Patient with a Solitary Pulmonary Mass Suspected of Being the Source of Probable Metastatic Disease

If the simpler techniques of sputum cytology and bronchoscopy are unsuccessful, needle aspiration biopsy of the pulmonary lesion demonstrating a bronchogenic carcinoma is considered sufficient evidence to institute radiotherapy to suspected cerebral or symptomatic bone metastases. Occasionally, the pulmonary abnormality is due to benign disease. A biopsy that shows the pulmonary lesion to be benign often prompts a complete re-evaluation of the patient.

The Patient with a Solitary Mass and a Known Extrathoracic Primary Malignancy

Frequently, full chest conventional tomography or computerized tomography is necessary to exclude other smaller metastases hidden behind the heart or diaphragm (see Chapter 5). If the mass is indeed solitary, needle aspiration biopsy should be performed after sputum cytology and bron-

Table 9-1
Indications for Needle Aspiration Biopsy

1. Inoperable patient with suspected bronchogenic carcinoma
2. Solitary pulmonary mass with extrathoracic metastases
3. Solitary pulmonary mass with known extrathoracic malignant disease
4. Solitary pulmonary mass—surgery refused
5. Multiple pulmonary masses
6. "Undiagnosed" solitary pulmonary mass
7. Pancoast tumors
8. Failure to respond to antituberculous therapy

choscopy. The clinical assumption that the solitary pulmonary mass is a metastasis can be misleading. In a study of 465 patients who either had a solitary pulmonary mass at the time an unspecified extrathoracic malignancy was discovered or developed a solitary pulmonary mass after an extrathoracic malignancy was diagnosed, 70 percent had a primary bronchogenic carcinoma. Twenty-eight percent had a solitary metastasis, and two percent had benign disease in their lungs.[16] In a study of 54 patients with colon carcinoma who developed a synchronous or metachronous solitary pulmonary mass, 25 (46 percent) had colon cancer metastases, and 29 (54 percent) had primary lung cancer.[17]

Some could argue that the survival rates of patients after removal of a solitary pulmonary metastasis are as good as or better than those for patients with a primary bronchogenic carcinoma,[17–19] and that establishing an exact diagnosis prior to thoracotomy is unnecessary. We believe that establishing a diagnosis of metastatic disease allows the primary physician to intensify his search for other metastases, to consider serial films to evaluate the doubling time of the metastasis, and to avoid mediastinoscopy in a patient with a solitary pulmonary metastasis.

If on the other hand, the needle aspiration biopsy demonstrates that the lesion is a primary bronchogenic carcinoma, a different approach to staging and therapy is indicated.

The Patient Who Refuses Surgery for a Solitary Pulmonary Mass Probably Due to Cancer

In this situation, an exact histologic or cytologic diagnosis is necessary for rational management by the radiotherapist or chemotherapist. Sputum cytology should be obtained and bronchoscopy should also be attempted before needle aspiration biopsy. Once a diagnosis of cancer was definitely established by needle aspiration biopsy, several of our patients reconsidered and opted to proceed with surgery. In other cases, the solitary pulmonary mass was due to benign disease.

The practice of treating the patient who refuses surgery for the presumptive diagnosis of tuberculosis is to be discouraged. Adverse reactions to varied antituberculous regimens range from 1 to 11 percent.[20] Several deaths due to isoniazid hepatitis have also been reported.[21] A needle aspiration biopsy diagnosis of tuberculosis provides a firm basis for the administration of these antibiotics.

The Patient with Multiple Pulmonary Lesions

Multiple new lesions, especially in patients with a documented extrathoracic malignant tumor, usually indicate metastatic spread to the lungs. The appearance of metastatic disease in the lungs prompts either chemotherapy or a change in the chemotherapeutic regimen. As chemotherapy is not without hazards, this important step is not justified without appropriate histologic or cytologic diagnosis of metastasis. Sputum cytology and bronchoscopy have a low priority in these situations, as the yield is low, whereas, needle aspiration biopsy has a high yield and a low morbidity (see Turner Needle—Results section).

The Patient with an Undiagnosed Solitary Pulmonary Mass

An extensive review of the solitary pulmonary mass is presented in another chapter (see Chapter 14). Below is a brief synopsis of how we use some of these features in patient selection for needle aspiration biopsy. Bronchogenic carcinoma is exceptionally rare in patients under the age of thirty.[22] A solitary pulmonary mass in a patient below thirty years of age is observed without further work-up.

A positive skin test is of no value in differentiating tuberculosis from cancer, as 11 percent of patients with lung cancer will have a positive skin test.[23] A negative tuberculin skin test increases the likelihood of a diagnosis of lung cancer; however, it may also indicate that the patient has a nontuberculous benign lesion.

We believe that a work-up is unnecessary when there is radiologic evidence that the mass is completely stable for a minimum of two years. These patients are followed by serial annual or semiannual chest radiographs.

If the chest radiograph or tomography shows diffuse speckled calcification, a large central calcification, or laminar calcification, this indicates that the mass is a granuloma. These patients are not evaluated but are followed. Demonstration of classic popcorn-like calcification in a hamartoma also precludes the need for a tissue diagnosis; however, in our experience, which is similar to Fraser and Pare's, hamartomas calcify much less frequently than the often-quoted 25–30 percent.[24] One small fleck of calcium does not preclude the need for a tissue diagnosis, as bronchogenic carcinoma may engulf pre-existing calcifications within the lung. In a series of

887 resected solitary pulmonary masses, 3.7 percent of lung cancers had films read as showing calcification within the mass. Many of these areas of calcification were confirmed at thoracotomy.[23]

Without radiologic evidence of complete stability for two years or classic benign calcification demonstrated by films or tomography, a tissue diagnosis is indicated in all patients over the age of thirty. The patient's age, history, skin tests, previous films, if available, radiographic appearance of the mass on the plain films and chest tomography are all analyzed. Benign lesions tend to occur in younger patients and tend to appear as smaller, sharply marginated pulmonary masses, whereas lung cancer is more common in the older age groups and tends to appear as larger masses with ill-defined spiculated margins. It is very important to note that these radiologic features of noncalcified pulmonary masses (margin, size, etc.) are not a substitute for a histologic or cytologic diagnosis but are only used to decide *what type* of needle should be employed (see section on Needle Selection) and *when* in the course of the work-up needle aspiration biopsy is indicated.

Our position is intermediate between Pearson's approach,[25] which consists of a needle aspiration biopsy on the morning of admission, and the approach of others who reserve needle aspiration biopsy for cases of inoperable bronchogenic carcinoma. In most cases, the choice of needle aspiration biopsy comes after a careful history and physical examination, search for old films, tomography to demonstrate calcium within the mass, sputum cytologies, and fiberoptic bronchoscopy. If the conventional work-up fails to reveal a definite diagnosis, the patients generally fall into one of three categories.

In the first category is the patient who probably has bronchogenic carcinoma and is operable. Although we believe that needle aspiration biopsy should be performed in these patients to give an exact cell type and to exclude an oat cell carcinoma or the remote possibility of benign disease, in this institution the patient is usually staged and has a thoracotomy without confirmation by needle aspiration biopsy. In this institution a possible exception to proceeding directly to a thoracotomy is the case of a patient who has extreme anxiety concerning major surgery without a definite diagnosis. In such cases, needle aspiration biopsy is performed.

In the second category are patients who probably have bronchogenic carcinoma but also have a borderline cardiopulmonary reserve. In this situation, needle aspiration biopsy definitely establishes the diagnosis, confirming the need for thoracotomy and allowing the surgeon to discuss the increased risk of surgery with the patient. In addition to the cancer's size and location, knowledge of its cell type may influence the surgeon to perform mediastinoscopy[26] (see Chapter 10).

The third category includes patients who probably have benign disease. Any clinical or radiologic feature of the mass that suggests benign disease takes precedence over other features that suggest malignant disease and strengthen the indication for needle aspiration biopsy. Every effort should be made to establish a diagnosis by needle aspiration biopsy and thus avoid thoracotomy. Where there is a clinical and/or radiologic suspicion that the solitary pulmonary mass is benign (provided the mass is easily accessible to percutaneous techniques), we have avoided the conventional work-up and proceeded directly to needle aspiration biopsy. Bronchoscopy with transbronchial biopsy using the standard 3-mm forceps usually does not provide enough tissue to diagnose granulomatous disease or hamartomas (see Chapter 8).

The Patient with a Superior Sulcus Tumor (Pancoast Tumor)

Several reports have indicated a better resectability and survival rate for patients with Pancoast tumors if preoperative radiotherapy is given.[27,28] Because benign conditions may mimic a superior sulcus tumor, radiotherapy is not indicated without a histologic or cytologic diagnosis.[29] Our experience agrees with that of Walls et al., who state that these tumors are frequently not diagnosed by sputum cytology, bronchoscopy, and/or supraclavicular node biopsy although they are easily and safely diagnosed by needle aspiration biopsy.[30] In a patient with a suspected Pancoast tumor, needle aspiration biopsy is generally the first procedure of choice.

The Patient Who Fails to Respond to Appropriate Antituberculosis Therapy

The association of lung cancer and tuberculosis is well known.[31,32] The obvious radiographic abnormality may not be the source of a sputum showing microscopic or culture evidence of tuberculosis.

CONTRAINDICATIONS

Our contraindications are listed in Table 9-2.

Bleeding Diathesis or Anticoagulation Therapy

If a precise diagnosis of the pulmonary abnormality is of paramount importance in the management of these patients, needle aspiration biopsy can be performed without serious sequelae after vitamin K therapy, infusion of platelets or other intravenous hemostatic agents, or the cessation of the anticoagulation therapy.

Table 9-2
Contraindications to Needle Aspiration Biopsy

1. Bleeding diathesis or anticoagulation therapy
2. Suspected vascular lesions
3. Blebs in the area
4. Echinococcus cyst
5. Uncooperative patient or uncontrollable cough
6. Pulmonary hypertension
7. Severely dibilitated patients
8. Contralateral pneumonectomy

Suspected Vascular Lesions

Even though vascular structures and arteriovenous malformations of the lung have been punctured and even purposely opacified by the injection of contrast agents by the transthoracic technique,[33] we do not puncture suspected vascular lesions. These lesions can usually be excluded by history and physical examination, pulmonary function tests to determine shunting, tomography, and fluoroscopy. In rare instances, we have resorted to pulmonary angiography and thoracic aortography.

Blebs in the Area of the Needle Aspiration Biopsy

If a bleb is directly in the only practical anticipated course of the needle, needle aspiration biopsy is not performed. Blebs in other areas of the lung and clinical or radiologic evidence of emphysema are not considered contraindications to needle biopsy. However, these patients have a higher incidence of pneumothorax. If the patient has signs of chronic obstructive pulmonary disease, often a smaller needle is selected, and the patient is scheduled only as an inpatient.

Suspected Echinococcus Cyst

Aspiration of a hydatid cyst with the release of fluid into the tracheobronchial tree can cause anaphylaxis. We consider the possibility of hydatid disease an absolute contraindication. This arises if the radiographic abnormalities suggest hydatid disease and the patient has a history of residence or travel in an endemic area. Nearly 90 percent of patients with echinococciasis will have either a positive skin test (Casoni's or substitute antigen) or a positive hemagglutination reaction.[34]

Uncooperative Patient or Uncontrollable Cough

This can be overcome by general anesthesia.

Pulmonary Hypertension

Pulmonary hypertension is a relative contraindication. A peripheral lesion is biopsied if the pulmonary hypertension is mild or moderate; a central lesion in a patient with mild pulmonary hypertension is not biopsied because of the potential of serious bleeding.

Debilitated Patients

There are three groups of patients who should be considered debilitated.

1. Patients in whom it is unlikely that determining the etiology of the solitary pulmonary mass will significantly change their management.
2. Patients who are too weak to clear secretions. Since there is a possibility of bleeding into the tracheobronchial tree after needle biopsy, we believe that patients should be strong enough to cough out the blood. If it is retained in the lungs, blood may promote atelectasis and pneumonia, or it may even asphyxiate the patient.
3. Patients with poor cardiopulmonary reserve, in whom it is likely that intermittent positive pressure breathing will be necessary within 24 hours after the procedure.

Contralateral Pneumonectomy

A pneumothorax or severe intrapulmonary hemorrhage in the remaining lung may create a life threatening situation.

PRE-BIOPSY PROCEDURE

The indications and contraindications are reviewed in each case. Each patient has a bleeding screen which consists of a platelet count and a prothrombin time. The patient is considered suitable for needle aspiration biopsy only if the platelet count is over 100,000/mm^3 and the prothrombin time is within 3 seconds of the control.

The procedure is carefully explained to the patient on the day prior to the percutaneous lung biopsy. After a careful explanation, sedation is generally not required. Mild sedation with phenobarbital or diazepam is administered intramuscularly one hour before the biopsy upon the request of either the patient or the referring physician.

The approach is planned by reviewing the P-A and lateral chest radiographs and other available radiographic studies. Tomography is not considered a prerequisite for needle aspiration biopsy; however, we have found lateral tomography to be very helpful in localizing small (less than 2 cm) upper-lobe lesions. These lesions are often well visualized under A-P fluoroscopy but impossible to see under lateral fluoroscopy. Here, we obtain lateral tomography. The tomographic cut best delineating the mass is superimposed on the midline tomographic cut, and the mass's relationship to the trachea and thoracic spine (structures usually identified at lateral fluoroscopy) is ascertained. Although this localization technique is not perfect, this maneuver, in addition to the usual ones of tactile sensation when engaging the mass and parallax, have improved our diagnostic rate. If there is a question of whether the patient's mass can be visualized under either fluoroscopic projection or if lateral tomography may be necessary before the procedure, a preliminary chest fluoroscopy is done the day before the scheduled needle aspiration biopsy.

BIOPSY PROCEDURE

All patients are biopsied in the recumbent position to avoid the possibility of air embolism. An approach allowing us to traverse the smallest amount of normal lung is selected. Most patients are biopsied in the supine or prone position; however, several have been biopsied in the oblique and lateral decubitus positions to permit a shorter passage through normal lung. All patients are biopsied using the Siemens' Orbiskop (Siemens Corporation, Iselin, New Jersey). This fluoroscope has a C-arm which allows monitoring the patient through a 90-degree arc.

We perform all of our biopsies under biplane fluoroscopic control. Although we feel biplane fluoroscopic visualization is necessary for small and/or deep lesions, single-plane fluoroscopy may be used for larger peripheral lesions. Here, the increased resistance felt when entering the mass, moving the needle with subsequent movement of the mass and parallax, may be used in localization.

During preliminary fluoroscopy, the approach is thoroughly planned. Care is taken to align a metal marker on the skin, the intercostal space, and the precise portion of the mass to be biopsied in one straight line. The importance of this thorough preliminary localization cannot be over-stressed. The intercostal space should be traversed in its lower half to avoid the upper intercostal neurovascular bundle. The skin incision and needle should not be placed immediately over the lower rib, as the needle may become trapped and lacerate the lung. All apical lesions located above the first rib anteriorly are biopsied from the posterior approach to avoid the anteriorly located subclavian artery and vein.

Sometimes osseous structures impose a barrier to a direct approach by needle aspiration biopsy. The most common problem is the overlying scapula in patients with posterolaterally positioned upper-lobe lesions. The scapula is rotated out of the needle path by having the patient lie prone and placing his right hand under his abdomen grasping his left flank and with his left hand grasping his right flank as if he were hugging a pillow or experiencing severe abdominal pain. Where this positioning is considered necessary on the basis of either the chest radiograph or preliminary fluoroscopy, the patient is asked to do exercises for both his shoulders and neck the morning before the procedure, thus avoiding patient discomfort during the biopsy.

In small, laterally positioned masses, the mass may be obscured by an overlying rib during the entire normal respiratory cycle. In this case, the appropriate interspace is selected where the mass is free of the rib during forced inspiration or expiration. Anesthesia and the needle aspiration biopsy are performed in the preselected phase of the respiratory cycle. Hyperventilation with supplemental oxygen immediately prior to the needle aspiration biopsy often allows the patient to suspend respiration for the period of time necessary for the biopsy.

After the preliminary fluoroscopy, the skin at the planned site of entrance is indented with a Kelley clamp. The area is then prepped first with alcohol and then with iodine. Sterile towels are placed over the patient. In those to be biopsied in the supine position, a sterile towel is placed over the face so that the patient cannot view the procedure. The patient's fears are allayed by frequent communication and sufficient warning before any anesthesia is injected or manipulations are performed. The biopsy site is then relocalized under fluoroscopy with a sterile Kelley clamp. One percent Xylocaine is used as the local anesthetic and is liberally infiltrated into the skin, subcutaneous tissues, and the pleura. The biopsy site is again relocalized under fluoroscopy with a one-half-inch, 25-gauge needle in the skin. All cutaneous localizing devices are placed in the center of the fluoroscopic screen to avoid errors due to parallax.

A small incision (0.2–0.3 cm) into the skin and subcutaneous tissue is made with a No. 11 scalpel blade. This permits free passage of the needle through the skin and allows greater appreciation of increased resistance when the needle tip touches the pulmonary mass. The preselected needle is then inspected. Qualities looked for are (1) excellent fit between the inner stylet and the outer biopsy needle, (2) sharp honed edges, and (3) easy, friction-free removal of the inner stylet.

Whenever possible, we perform the biopsy with the needle exactly perpendicular to the patient and the table just as we have localized the mass. A nurse stationed at the head of the table is asked to comment as to slight medial or lateral angulation that may not be recognized by the physician. The patient is instructed to momentarily hold his breath while the needle is passed through the pleura. For the remainder of the procedure, the patient is asked to breathe quietly. The needle is advanced in one- to two-centimeter increments with frequent monitoring under biplane fluoroscopy. The monitoring is done when the radiologist's hands are not in the fluoroscopic field. Occasionally, the needle is held by a long sterile clamp.

Once the mass is encountered, usually a slight increased resistance is felt. Engagement of the mass is documented by biplane fluoroscopy, parallax, and movement of the needle tip with the mass during shallow respiration. Small masses (less than 1.5 cm in diameter) and exceptionally hard masses (healed granulomas and hamartomas) often present a problem in engagement. These are best biopsied with smaller bore needles and can be penetrated by a swift rapid advancement. Often momentary suspension of respiration and/or constant fluoroscopic monitoring (90 degrees to the operator's hands) is necessary to engage these small lesions, especially if they are in a lower lobe.

When the needle is in position, the inner stylet is removed. The operator's thumb is placed over the open hub to avoid air embolism while a 30-cc disposable syringe is attached. Tissue is obtained by simultaneously advancing and rotating the needle while maintaining constant suction. Two or three short thrusts are made into the mass. Whenever possible, we biopsy the periphery rather than the center of a mass; the center of a primary bronchogenic carcinoma is frequently necrotic and the center of a granuloma is often fibrotic. The entire needle is then quickly removed from the chest as the operator maintains constant suction. This ensures retrieval of all the tissue and theoretically reduces the chances of local tumor spread along the needle tract. The patient is questioned about any pain, and his chest is reexamined by fluoroscopy to look for complications. A pneumothorax is usually evident by visualization of the visceral pleura or may be suspected if the mass is seen to move downward and/or medially.

Should pus be present in the syringe, a portion of the material is transferred immediately to anaerobic culture media. In the usual situation where only small fragments of tissue and blood are in the needle, the specimen is aspirated into the syringe by applying a gentle suction with the needle tip placed in Hanks' solution (Microbiological Associates, Walkersville, Maryland). Any air in the needle or syringe is expelled with the needle tip in a sterile test tube to prevent loss of any of the specimen. Once all the material is withdrawn into the syringe, the needle is removed, and the syringe is emptied into a 30-cc, sterile plastic medicine cup. The syringe is checked for retained material and often is reflushed with an additional 5 to 10 cc of Hanks' solution. The adequacy of the specimen can be determined by visual inspection.

To ensure adequate material for all diagnostic laboratories and representative samplings from different portions of the mass, frequently a second and occasionally a third aspirate is obtained. If the first specimen contains mostly blood, subsequent aspirations are made with 1–2 cc of heparin (1,000 units per ml) in the syringe. Additional aspirations are not performed if there is (1) chest discomfort, (2) fluoroscopic evidence of a pneumothorax, (3) hemoptysis, or (4) intrapulmonary hemorrhage extensive enough to obscure the mass.

POST-BIOPSY PROCEDURE

Patient Care

Once adequate amounts of tissue have been obtained or a complication is evident or suspected, a small Band-aid is placed over the skin incision. Auscultation of the chest is performed and then the patient is sent by stretcher for an immediate sitting P-A chest radiograph in inspiration and expiration, as well as a lateral chest radiograph in inspiration. The patient is readvised as to the symptoms of a pneumothorax. In the absence of an immediate pneumothorax, the patient is placed on complete bedrest and returned to his hospital bed for the next three hours, after which time repeat P-A and lateral chest radiographs are obtained. If no delayed pneumothorax has developed, the patient is given bathroom privileges for the rest of the evening. A repeat physical examination and chest radiographs are obtained twenty-four hours after the procedure. If these are normal, the patient is allowed to resume usual hospital activity.

Should an immediate pneumothorax be evident, the patient is treated with 100 percent oxygen by mask and kept in the radiology department where he is followed clinically and radiologically at intervals dictated by the symptoms and the radiologic estimate of the degree and progression of the pneumothorax.

Outpatients are followed in the department for a minimum of six hours. Should a pneumothorax occur after a needle aspiration biopsy is done in an outpatient, the patient is admitted to the hospital for observation.

The discomfort with needle aspiration biopsy is usually minimal. Post-procedure analgesics are generally not necessary. If a repeat needle aspiration biopsy is necessary, it is usually not difficult to convince the patient to consent to a second procedure.

Specimen Handling

All the specimens are handled with a sterile technique. The fragments of tissue are left in the plastic medicine cups containing Hanks' solution until the end of the procedure. The larger tissue fragments settle to the bottom of the cups which can be compressed into a funnel. The supernate is decanted into test tubes and sent for tuberculosis and fungal culture and staining. The smaller fragments are poured into other test tubes and sent for cytologic evaluation. These are poured through a Millipore filter and then stained with standard Papanicolaou's stain. The larger fragments, which often remain in the bottom of the cup, are transferred by pouring 5–10 cc of formalin into the plastic cup, mixing the material, and then rapidly pouring the contents back into the jar of formalin. These fragments are stained with eosin immediately upon their arrival in the pathology department, thus allowing them to be more readily identified during the subsequent processing (see Chapter 7).

Sometimes, a few of the smaller fragments collected in this manner were lost in processing. In an attempt to decrease this loss, we have recently been employing a thrombin-clot technique. Once the minute fragments have been decanted off for cytologic evaluation, the larger cores are removed from the medicine cup with a needle or tissue forceps and placed into a bottle of formalin. The remaining smaller fragments are transferred to a glass medicine cup and allowed to settle. The fluid is slowly removed with a needle and 10-cc syringe and sent to cytology. The smaller fragments with about 0.5 cc of Hanks' solution are left in the bottom of the glass medicine cup. To this, 1 ml of human plasma anticoagulated with CPD, 0.2 ml of 0.025 M $Ca^{++}Cl_2^-$, and 0.2 ml of thrombin (50 NIH units per ml) are added, and the entire solution is gently agitated to ensure complete mixing. Two minutes later the gelatinous fibrin clot containing the small tissue fragments is poured onto filter paper. Within one or two minutes, the fluid is absorbed leaving a thin fibrin film in which the small fragments of tissue are embedded. This is rolled up and then compressed into an ovoid about 4 × 4 × 2 mm and placed into a separate jar of formalin.

Bloody material presents a special problem in handling. Every effort should be made to identify any small white cores of tissue. These should be removed and sent to the pathology laboratory in a separate jar of formalin; otherwise, they may be lost in sectioning, as the technologists will choose the larger more obvious blood clots in the paraffin block for preparation of the slides. Material that appears to consist only of blood should never be discarded, as frequently small fragments of tissue and clusters of cells may be embedded in the blood clot and may be readily identified upon histologic or cytologic evaluation.

NEEDLE SELECTION

Aspirating Needles Capable of Obtaining a Histologic Diagnosis

TUMOR BIOPSY NEEDLE "TURNER NEEDLE"
(Cook Catheter Corporation, Bloomington, Indiana)

In 1968 Turner developed an aspirating needle for percutaneous needle aspiration biopsy.[35] We have used this needle almost exclusively for patients with single or multiple discrete pulmonary masses. This thin-walled needle, fitted with an inner stylet, has a circumferentially sharpened 45-degree cutting edge as opposed to the spinal needle which has a long bevel (Figs. 9-1A and 9-1B). Both the spinal needle and the Turner needle obtain excellent material for cytologic preparation. The modification of a cutting edge on an aspirating needle allows tissue fragments large enough for conventional histologic staining to be obtained. We believe a histologic as well as a cytologic evaluation is often helpful in patients with either solitary or multiple pulmonary masses. If the lesion is benign, the definitive diagnosis of granulomatous disease, hamartoma, etc., can be only made by histologic criteria. If a lesion proves to be malignant the additional histologic classification as to cell type is often helpful. The Turner needle is manufactured in both 18 and 16 gauges. All large masses near the periphery of the lung were biopsied with the 16-gauge needle, whereas all deep lesions were biopsied with an 18-gauge needle. For lesions intermediate in depth, the 16-gauge needle is used when we anticipate the lesion to be benign, and an 18-gauge needle is used when we suspect that the lesion is malignant. Rarely, the 18-gauge needle does not obtain enough material for histologic evaluation. The material sent for cytologic evaluation in those cases has been excellent. Sometimes small peripheral lesions are biopsied with an 18-gauge needle, as it may be difficult to engage a small mass with the larger needle which tends to displace the lesion. Although the manufacturer states that these needles can be resharpened and resterilized, we prefer to use a new needle for each patient. Each needle costs $28.00.

The needles are manufactured in 6-inch and 8-inch lengths; recently, we have had 3½-inch lengths manufactured to afford us better control in patients with peripheral masses.

Results. The results of our first 200 patients undergoing Turner needle aspiration biopsy with a localized pulmonary mass or masses are listed in Table 9-3. One hundred and fifty-four patients presented with a solitary pulmonary mass. Definite histologic and/or cytologic evidence of malignant disease was established by needle aspiration biopsy in 93 of 109 patients (85 percent) with proven malignant disease. Five patients had cytologic material strongly suggestive of cancer. All of these latter five had cancer confirmed at surgery. The diagnostic rate, therefore, of cancer, or of those having a strong suspicion of cancer, is 98 out of 109 patients, or 90 percent.

Eleven of 109 (10 percent) patients with malignant disease were not diagnosed by needle aspiration biopsy. Malignant lesions not diagnosed fell into three categories: (1) small lesions that could not be seen in both fluoroscopic projections, (2) those patients in which the procedure was terminated after only one aspiration, and (3) aspiration of a pneumonia distal to a bronchogenic carcinoma. In this latter situation, we biopsied two patients in which the specimen showed only nonspecific inflammation. In both of these, the previous bronchoscopy had demonstrated bronchial narrowing strongly suggestive of bronchogenic carcinoma. These two patients were operated on within a week of the needle aspiration biopsy, and the diagnosis of cancer was confirmed. With this high diagnostic rate, we now feel that if the needle can be seen to enter the mass in both fluoroscopic projections, two or three passes can be made, and if the material is not diagnosed as ma-

Table 9-3
Results of the First 200 Patients Undergoing Needle Aspiration Biopsy—Turner Needle

Solitary Pulmonary Masses–154				
Malignant	109			
Diagnosed by needle aspiration biopsy		93	(85.3%)	90%
Suspicious by needle aspiration biopsy		5	(4.6%)	
Benign	36			
Diagnosed by needle aspiration biopsy		20	(55%)	
Diagnosed by surgery		7		
Decreased in size after needle aspiration biopsy		5		
Stable for two years		4		
Being followed	8			
Lost to follow-up	1			
Multiple Pulmonary Masses–46				
Malignant	33			
Diagnosed by needle aspiration biopsy		31	(94%)	97%
Suspicious by needle aspiration biopsy		1	(3%)	
Diagnosed by surgery		1		
Benign	13			
Diagnosed by needle aspiration biopsy		9	(69%)	
Decreased or stable for two years		4		

lignant disease or as strongly suspicious of cancer, then the likelihood that the mass is malignant is extremely small. In the older age group with an inconclusive needle aspiration biopsy, the chance that the mass is malignant is less than the operative mortality, as in most large series, the operative mortality is approximately 5 percent for a lobectomy and approximately 10 percent for a pneumonectomy.[36]

A definite diagnosis was made by needle aspiration biopsy in 20 of 36 patients (55 percent) having a benign solitary pulmonary mass. We accepted only the histologic diagnosis of active granulomatous infection, a hamartoma, amyloidosis, or material suggestive of an abscess or rheumatoid nodule as a definite benign diagnosis. Nonspecific inflammation and/or fibrosis was not tabulated as a definite benign diagnosis. The needle biopsy diagnosis of nonspecific inflammation or fibrosis, however, when coupled with the radiographic, bronchoscopic and clinical findings, allowed us to follow many of these patients rather than operate on them. Only 3 of the 20 patients with benign disease proven by needle aspiration biopsy have undergone surgery. These three patients in whom the needle aspiration biopsy definitively established a benign diagnosis (rheumatoid nodule, hamartoma, and chronic granulomatous inflammation) were seen early in our experience. Seven patients with benign disease who were not diagnosed by needle aspiration biopsy had their diagnosis made at thoracotomy. The remaining nine patients are classified as having benign disease either because the mass has disappeared or markedly decreased (5 patients) or remained stable for two years (4 patients).

At present we are following eight patients in whom the needle aspiration biopsy diagnosis was focal nonspecific inflammation and fibrosis. They are not classified as either benign or malignant. In a follow-up period ranging from three to nineteen months, only one patient's pulmonary lesion grew slightly. He has refused further evaluation. One patient has been lost to follow-up.

Forty-six of the initial 200 patients had multiple pulmonary masses. Malignant disease was definitely diagnosed in 31 of 33 patients (94 percent). Benign disease was diagnosed in 9 of 13 patients (69 percent). The higher success rate with multiple chest masses can be explained by a number of factors. (1) A large peripheral lesion can be selected, seen in both fluoroscopic projections, and biopsied with the 16-gauge Turner needle. (2) Multiple lesions are often metastases. Malignant disease can be easily diagnosed even with small tissue fragments sent for cytologic evaluation. One patient with lymphoma had histologic and cytologic material strongly suggestive of, but not diagnostic of, lymphoma. The one patient with malignant disease that we failed to diagnose by needle aspiration biopsy had only two small deep lesions.

Of the initial 200 patients, 26 (13 percent) had repeat needle aspiration biopsies (23 with a solitary pulmonary mass and three with multiple pulmonary masses). The repeat needle aspiration biopsy established a definite diagnosis in 14. In the remaining 12 patients, cells suspicious of cancer prompted surgery, whereas in others, additional material showing only nonspecific inflammation and fibrosis often gave us further confidence to follow the patients rather than operate on them.

From Table 9-3 the reader will note that among our first 200 patients, a definite diagnosis of malignant disease was established in 124 of 142 (87 percent) while benign disease was diagnosed in 29 of 49 (59 percent). Needle aspiration biopsy was also helpful in another six patients with material suspicious for malignant disease, and in an additional 13 patients that were not operated on after the needle aspiration biopsy diagnosis of nonspecific inflammation and/or fibrosis. There have been no false-positive diagnoses of cancer or definitive benign disease in this group of patients or in those undergoing subsequent needle aspiration biopsies.

Complications. Two recent excellent reviews of the complications of needle biopsy procedures have been compiled by Sinner[37] and Herman and Hessel.[38] Our complications are listed in Table 9-4. The complications were tabulated per patient rather than per procedure. For example, if a patient had two separate needle aspiration biopsies and a pneumothorax occurred after each one, only one pneumothorax was recorded. Conversely, if a patient underwent a repeat needle aspiration biopsy and sustained a pneumothorax only at the second procedure, one pneumothorax also was recorded.

Table 9-4
Complications, First 200 Patients Undergoing Needle Aspiration Biopsy—Turner Needle

Solitary Pulmonary Masses	
Pneumothorax	29%
Chest tube	6%
Hemoptysis	19%
Hemothorax	1%
Subcutaneous emphysema and pneumomediastinum	1%
Multiple Pulmonary Masses	
Pneumothorax	20%
Chest tube	2%
Hemoptysis	17%

Pneumothorax was our most frequent complication, occurring in 29 percent of patients with a solitary pulmonary mass and in 20 percent of patients with multiple pulmonary lesions. The pneumothorax was often small and asymptomatic. Six percent of patients with a solitary pulmonary mass, and 2 percent of those with multiple lesions required a chest tube. We feel this is an acceptable chest tube rate. Pneumothorax appeared to occur more frequently in (1) older patients, (2) those with deeper lesions, (3) those with smaller lesions, and (4) when the needle aspiration biopsy was done by a relatively inexperienced radiologist. We have not adopted the blood patch seal method as described by McCartney et al.[39] as an attempt to decrease our pneumothorax rate, as the outer Teflon sheath would have to be very large to accommodate a 16-gauge needle and the possibility of lacerating the sheath exists when the biopsy needle is advanced.

Hemoptysis was our second most common complication, occurring in 19 percent of patients with a solitary pulmonary mass and 17 percent of those with multiple lesions. Hemoptysis was always mild and transitory. Neither a transfusion nor an operative procedure was required. Hemoptysis usually ceased spontaneously two to three hours after the procedure. One patient coughed up a well-formed blood clot four days after the percutaneous lung biopsy.

Two patients had focal pleural collections, presumably blood, after the procedure; however, neither of these required tube drainage. One patient experienced subcutaneous emphysema and pneumomediastinum.

There were no deaths in this series or in our subsequent needle aspiration biopsies. Using the Turner needle, two deaths have been reported.[40] Both deaths were of extremely debilitated patients.

Local tumor spread was not evident in our experience. In many of the larger series, no evidence of local tumor spread has been reported.[3,40,41–43] In one series, which included 2726 patients who underwent percutaneous transthoracic needle biopsy, only one patient subsequently developed local tumor spread.[44] The incidence of local tumor spread is extremely rare and should not be used as an argument against percutaneous needle aspiration biopsy.

Case 1: Poor Surgical Risk and Suspicion of Metastasis. A 68-year-old white male whose initial symptom was recurrent headaches had P-A and lateral chest radiographs (Figs. 9-2A and 9-2B) that demonstrated a $1\frac{1}{2}$-cm mass in the left upper lobe. A brain scan and spinal tap were within normal limits. Bronchoscopy was nondiagnostic. Percutaneous lung biopsy with an 18-gauge Turner needle revealed small cell undifferentiated carcinoma (Fig. 9-2C H&E and Fig. 9-2D Cytology). *Comment:* Small cell carcinoma comprises 15–25 percent of primary bronchogenic carcinomas.[45] We, as others, believe that a diagnosis of small cell undifferentiated carcinoma is a contraindication to thoracotomy even without definite evidence of mediastinal or extrathoracic spread.[46]

Case 2: Undiagnosed Solitary Pulmonarry Mass—Benign Disease Possible. The patient is a 56-year-old white male, heavy smoker, who had hemoptysis and a low-grade fever. A 6-cm mass in the left upper lobe and a small ill-defined infiltrate in the right lower lobe were evident on his chest radiograph (Figs. 9-3A and 9-3B). Sputum cytology and bronchoscopy were nondiagnostic. Needle aspiration biopsy showed active granulomatous disease (Fig. 9-3C) with tuberculosis demonstrated on stain and culture. The patient was treated for tuberculosis. Follow-up of $1\frac{1}{2}$ years has shown no evidence of carcinoma. *Comment:* The history of heavy smoking and the size of the mass made bronchogenic carcinoma the most likely diagnosis. The low-grade fever and ill-defined infiltrate in the contralateral lung suggested that this patient might also have an infection. These features suggesting benign disease took precedence; needle aspiration biopsy established the definite diagnosis of benign disease in this patient. We suspect that he might have been subjected to thoracotomy in centers where needle aspiration biopsy is not employed.

Case 3: Undiagnosed Solitary Pulmonary Mass—Benign Disease Possible. A 45-year-old asymptomatic white male, heavy smoker, who presented with a sharply defined mass in the lingula. (Figs. 9-4A and 9-4B) Bronchoscopy was within normal limits. Needle aspiration biopsy with a 16-gauge Turner needle demonstrated a hamartoma. (Figs. 9-4C and 9-4D) In a follow-up of two years, the hamartoma has grown only 1 mm in each direction. *Comment:* Again lung cancer was the admitting diagnosis. Needle aspiration biopsy established the definitive diagnosis of benign disease in this patient. Hamartomas are frequently diagnosed only at thoracotomy.[47] Even though this benign neoplasm may continue to grow, it is our current policy to follow rather than operate on patients with hamartoma of the lung.

Case 4: Failure to Respond to Antituberculosis Treatment. The patient is a 63-year-old asymptomatic white male. The initial chest radiograph showed a sharply defined mass in the middle lobe (Fig. 9-5). His skin test was positive for tuberculosis. One bronchoscopic washing yielded a light growth of atypical tuberculosis. The patient was treated for tuberculosis with two drugs for two months. The mass increased slightly in size. Repeat bronchoscopy was nondiagnostic. Needle aspiration biopsy with a 16-gauge Turner needle demonstrated poorly differentiated adenocarcinoma. *Comment:* Needle aspiration biopsy is a safe, accurate method of establishing a definitive diagnosis in a patient with a solitary pulmonary mass.

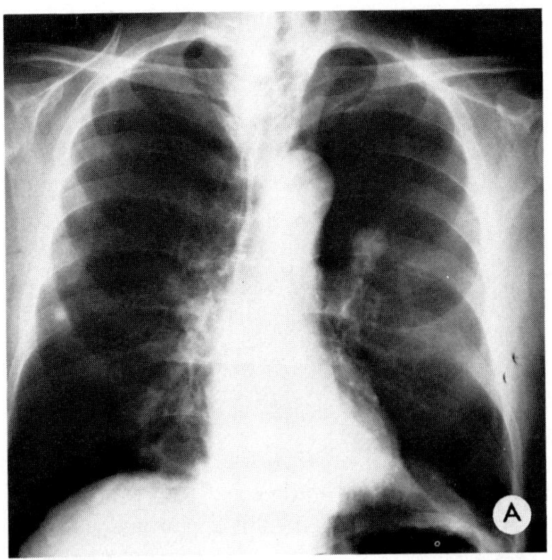

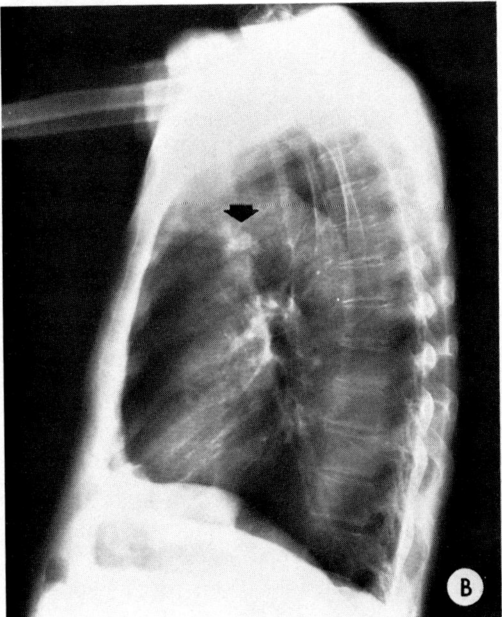

Fig. 9-2. *Case 1—Inoperable bronchogenic carcinoma proven by Turner needle biopsy.* Needle aspiration biopsy with an 18-gauge Turner needle showed oat cell carcinoma. The 18-gauge needle was selected due to the central location of the mass (arrow lateral view). (A) P-A view; (B) Lateral view; (C) Histology (H&E original magnification 300×); (D) Cytology (Papinicolaou's stain original magnification 2278×).

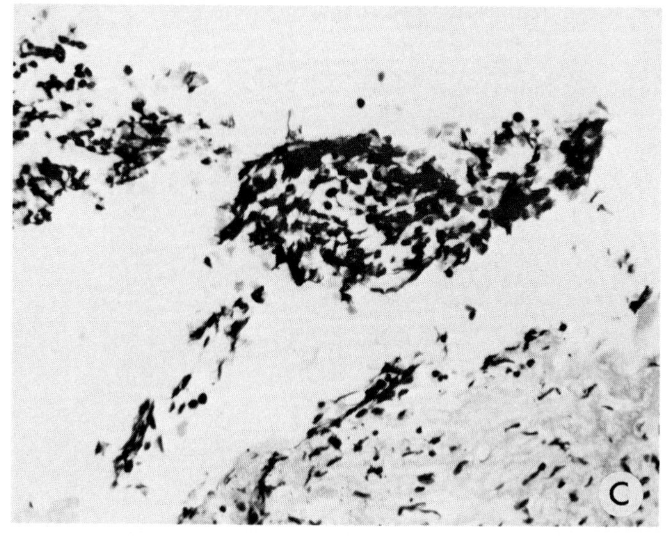

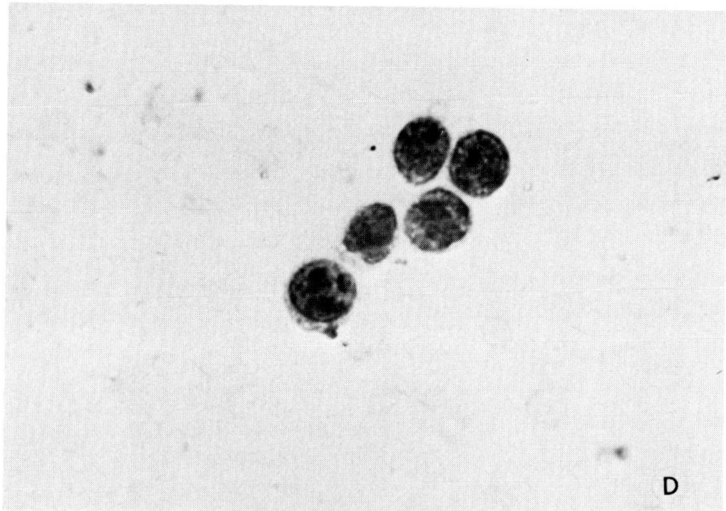

Figs. 9-2C and D.

Pleural Disease—Turner Needle. We have used the Turner needle in evaluating 18 patients with pleural masses or focal collections of pleural fluid. We have established the diagnosis in all but one. That patient had a lipoma from which fat and muscle were obtained by needle aspiration biopsy, but this material was not considered diagnostic. Three patients sustained small pneumothoraces which did not require chest tube drainage. At this time, we feel that peripheral pleural masses or focal collections of fluid are best approached under ultrasound guidance. Aspiration of intralobar collections of fluid is still an indication for fluoroscopic guidance.

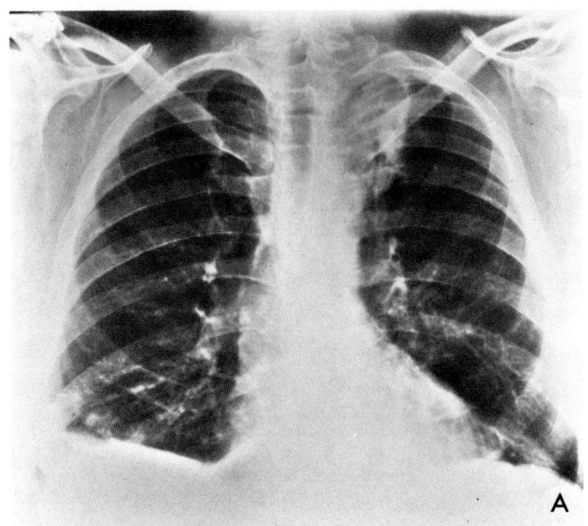

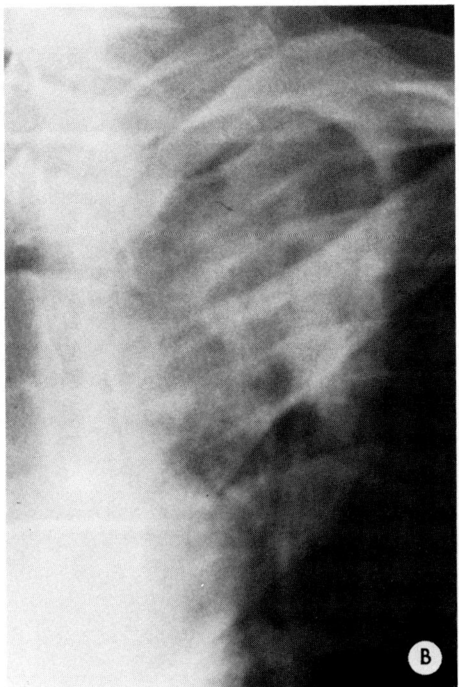

Fig. 9-3. *Case 2—Tuberculosis proven by Turner needle biopsy.* A 16-gauge Turner needle demonstrated active granulomatous infection in this patient. Special stains and culture showed tuberculosis. (A) P-A view; (B) Close-up of the left upper lobe; (C) Histology—Three large granulomata are in the center of the core. Several giant cells are seen scattered throughout the specimen (H&E original magnification 85×).

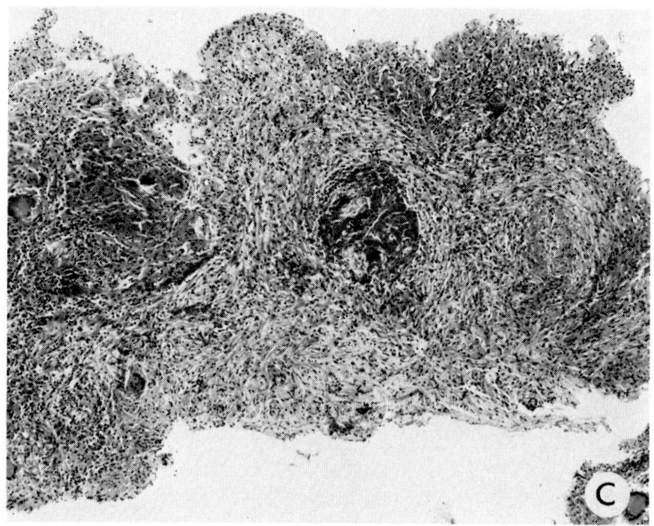

Fig. 9-3C.

Case 5: A 42-year-old black male had left lower lobe pneumonia and empyema, both of which responded to antibiotics and pleural drainage through a chest tube, but a large collection of fluid in the major fissure persisted (Fig. 9-6). Needle aspiration removed 170 cc of sterile fluid. The collection of fluid did not recur. The aspiration was performed with a 16-gauge Turner needle to ensure that the viscous fluid could be easily aspirated.

Diffuse Disease—Turner Needle. We have used the Turner needle in only four patients with diffuse disease. Although the diagnosis was made in three of these and was suggested in the fourth, most patients with diffuse disease are diagnosed by transbronchial biopsy, open biopsy, or closed biopsy with the larger cutting needles.

Case 6: A 48-year-old black female had fever and weight loss. A nodular infiltrate was present throughout both lungs (Fig. 9-7). Needle aspiration biopsy (16-gauge Turner needle into the right upper lobe) showed granulomatous inflammation on histology. Tuberculosis was identified on stain and culture.

OTHER ASPIRATING NEEDLES CAPABLE OF OBTAINING A HISTOLOGIC DIAGNOSIS

The Unique Needle. Lee has described a needle that employs an inner sharpened stylet to cut off small pieces of tissue that are then aspirated into a syringe.[48] Multiple specimens can be taken through the inner needle while the outer needle is left in place. We have evaluated the disposable version of this needle (Lee needle, B.D., Rutherford, New Jersey) (Fig. 9-1C) in a limited number of patients and have found it to be slightly cumbersome.

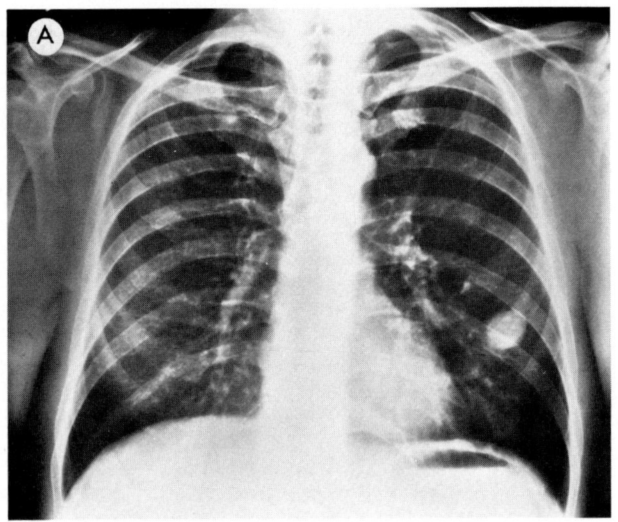

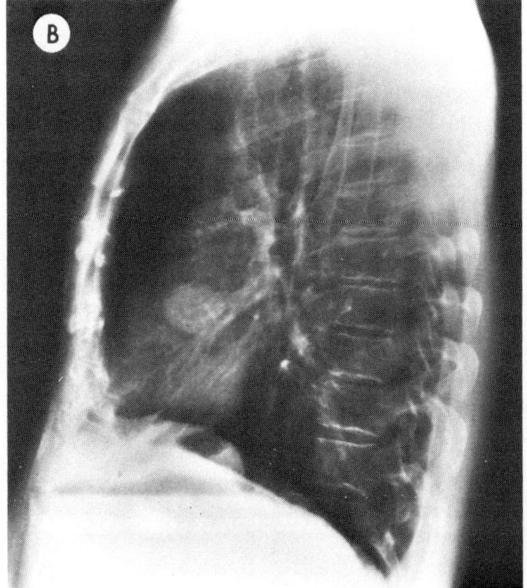

Fig. 9-4. *Case 3—Hamartoma proven by Turner needle biopsy.* A 16-gauge Turner needle was used in this patient as the sharply defined margins suggested benign disease. (A) P-A view; (B) Lateral view; (C) Glass slide from the histologic preparation showing a large core of material. Hamartomas are often difficult to engage, but once they are engaged provide the largest continuous core of tissue; (D) Histology—Cartilage in different degrees of differentiation can be seen at this low power of the core. (H&E original magnification 65×)

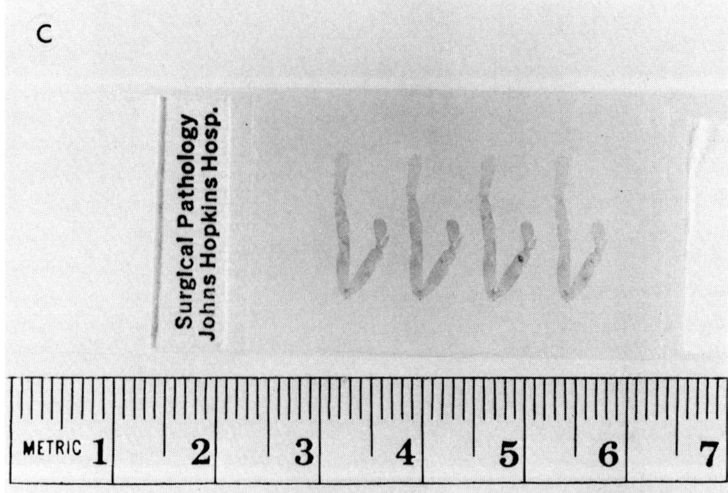

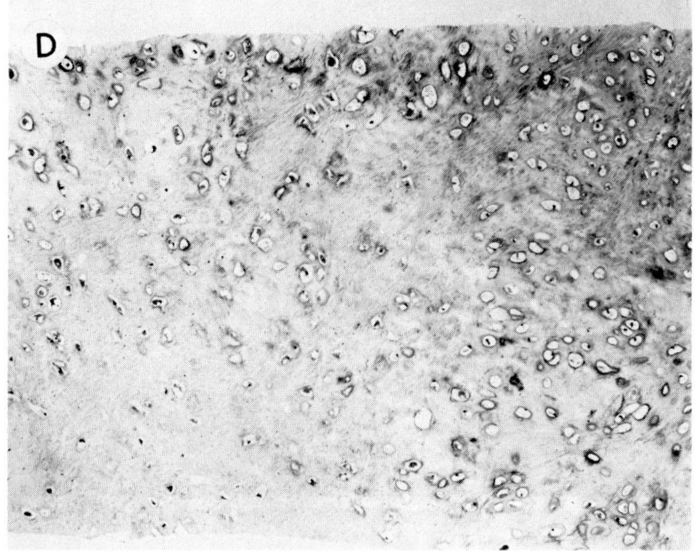

Figs. 9-4C and D.

The material obtained is satisfactory and is comparable to that obtained with an 18-gauge Turner needle.

Modified Franceen Needle. We have not had any personal experience with the modified Franceen needle. The material shown by physicians who have used it appears to be adequate and similar to that obtained with the 18-gauge Turner needle.[49,50]

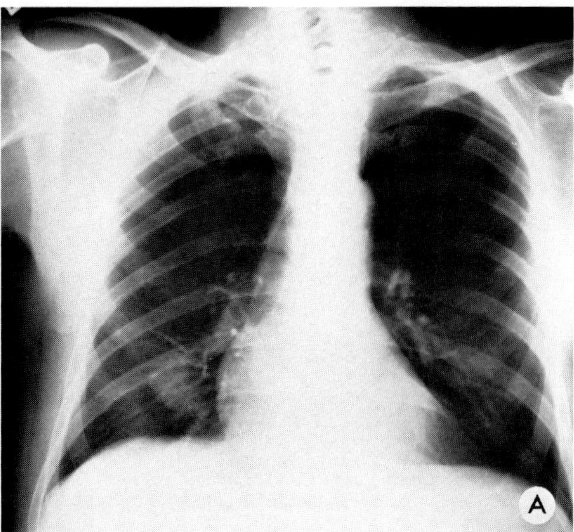

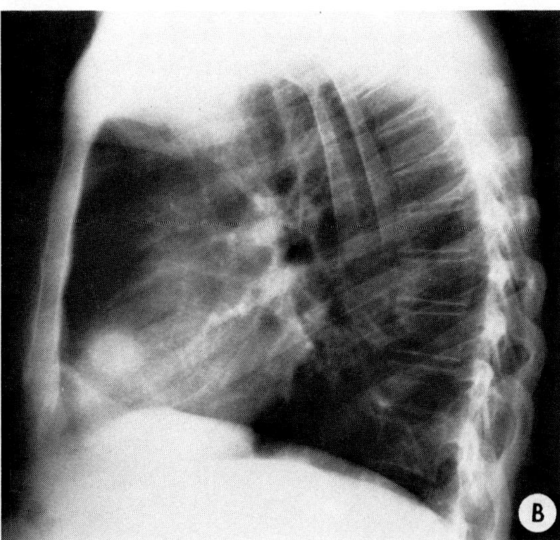

Fig. 9-5. *Case 4—Carcinoma of the lung in a patient with suspected tuberculosis failing to respond to adequate therapy—Turner needle.* Needle aspiration biopsy in this patient with a 16-gauge Turner needle showed adenocarcinoma of the lung. (A) P-A view; (B) Lateral view.

Spinal Needle

In most of the larger series of needle aspiration biopsy, the aspiration has been performed with a spinal type needle.[3,12,41] Many modifications in the basic design and numerous instruments such as brushes and screw-type devices, that can be passed through the spinal needle have been reported to increase the amount of material obtained.[51–53] These smaller needles (18 to

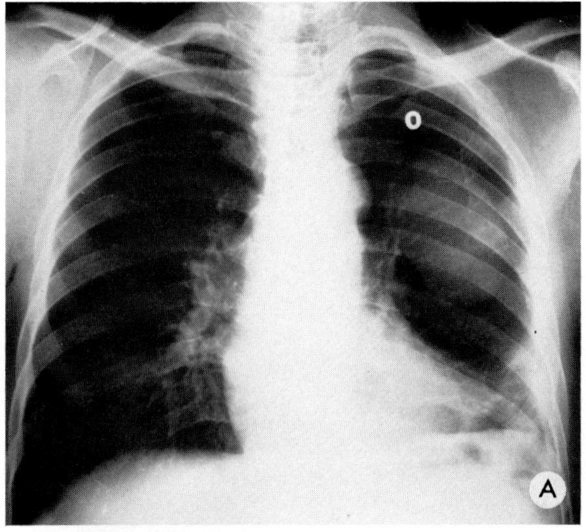

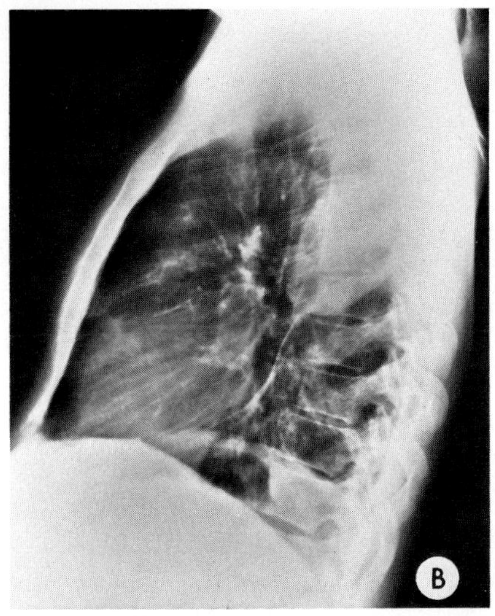

Fig. 9-6. *Case 5—Aspiration of a loculated intralobar collection of fluid with Turner needle.* A 16-gauge Turner needle was used in this case to ensure that the viscous material could be adequately aspirated. (A) P-A view; (B) Lateral view.

21 gauge) generally obtain insufficient amounts for histologic examination. The material is usually evaluated by cytologic and microbiologic techniques. Although this may sometimes be adequate to establish a diagnosis of benign disease, we prefer in most instances to make the diagnosis of benign disease by histologic criteria. We perform needle aspiration biopsy with the spinal needle in three clinical settings: obvious central bronchogenic carcinoma, pulmonary lesions difficult to separate from the mediastinal structures, and definite mediastinal masses.

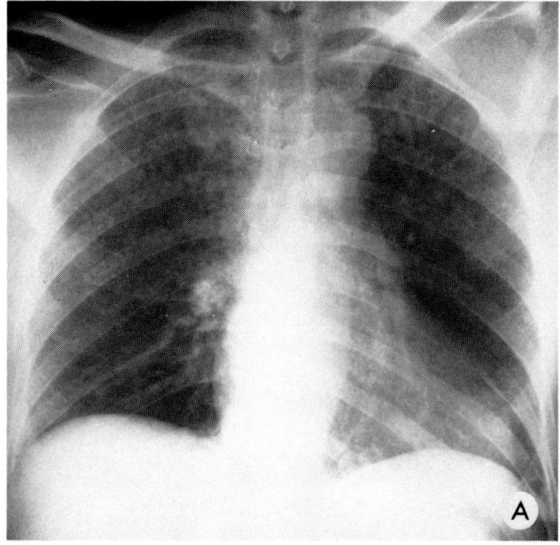

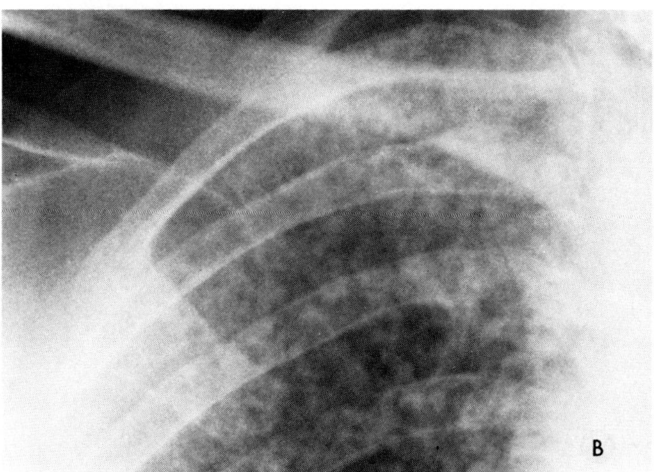

Fig. 9-7. *Case 6—Diffuse disease diagnosed by Turner needle aspiration biopsy.* Three passes with a 16-gauge Turner needle were made into the infiltrate in the right upper lobe. Tuberculosis was demonstrated on histologic sections and on culture. (A) P-A view; (B) Close-up right upper lobe.

OBVIOUS CENTRAL BRONCHOGENIC CARCINOMA

We use a spinal needle in patients with deep central lesions, poor pulmonary reserve, and a strong suspicion that the mass is malignant (history of heavy smoking, radiographic appearance of the mass, brain scan suggesting metastases). In an effort to decrease the pneumothorax rate, we use a 20- or 21-gauge spinal needle. By the same technique described earlier, one pass is made into the periphery of the mass. A portion of the material is transferred onto a glass slide, immediately fixed by a cytologic technologist in a 95 percent alcohol solution and then carried to the cytopathology department where it is stained and interpreted. This entire "quick reading" takes only 20 minutes. If the initial evaluation by the cytopathologist is cancer or material strongly suggestive of cancer, the procedure is terminated and the remaining material is sent to the cytopathology laboratory for routine processing. If the initial evaluation is inadequate (e.g., necrosis) a repeat aspiration is performed. In this clinical setting, we have used the spinal needle in 20 patients and have established the diagnosis of cancer in all 20. Eight sustained a pneumothorax (two required a chest tube) and one had mild transitory hemoptysis. There were no other complications.

Case 7: The patient is a 66-year-old white male who had a slowly growing left upper lobe mass (Fig. 9-8). His pulmonary function was markedly reduced because of chronic obstructive pulmonary disease and severe kyphoscoliosis. Sputum cytology and two bronchoscopies had failed to reveal the diagnosis. Needle aspiration biopsy with a 20-gauge spinal needle showed large cell undifferentiated carcinoma both on the quick reading and on the final evaluation. Combined chemotherapy and radiotherapy were begun.

PULMONARY LESIONS DIFFICULT TO SEPARATE FROM THE MEDIASTINUM

In the situation illustrated by the following case report, we use the spinal needle.

Case 8: A 51-year-old black female had experienced a recent twenty-pound weight loss. Chest x-ray (Fig. 9-9) showed an ill-defined mass adjacent to the aortic arch that could not be separated from the arch at fluoroscopy. Needle aspiration biopsy with a 20-gauge spinal needle showed giant cells, histiocytes, and fibroblasts on cytologic evaluation suggesting granulomatous disease. The referring physician did not consider this adequate evidence of benign disease and recommended a thoracotomy. The patient refused surgery and was treated for tuberculosis. Seven months later the infiltrate had markedly decreased.

MEDIASTINAL MASSES

Most discrete anterior mediastinal masses go to thoracotomy after a substernal thyroid or a diffuse lymphoma have been excluded. Mediastinal masses presumed to be due to adenopathy from lung cancer generally are diagnosed by mediastinoscopy. (See Chapter 10.) The transcervical approach may not give the diagnosis, especially if the nodes are in the posterior or inferior portion of the hilum. When needle aspiration biopsy is done in this situation, we use a 21- or 23-gauge spinal needle. An oblique course is taken into the hilum to avoid the heart and great vessels. Once the needle tip is in the hilum, the inner stylet is removed and checked for the return of blood. If blood is returned through the needle it is repositioned. Although our experience in the mediastinum is limited, it is in agreement with Zelch

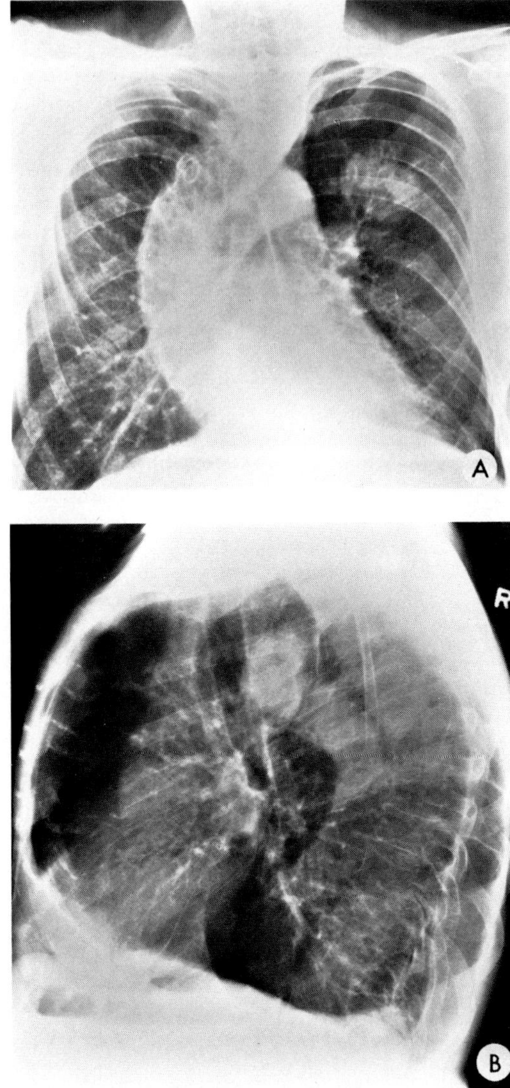

Fig. 9-8. *Case 7—Central bronchogenic carcinoma diagnosed by spinal needle biopsy.* A single pass with a 20-gauge spinal needle demonstrated large cell undifferentiated carcinoma. (A) P-A view; (B) Lateral view.

and Lalli's contention that there is no danger of inadvertently puncturing the central pulmonary arteries or the aorta with these very small needles.[33]

Case 9: A 62-year-old white male, heavy smoker, had experienced a recent weight loss. The chest x-ray demonstrated moderate right hilar adenopathy primarily of the posterior and inferior nodes (Fig. 9-10). Sputum cytology, broncho-

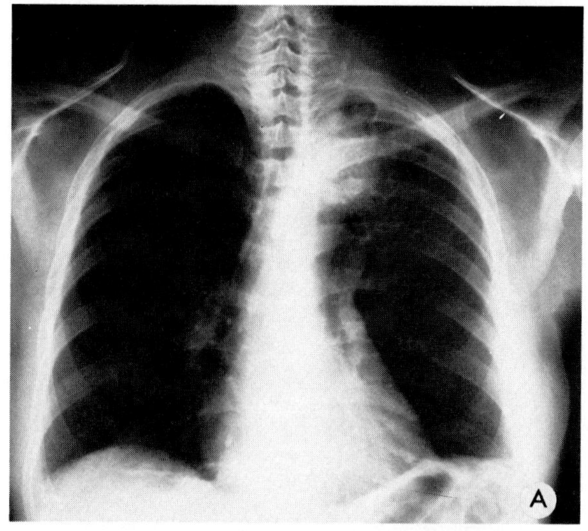

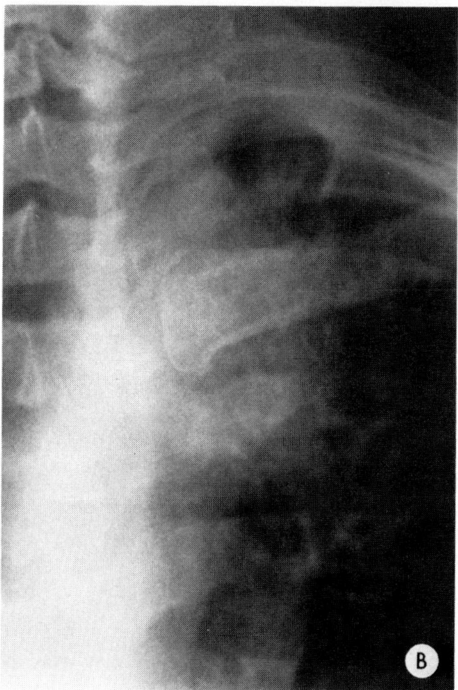

Fig. 9-9. *Case 8—Spinal needle biopsy of a mass adjacent to mediastinal structures.* Two aspirations with a 20-gauge spinal needle showed evidence suggestive of tuberculosis in this patient. The spinal needle was chosen as the mass was difficult to separate from the aortic arch. (A) P-A view; (B) Close-up left upper lobe.

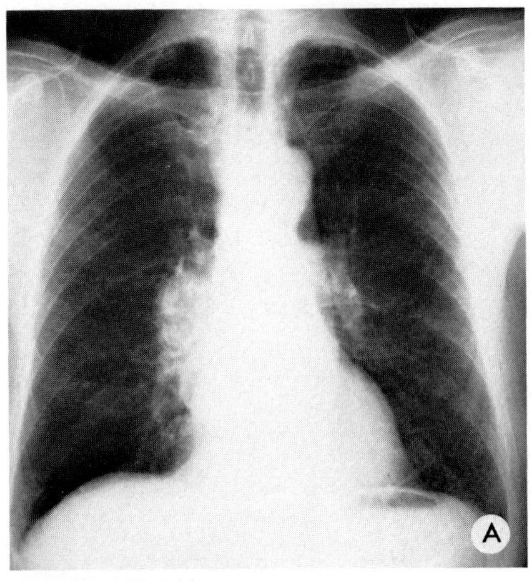

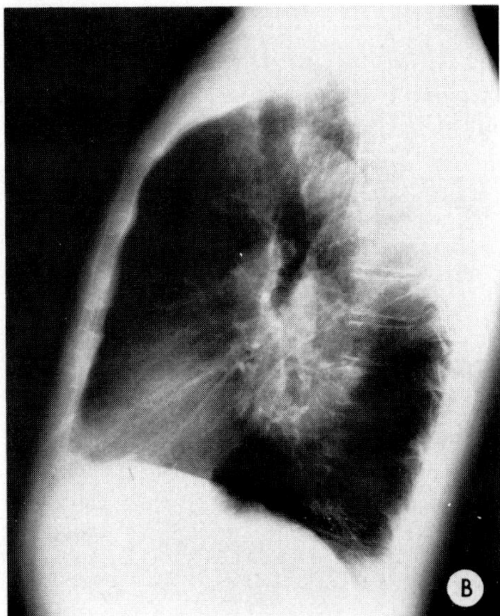

Fig. 9-10. *Case 9—Spinal needle biopsy of hilar adenopathy.* Two passes with a 20-gauge spinal needle into the right hilar adenopathy demonstrated large cell undifferentiated carcinoma. (A) P-A view; (B) Lateral view.

scopy, and mediastinoscopy did not establish a diagnosis. Needle aspiration biopsy with a 21-gauge spinal needle of the right posterior hilar nodes showed undifferentiated carcinoma. Radiotherapy was begun.

OTHER USES OF THE SPINAL NEEDLE

Rarely we have used this needle in patients with small, deep, multiple lesions where there is a strong clinical suspicion of metastasis. We biopsy all children with spinal needles. In children, the biopsy is performed either under general anesthesia or under heavy sedation with a general anesthesia standby.

Cutting Needles

In the 1950s and 1960s large cutting needles (Vim-Silverman, Vim-Franklin) were used extensively to diagnose patients with both localized and diffuse pulmonary disease. These needles obtain larger fragments of tissue than the aspirating needles, but a higher incidence of complications results. We believe that discrete pulmonary lesions should be aspirated. Cutting needles and air-trephine drill biopsies[54–58] still play a role in patients with diffuse infiltrative disease. Although most of our patients with diffuse disease are evaluated by transbronchial biopsy or open-lung biopsy, we have studied eight patients with diffuse disease. Biopsy with the Tru-Cut needle (Travenol Laboratories, Inc., Morton Grove, Illinois) (Fig. 9-1D) established the diagnosis in all eight. Two sustained a pneumothorax and one of these required a chest tube. Hemoptysis occurred in two patients, with one patient having fairly brisk hemoptysis. He coughed up blood-tinged sputum for four days. No specific therapy or transfusion was required. There were no deaths or cases of local tumor spread in this small series.

We prefer to perform cutting or drill biopsies in the radiology department under careful fluoroscopic control. This permits us to select the area of lung most likely to give the diagnosis and allows us to avoid the heart, the larger pulmonary arteries, and the diaphragm. In our department, there is a team of nurses and technologists who are accustomed to handling biopsy material and in helping in the post-biopsy management.

Case 10: A 62-year-old white male experienced a recent thirty-pound weight loss. His chest radiograph showed many small linear interstitial infiltrates scattered throughout both lungs (Fig. 9-11). Biopsy of the right lower lobe with a Tru-Cut needle showed metastatic adenocarcinoma.

Case 11: A 67-year-old black male had increasing dyspnea. His chest radiograph showed a diffuse interstitial infiltrate (Fig. 9-12). A chest radiograph three years earlier had been normal. Past occupational history included employment in a steel mill. Percutaneous lung biopsy with a Tru-Cut needle showed a pneumoconiosis probably caused by iron oxide.

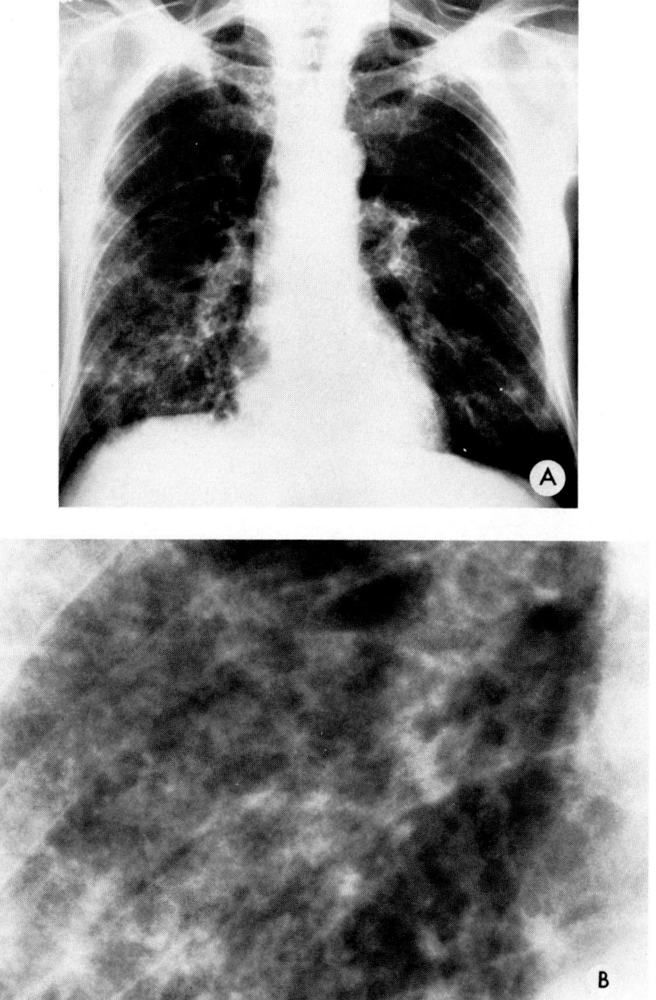

Fig. 9-11. *Case 10—Malignant diffuse disease diagnosed by a Tru-Cut biopsy.* One cutting biopsy with the Tru-Cut needle demonstrated metastatic adenocarcinoma in this patient's right lower lobe. (A) P-A view; (B) Close-up right lower lobe.

SUMMARY

Needle aspiration biopsy can play an important role in the diagnosis and management of patients with a discrete pulmonary mass or masses. As long as the indications and contraindications are strictly adhered to, the procedure is safe with no mortality, acceptable morbidity, and an insignificant chance of local tumor spread. In most patients with localized pulmonary disease, we feel that the aspirate should be done with a needle capable of

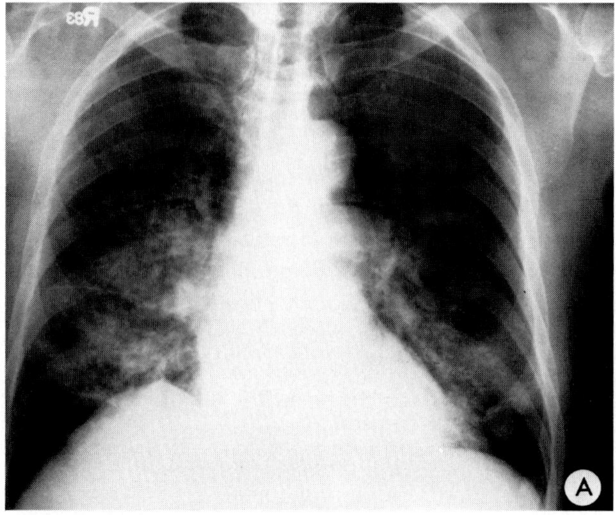

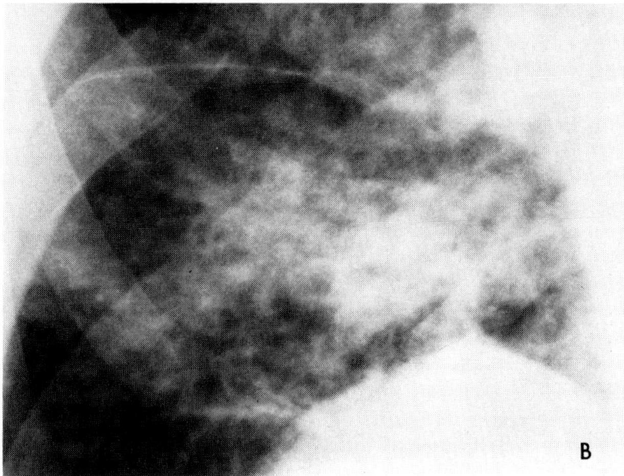

Fig. 9-12. *Case 11—Benign diffuse disease diagnosed by a Tru-Cut biopsy.* A single cutting biopsy in this patient demonstrated a pneumoconiosis in his right lower lobe. (A) P-A view; (B) Close-up right lower lobe.

obtaining material for histologic examination such as the Turner needle. Although there are only a few large series in the literature[40,59,60] in which this needle has been used, we feel it is ideal for most patients. A definitive diagnosis of benign disease can be established with the morphology obtained by histologic examination. The availability of an experienced cytopathologist is not as critical, and therefore, needles of this type may be used in small medical centers.

Needle aspiration biopsy is complementary to sputum cytology and bronchoscopy in the evaluation of patients with a solitary pulmonary mass. Sputum cytology and bronchoscopy frequently do not establish the diagnosis in (1) very peripheral lesions, (2) benign disease, (3) large bronchogenic carcinomas that have produced extrabronchial compression, and (4) Pancoast tumors. In these situations, needle aspiration biopsy is a safe, simple, reliable, cost-effective procedure. Needle aspiration biopsy is often the first procedure performed in such patients.

Aspiration biopsy with the spinal needle is of value in establishing the diagnosis in a patient with lung cancer where the disease is centrally located and/or there is poor pulmonary reserve. Use of this needle makes the availability of an experienced cytopathologist mandatory, however.

Cutting needles should not be used for diagnosing discrete pulmonary masses. The cutting needle and drill biopsy may still play a role in diffuse disease where transbronchial techniques are not available or after they have been tried and have failed to give a diagnosis.

REFERENCES

1. Leyden H: Üeber infectiöse pneumonie. Deutsch Med Wochnschr 9:52–54, 1883
2. Ménétrier P: Cancer primitif du poumon. Bull Soc Anat Paris 4:643, 1886
3. Lauby VW, Burnett WE, Rosemond GP, et al: Value and risk of biopsy of pulmonary lesions by needle aspiration. Twenty-one years' experience. J Thorac Cardiovasc Surg 49:159–172, 1965
4. Woolf CR: Applications of aspiration lung biopsy with review of the literature. Dis Chest 25:286–301, 1954
5. Meyer JE, Ferrucci JT Jr, Janower ML: Fatal complications of percutaneous lung biopsy. Radiology 96:47–48, 1970
6. Youmans CR Jr, DeGroot WJ, Marshall R, et al: Needle biopsy of the lung in diffuse parenchymal disease: An analysis of 151 cases. Am J Surg 120:637–643, 1970
7. Adamson JS Jr, Bates JH: Percutaneous needle biopsy of the lung. Arch Intern Med 119:164–169, 1967
8. Smith WG: Needle biopsy of the lung. Lancet 2:318, 1964
9. Dutra FR, Geraci CL: Needle biopsy of the lung. JAMA 155:21–24, 1954
10. Aronovitch M, Chartier J, Kahana LM., et al: Needle biopsy as an aid to the precise diagnosis of intrathoracic disease. Can Med Assoc J 88:120–127, 1963
11. Wolinsky H, Lischner MW: Needle track implantation of tumor after percutaneous lung biopsy. Ann Intern Med 71:359–362, 1969
12. Dahlgren S, Nordenstrom B: Transthoracic Needle Biopsy. Chicago: Year Book Medical Publishers, Inc., 1966
13. Weiss W: Operative mortality and fivc-year survival rates in men with bronchogenic carcinoma. Chest 66:483–487, 1974
14. Fontana RS, Miller EW, Beabout JW, et al: Transthoracic needle aspiration of

discrete pulmonary lesions: Experience in 100 cases. Med Clin North Am 54:961–971, 1970

15. Berger RL, Dargan EL, Huang BL: Dissemination of cancer cells by needle biopsy of the lung. J Thorac Cardiovasc Surg 63:430–432, 1972
16. Cahan WG, Shah J: Benign solitary lung lesions found with an extrathoracic cancer: A report of 12 cases. Chest 62:360, 1972 (Abstract)
17. Cahan WG, Castro EB, Hajdu SI: The significance of a solitary lung shadow in patients with colon carcinoma. Cancer 33:414–421, 1974
18. Neifeld JP, Michaelis LL, Doppman JL: Suspected pulmonary metastases correlation of chest x-ray, whole lung tomograms, and operative findings. Cancer 39:383–387, 1977
19. Thomford NR, Woolner LB, Clagett OT: The surgical treatment of metastatic tumors in the lungs. J Thorac Cardiovasc Surg 49:357–363, 1965
20. Newman R, Doster BE, Murray FJ, et al: Rifampin in initial treatment of pulmonary tuberculosis. A U.S. Public Health Service Tuberculosis Therapy Trial. Am Rev Respir Dis 109:216–232, 1974
21. FDA/HEW: Isoniazid. Labeling revision. Fed Reg 43:3763–3766, (Jan. 27) 1978
22. Nathan MH: Management of solitary pulmonary nodules. An organized approach based on growth rate and statistics. JAMA 227:1141–1144, 1974
23. Steele JD: The solitary pulmonary nodule. Report of a cooperative study of resected asymptomatic solitary pulmonary nodules in males. J Thorac Cardiovasc Surg 46:21–39, 1963
24. Fraser RG, Pare JP: Diagnosis of Diseases of the Chest, vol. 2, 2nd ed. Philadelphia: W. B. Saunders, 1978
25. Pearson FG: Cancer of the lung: Assessment of operability and resectability. Surgical Grand Rounds, Johns Hopkins Medical Institutions, April 16, 1977
26. Whitcomb ME, Barham E, Goldman AL, et al: Indications for mediastinoscopy in bronchogenic carcinoma. Am Rev Respir Dis 113:189–195, 1976
27. Paulson D: The role of preoperative radiation therapy in the surgical management of carcinoma in the superior pulmonary sulcus. Front Radiation Ther Oncol 5:177–187, 1970 (Karger, New York)
28. Hilaris BS, Martini N, Luomanen RKJ, et al: The value of preoperative radiation therapy in apical cancer of the lung. Surg Clin North Am 54:831–840, 1974
29. Pancoast H: Superior pulmonary sulcus tumor; tumor characterized by pain, Horner's syndrome, destruction of bone, and atrophy of hand muscles. JAMA 99:1391–1396, 1932
30. Walls WJ, Thornbury JR, Naylor B: Pulmonary needle aspiration biopsy in the diagnosis of Pancoast tumors. Radiology 111:99–102, 1974
31. Gopalakrishnan P, Miller JE, McLaughlin JS: Pulmonary tuberculosis and coexisting carcinoma: A 10-year experience and review of the literature. Am Surg 405–408, 1975
32. Steinitz R: Pulmonary tuberculosis and carcinoma of the lung. A survey from two population-based disease registers. Am Rev Respir Dis 92:758–766, 1965
33. Zelch JV, Lalli AF: Diagnostic percutaneous opacification of benign pulmonary lesions. Radiology 108:559–561, 1973
34. Wintrobe MM et al (eds): Harrison's Principles of Internal Medicine, ed 6, New York: McGraw-Hill, 1970

35. Turner AF, Sargent EN: Percutaneous pulmonary needle biopsy:An improved needle for a simple direct method of diagnosis. Am J Roentgenol Radium Ther Nucl Med 104:846–850, 1968
36. Baker RR, Stitik FP, Summer WR: Preoperative evaluation of patients with suspected bronchogenic carcinoma. Current Problems in Surgery. Chicago: Year Book Medical Publishers, Inc., 1974
37. Sinner WN: Complications of percutaneous transthoracic needle aspiration biopsy. Acta Radiol [Diagn] 17:813–828, 1976.
38. Herman PG, Hessel SJ: The diagnostic accuracy and complications of closed lung biopsies. Radiology 125:11–14, 1977
39. McCartney R, Tait D, Stilson M, et al: A technique for the prevention of pneumothorax in pulmonary aspiration biopsy. Am J Roentgenol Radium Ther Nucl Med 120:872–875, 1974
40. Sargent EN, Turner AF, Gordonson J, et al: Percutaneous pulmonary needle biopsy: Report of 350 patients. Am J Roentgenol Radium Ther Nucl Med 122:758–768, 1974
41. Lalli AF, McCormack LJ, Zelch M, et al: Aspiration biopsies of chest lesions. Radiology 127:35–40, 1978
42. Sanders DE, Thompson DW, Pudden BJE: Percutaneous aspiration lung biopsy. Can Med Assoc J 104:139–142, 1971
43. Stevens GM, Weigen JF, Lillington GA: Needle aspiration biopsy of localized pulmonary lesions with amplified fluoroscopic guidance. Am J Roentgenol Radium Ther Nucl Med 103:561–571, 1968
44. Sinner WN, Zajicek J: Implantation metastasis after percutaneous transthoracic needle aspiration biopsy. Acta Radiol [Diagn] 17:473–480, 1976
45. Matthews MJ, Gordon PR: Morphology of Pulmonary and Pleural Malignancies. In Straus MJ. (ed): Lung Cancer Clinical Diagnosis and Treatment. New York: Grune & Stratton, pp. 49–69, 1977
46. Mountain CF: Biologic, physiologic, and technical determinants in surgical therapy for lung cancer. In Straus MJ (ed): Lung Cancer Clinical Diagnosis and Treatment. New York: Grune & Stratton, pp 185–198, 1977
47. Bateson EM: So-called hamartoma of the lung—A true neoplasm of fibrous connective tissue of the bronchi. Cancer 31:1458–1467, 1973
48. Lee LH: Percutaneous lung biopsy. Appl Radiol 5:59–61, 1976
49. Arnston TL, Boyd WR: Percutaneous biopsy using a safe, effective needle. Radiology 127:265, 1978
50. Ballard GL, Boyd WR: A specially designed cutting aspiration needle for lung biopsy. Am J Roentgenol Radium Ther Nucl Med 130:899–903, 1978
51. Nordenstrom B: A new technique for transthoracic biopsy of lung changes. Br J Radiol 38:550–553, 1965
52. Hayata Y, Oho K, Ichiba M, et al: Percutaneous pulmonary puncture for cytologic diagnosis—Its diagnostic value for small peripheral pulmonary carcinoma. Acta Cytol 17:469–475 1973
53. House AJS, Thomson KR: Evaluation of a new transthoracic needle for biopsy of benign and malignant lung lesions. Am J Roentgenol Radium Ther Nucl Med 129:215–220, 1977
54. Vitums VC: Percutaneous needle biopsy of the lung with a new disposable needle. Chest 62:717–719, 1972

55. Tukiainen P: Needle biopsy in diffuse lung manifestations—An analysis of 145 consecutive cases. Scand J Respir Dis (Suppl) 94:1–100, 1975
56. Steel SJ, Winstanley DP: Trephine biopsy for diffuse lung lesions. Br Med J 3:30–32, 1967
57. Castillo G, Ahmad M, VanOrdstrand HS, et al: Trephine drill biopsy of the lung—Cleveland Clinic experience. JAMA 228:189–191, 1974
58. Boylen CT, Johnson NR, Richters V, et al: High speed trephine lung biopsy: Methods and results. Chest 63:59–62, 1973
59. Sagel SS, Forrest JV: Fluoroscopically assisted lung biopsy techniques. Saunders Monographs in Clinical Radiology 8:22–68, 1976
60. Dick R, Heard BE, Hinson KFW, et al: Aspiration needle biopsy of thoracic lesions: An assessment of 227 biopsies. Br J Dis Chest 68:86–94, 1974

R. Robinson Baker, M.D.

10

Mediastinoscopy

INTRODUCTION

Mediastinoscopy is defined as exploration of the mediastinum. At The Johns Hopkins Hospital we currently employ two techniques to explore the mediastinum—transcervical mediastinoscopy and parasternal exploration. Transcervical mediastinoscopy explores the midmediastinum and those structures lateral and anterolateral to both sides of the trachea (Fig. 10-1). Parasternal exploration (mediastinotomy) explores the anterior mediastinum and hilar areas. The latter procedure permits examination of only one side of the anterior mediastinum, bilateral explorations require bilateral incisions on either side of the sternum. The posterior mediastinum cannot be explored by either of these procedures. The posterior mediastinum can only be explored through an anterolateral or posterolateral thoracotomy.

Both transcervical mediastinoscopy and parasternal exploration or mediastinotomy are usually undertaken to biopsy or excise mediastinal lymph nodes. In the majority of cases, the mediastinal lymph nodes are of concern because of x-ray evidence of a lesion in the hilum or in the parenchyma of the lung. The lymphatic drainage of the lungs is thus of crucial importance in any consideration of transcervical mediastinoscopy or mediastinotomy.

ANATOMY

The lymphatic drainage of the lungs can be divided into multiple interconnecting groups of lymph nodes (Fig. 10-2). The most proximal group of lymph nodes lies within the pulmonary parenchyma. These nodes drain the

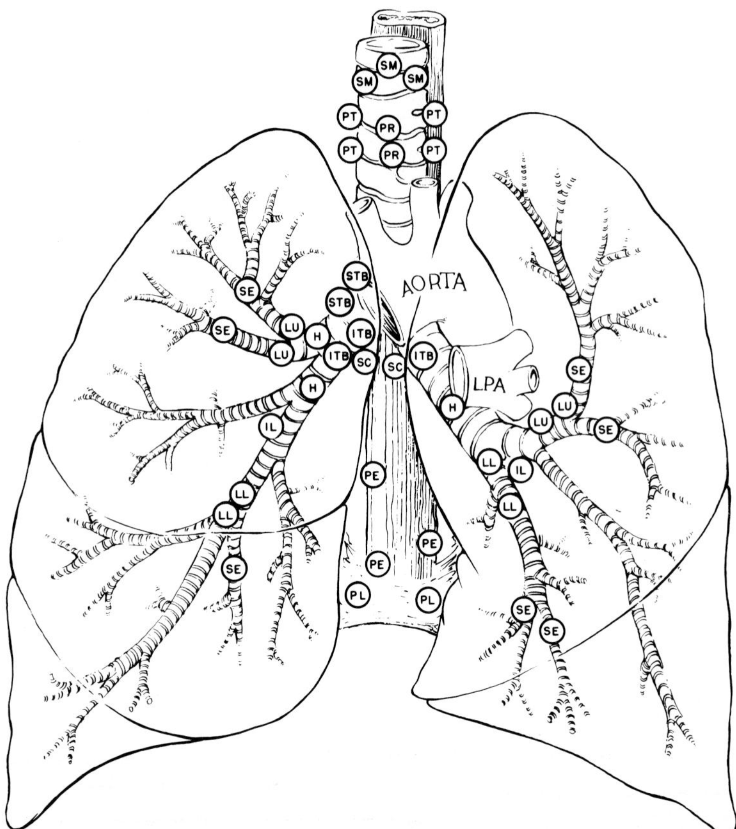

Fig. 10-1 Diagram of thoracic lymph nodes. (1) "H" = hilar or bronchopulmonary nodes, (2) "ITB" = inferior tracheal bronchial lymph nodes; (3) "LPA" = left pulmonary artery; (4) "LL" = lower lobe lobar bronchial nodes; (5) "LU" = upper lobe lobar bronchial nodes; (6) "PE" = paraesophageal lymph nodes; (7) "PL" = nodes of inferior pulmonary ligament; (8) "PR" = pretracheal lymph nodes; (9) "PT" = paratracheal lymph nodes; (10) "SC" = subcarinal lymph nodes; (11) "SE" = segmental nodes; (12) "SM" = superior mediastinal nodes; (13) "STB" = superior tracheal bronchial lymph nodes.

pulmonary parenchyma and communicate with lymph nodes lying in a cuff around the segmental bronchi. These segmental nodes drain in turn into a similar group of nodes around the lobar bronchus. The lobar bronchial nodes communicate with bronchopulmonary lymph nodes, which are located in the hilum of each lung surrounding the main stem bronchi. These bronchopulmonary lymph nodes have lymphatic connections to the posterior mediastinal lymph nodes lying along the esophagus and in the inferior pulmonary ligament and also with the inferior and superior tracheobronchial lymph nodes, the paratracheal lymph nodes, and the subaortic and anterior mediastinal lymph nodes. The inferior tracheobronchial lymph nodes lie in

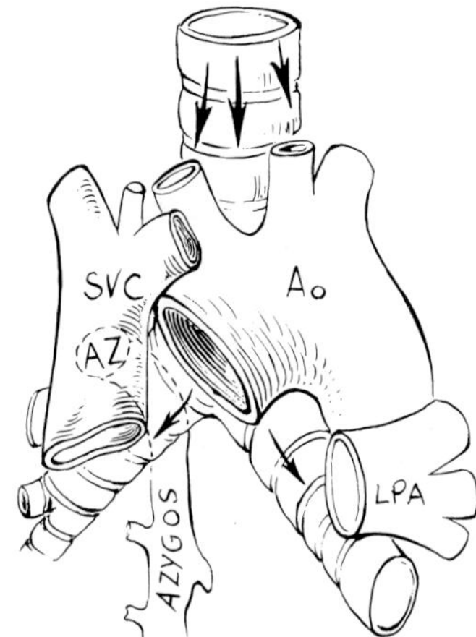

Fig. 10-2. Diagram of approach during transcervical mediastinoscopy. "Ao" = aorta; "AZ" = azygos vein; "LPA" = left pulmonary artery; "SVC" = superior vena cava.

the subcarinal area in the angle between the left and right main stem bronchi. The superior tracheobronchial lymph nodes lie anterior and superior to these subcarinal nodes in the angle between the trachea and the anterolateral wall of the major bronchi. The paratracheal nodes are located along the anterolateral wall of the trachea and communicate with the scalene nodes, which lie behind the clavicle on the anterior scalene muscles. The anterior mediastinal lymph nodes lie anterior to the aorta in the loose areolar tissue of the anterior mediastinum. These nodes have lymphatic connections to the internal mammary nodes, which in turn communicate with the anterior scalene nodes. The subaortic nodes lie along the inferior border of the aortic arch. The most significant group of subaortic nodes lies between the arch of the aorta and the left main pulmonary artery, the so-called aortic pulmonary window. It should be emphasized that normal lymphatic flow is altered by obstruction and that lymphatic blockage by metastatic tumor or scarring frequently results in rerouting and retrograde lymphatic flow.

There is general agreement that the lymphatic drainage of the right lung is predominantly to the right inferior and superior tracheobronchial nodes and to the right paratracheal nodes. Lymphatic drainage of the left lung is variable. In 1932 Rouviere, following an autopsy study in infants, first suggested that there was contralateral drainage of the left lower lobe to the right paratracheal area.[1] Subsequent clinical experience with mediastinoscopy indicates an appreciable incidence of contralateral metastases in patients with bronchogenic carcinoma in the left lower lobe. Vanderhoft[2] reports a 50 percent incidence of positive biopsies from the right paratracheal nodes in patients with left-sided bronchogenic carcinoma, and Nohl-Oser[3] describes a 28 percent incidence of such metastases. The experience at Johns Hopkins also supports this concept of primary lymphatic drainage of the left lower lobe to the right paratracheal area. We have also encountered patients with lesions of the left lower lobe who have metastases solely to the right paratracheal area.

In contrast to lesions of the left lower lobe, which drain to either the ipsilateral or contralateral paratracheal regions, lesions of the left upper lobe, and lesions arising in the left main stem bronchus have a high incidence of metastases to the anterior mediastinal and subaortic lymph nodes. Pearson et al.[4] report that 100 patients with x-ray evidence of lesions in the left upper lobe and left hilum had negative transcervical mediastinoscopies.[4] Twenty-two of these patients, however, had mediastinal lymph node metastases at operation; in 11 patients anterior mediastinal lymph node metastases were present, and in 12 patients subaortic lymph node metastases were present. A similar experience has been reported by Carlens and Jepson,[5] Jolly et al.,[6] Shah et al.,[7] and Stemmer et al.[8]

TECHNIQUE OF TRANSCERVICAL MEDIASTINOSCOPY

The technique of mediastinoscopy from the cervical approach or, more precisely, a midline superior mediastinal exploration, was first described by Carlens in 1959.[9] Although the procedure is usually performed under general anesthesia with an endotracheal tube, some authors prefer a local anesthetic.[10,11] A 3–4-cm transverse incision is made 2 cm above the sternal notch. The platysma muscle is divided in line with the skin incision, and the midline cervical fascia is incised. The sternohyoid and sternothyroid muscles are retracted exposing the trachea below the thyroid isthmus. The pretracheal fascia is incised in the midline. It is extremely important to divide the pretracheal fascia and establish a plane of dissection deep to this fascia, otherwise the dissection would lead one anterior to the major vessels. The mediastinum is thus entered in a plane deep to the pretracheal fascia. By blunt dissection a tunnel is easily created down along the anterolateral wall of the trachea to the carina. After the tunnel has been created, a careful exploration of tissues anterior and lateral to the trachea is carried out with the index finger. Extensive mediastinal tumor involvement, either from direct extension of a primary tumor in the superior mediastinum or from carcinomatous replacement of the regional lymph nodes, is usually obvious at this time. Following palpation, the mediastinoscope, a hollow rigid tube approximately 2 cm in diameter and 8 cm in length (Fig. 10-3), is introduced and the carinal area is further examined. Dissection along the left main stem bronchus is limited by the pulmonary artery, and the azygous vein limits dissection along the right main stem bronchus (Fig. 10-1). Enlarged lymph nodes such as those encountered in patients with sarcoidosis and lymphomas can usually be enucleated by blunt dissection and excised intact with little danger of significant bleeding. Total excision is considerably more difficult if there is fibrosis around the capsule of the node such as that seen in some patients with tuberculosis or extension of metastatic tumor through the capsule. In these situations, multiple biopsies are performed,

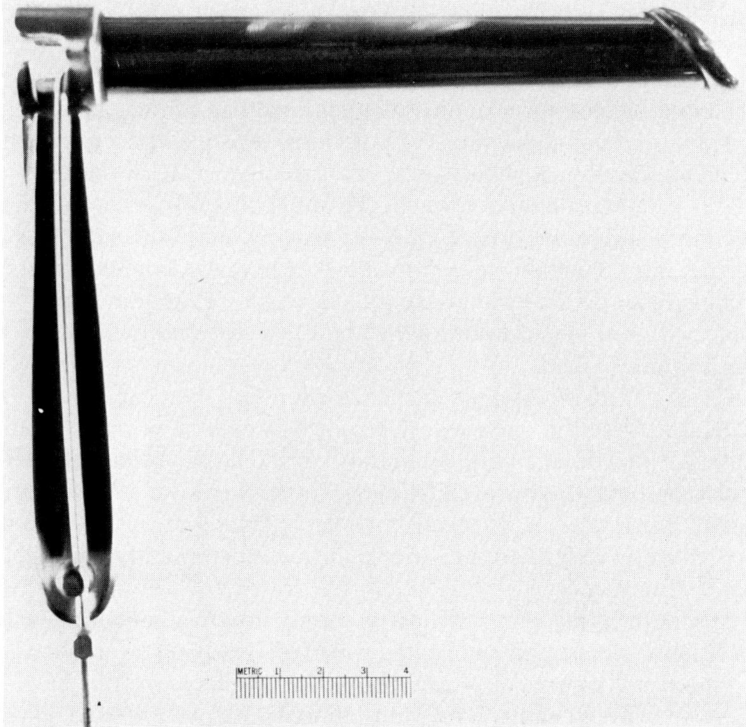

Fig. 10-3. Mediastinoscope.

and bleeding is controlled with the cautery. Hemorrhage from laceration of an artery or vein is the greatest hazard of mediastinoscopy. Vascular structures should always be identified by fine-needle aspiration, therefore, prior to any type of excisional biopsy.

If there is no gross primary or metastatic tumor in the operative field, the paratracheal and subcarinal regions are examined by dissecting the loose fatty tissue in these regions with small Alligator forceps or the tip of a metal suction cannula. Occasionally, small extranodal tumor implants are discovered during these maneuvers, and small involved nodes can be detected. Biopsy is performed with modified laryngeal biopsy forceps after appropriate fine-needle aspiration to identify adjacent blood vessels. Even when there is no apparent pathology in the mediastinum, an attempt is made to excise representative paratracheal nodes for microscopic examination. Unexpected intranodal tumor foci or histologic evidence of granulomatous disease are not uncommon findings following this maneuver. If an infectious process is suspected, representative samples of tissue should be obtained for bacteriologic stains and appropriate cultures as well as for histologic study.

If transcervical mediastinoscopy is being performed as a staging procedure in patients with bronchogenic carcinoma, both sides of the trachea should be examined because of the possibility of contralateral lymph node metastases. As previously noted, the incidence of contralateral metastases is considerably higher for lesions of the left lung than for lesions of the right lung. Transcervical mediastinoscopy performed as a staging procedure for bronchogenic carcinoma should only be carried down to the carina. Nodal metastases on the main stem bronchi are not necessarily a contraindication to resection, and the hazards of mediastinoscopy increase as the dissection extends out onto the main stem bronchi. The average length of trachea between the cricoid cartilage and the carina is 12 cm. Exploration beyond the reach of an 11-cm mediastinoscope should therefore be considered somewhat hazardous.

Following transcervical mediastinal exploration, hemostasis can usually be established with the cautery. If hemostasis cannot be established with the cautery, the wound can be temporarily packed, or at times the affected vessel can be occluded with metal clips. After hemostasis is established, the wound is irrigated and closed in layers. Drains are not left in place. The procedure is well tolerated, and significant postoperative discomfort is unusual.

Transcervical mediastinoscopy is rarely associated with significant complications. Jepsen, in a collected series of 4134 patients, reports a morbidity rate of 0.9 percent.[12] Foster et al., in a collected series of 3742 patients, reports three deaths, a mortality rate of 0.08 percent, and 66 complications—a morbidity rate of 1.6 percent.[13] In the series of Foster et al., the three deaths were due to respiratory insufficiency in two instances and, in one instance, to cardiac arrest. Hemorrhage from injury to a major vascular structure has also been reported as a cause of death. Significant complications directly attributable to the mediastinal exploration include bleeding, vocal cord paralysis, hemiparesis, and pneumothorax. Significant bleeding can be avoided by careful needle aspiration prior to biopsy. The left recurrent laryngeal nerve is at far greater risk to injury than the right recurrent laryngeal nerve. While the right recurrent laryngeal nerve comes off the vagus nerve high in the superior mediastinum at the level of the right subclavian artery, the left recurrent laryngeal nerve comes off the vagus nerve at the level of the obliterated ductus arteriosis and ascends in the tracheo-esophageal groove. Since the right recurrent laryngeal nerve is above the usual area of dissection and therefore at little risk, the right paratracheal area should always be examined initially in the course of a transcervical mediastinoscopy. Hemiparesis can occur secondary to occlusion of the innominate artery from pressure applied by the adjacent mediastinoscope. This complication can be avoided if the right radial pulse is constantly monitored during the mediastinoscopy. A pneumothorax is unusual and rarely requires insertion of a pleural tube. In over 200 transcervical mediastinoscopies, we have not encountered one significant infection.

INDICATIONS FOR TRANSCERVICAL MEDIASTINOSCOPY

It is important to emphasize that transcervical mediastinoscopy provides an accurate means of detecting paratracheal lymph node metastases and, to a lesser extent, inferior and superior tracheobronchial lymph node metastases. The procedure also provides a means of detecting direct extension of bronchogenic carcinoma to the paratracheal area. Transcervical mediastinoscopy does not provide access to the space between the aorta and the left main pulmonary artery or to the heart, pericardium, diaphragm, anterior mediastinum, or esophagus.

Patients with Proven or Suspected Bronchogenic Carcinoma

Because mediastinal lymph node metastases or direct extension of the tumor into the mediastinum usually means that the patient is incurable, transcervical mediastinoscopy has been extensively used as a staging procedure in patients with suspected or proven bronchogenic carcinoma. Some authorities[14,15] are opposed to the routine use of transcervical mediastinoscopy in patients with bronchogenic carcinoma, because they feel that the procedure is potentially hazardous, has a relatively low yield, and necessitates a second general anesthetic for the thoracotomy if the procedure does not demonstrate mediastinal lymph node metastases. In addition, mediastinal lymph node metastases are not thought to be contraindications to thoracotomy by some investigators.[16]

The argument that transcervical mediastinoscopy is potentially hazardous does not appear to be a valid one in view of the remarkably low morbidity and mortality figures referred to earlier in this chapter. Since transcervical mediastinoscopy will detect the presence of mediastinal lymph node metastases in 30–40 percent of the patients with bronchogenic carcinoma who appear to have otherwise resectable cancers, the argument of a low yield also does not appear to be valid. Exploratory thoracotomies are painful and potentially hazardous procedures. They accomplish nothing other than to establish the fact that the patient has incurable disease. If unnecessary thoracotomy can be avoided, the patients' interests are better served. It seems very reasonable therefore, to subject 100 patients to a low-risk diagnostic procedure (transcervical mediastinoscopy), if this type of management will avoid a major operative procedure in 30–40 percent of the patients. Transcervical mediastinoscopy can be performed immediately prior to thoracotomy. The surgeon can then proceed with thoracotomy under the same anesthesia if no evidence of mediastinal lymph node metastases is found on frozen section examination of the biopsy specimen. Therefore, the argument that mediastinoscopy requires a second anesthesia does not appear to be valid.

The significance of mediastinal lymph node metastases remains controversial. The clinical evidence gathered thus far indicates that mediastinal lymph node metastases are a poor prognostic sign.[17,18] Their presence indicates that the majority of patients have an incurable tumor, either because of local unresectability or because of the presence of distant although clinically occult metastases. However, patients with confined ipsilateral mediastinal lymph node metastases from squamous cell carcinomas without capsular invasion have some chance of survival.[19] On the other hand, patients with mediastinal lymph node metastases from large cell carcinomas and adenocarcinomas have almost no chance of survival. Metastatic tumor that has grown through the capsule of the lymph node (perinodal metastases) has a dismal prognosis regardless of histologic type.[20,21] The controversy concerning the significance of mediastinal lymph node metastases is concerned therefore with the management of patients with intranodal metastases from a squamous cell carcinoma. In the presence of such lesions some authors continue to advocate resection of the tumor combined with mediastinal lymph node dissection and postoperative irradiation. The argument in favor of this approach is based on a relatively small number of patients described by Kirsh.[19] He has reported a five-year survival rate of 30 percent in 17 patients with squamous cell carcinoma of the lung and mediastinal lymph node metastases who were treated by resection of the tumor, mediastinal lymph node dissection, and postoperative irradiation. Similar results have been reported in small numbers of cases by Ramsey et al.,[22] Konrad and Schulte,[23] and Bell.[24] In some of these latter reports, postoperative irradiation was not employed. These studies indicate that a five-year survival following curative resection is possible in a selected group of patients—i.e., patients with squamous cell carcinoma of the right lung demonstrating intranodal metastatic nodes located low on the right side of the trachea. These results should not be used as an argument against routine preoperative mediastinoscopy, because they apply only to a very small number of patients. If mediastinal lymph nodes are present in such patients, it would be preferable to detect them prior to operation. Preoperative irradiation is a more efficient means of destroying small foci of tumor than postoperative irradiation. If mediastinal lymph node metastases are detected preoperatively by transcervical mediastinoscopy, the mediastinum can be irradiated prior to resection of the tumor and the mediastinal lymph nodes.

In summary, transcervical mediastinoscopy is indicated in patients with proven or suspected bronchogenic carcinoma who have x-ray evidence of hilar or mediastinal lymphadenopathy. This procedure is also indicated in patients with peripheral lesions greater than 3 cm in diameter either with or without x-ray evidence of hilar or mediastinal lymph node metastases. Peripheral lesions less than 3 cm in diameter are rarely associated with mediastinal lymph node metastases. Transcervical mediastinoscopy is not indicated routinely, therefore, in these patients if there is no x-ray evidence of mediastinal widening. Transcervical mediastinoscopy is also employed in patients with lesions of the left hilum and left upper lobe. If exploration of the paratracheal area in these patients is negative, however, the anterior mediastinum and aortic pulmonary window should be explored by a parasternal incision.

Patients with Malignancies Other Than a Bronchogenic Carcinoma

Transcervical mediastinoscopy has been employed as a diagnostic and staging procedure in patients with a number of malignancies other than bronchogenic carcinoma. In an occasional patient with Hodgkin's disease, the first manifestation of the disease may be mediastinal widening detected by chest x-ray. The radiographic findings may or may not be associated with systemic symptoms. If no other nodes are palpable and the chest x-ray reveals mediastinal lymphadenopathy, a histologic diagnosis can usually be established by transcervical mediastinoscopy. Since distortion of the normal architecture of a lymph node is important in the differential diagnosis of lymphoma, it is helpful to the pathologist if the operator can dissect a lymph node out intact for histologic study. Some investigators have also used transcervical mediastinoscopy as a staging procedure in patients with Hodgkin's disease involving the neck who have no x-ray evidence of mediastinal involvement or equivocal x-ray evidence of mediastinal involvement.[25] Transcervical mediastinoscopy has also been employed in the United States and in Europe as a staging procedure in patients with carcinoma of the middle and lower thirds of the esophagus. Although most surgeons in the United States feel that the majority of patients with esophageal carcinoma are candidates for palliative resection regardless of the presence or absence of mediastinal lymph node metastases, other investigators feel that mediastinal lymph node metastases are a contraindication to surgical excision. Akovbiantz reports that 9 of 32 patients with lesions of the middle third of the esophagus and 2 of 14 patients with lesions of the lower third of the esophagus had positive transcervical mediastinoscopies.[26]

Transcervical mediastinoscopy has also been employed to detect metastatic breast cancer in patients with a history of treatment for a previous breast cancer and x-ray evidence of mediastinal lymphadenopathy. This procedure can also be employed to obtain tissue from localized metastatic mediastinal nodes for analysis for the presence of estrogen-binding protein in the cytoplasm of the breast cancer cells, an important consideration in the management of patients with metastatic breast cancer.

There are a number of other indications for transcervical mediastinoscopy in patients with x-ray evidence of mediastinal widening and a history of malignant tumors with a high incidence of mediastinal lymph node metastases. These tumors include thyroid cancer, hypernephroma, and certain testicular tumors.

Patients with Benign Disease

Transcervical mediastinoscopy is an excellent diagnostic procedure when there is x-ray evidence of paratracheal, superior mediastinal, or hilar lymphadenopathy. Clinical experience indicates that transcervical mediastinoscopy is not indicated in patients with diffuse pneumonic infiltrates and no evidence of mediastinal widening on the chest x-ray.

Contraindications to Transcervical Mediastinoscopy

There are no absolute contraindications to transcervical mediastinoscopy. In certain clinical situations, however, the risk of transcervical mediastinoscopy is considerably increased. Although a histologic diagnosis can usually be established by transcervical mediastinoscopy in patients with obstruction of the superior vena cava secondary to a primary bronchogenic carcinoma or to any other type of metastatic tumor, the venous congestion caused by the superior vena caval obstruction increases the risk of hemorrhage. Previous transcervical mediastinoscopy or irradiation of the mediastinum also increases the risk of this procedure, since normal tissue planes are obliterated and blood vessels are more difficult to identify. On one occasion, I attempted to mediastinoscope a patient who eventually proved to have mediastinal collagenosis. Tissue planes could not be developed in this patient. If mediastinal collagenosis is suspected after undertaking a transcervical mediastinoscopy, the procedure should be discontinued. The diagnosis is more safely established by an anterolateral thoracotomy.

Results of Transcervical Mediastinoscopy

IN PATIENTS WITH SUSPECTED OR PROVEN BRONCHOGENIC CARCINOMA

In unselected patients with suspected or proven bronchogenic carcinoma, transcervical mediastinoscopy will detect histologic evidence of mediastinal lymph node metastases in 30–40 percent of the cases.[27–31] The incidence of a positive mediastinoscopy varies with the particular histologic type of tumor encountered, the location of the tumor within the lung, the size of the primary tumor, and the presence or absence of mediastinal lymphadenopathy on x-ray (either plain films or tomograms of the mediastinum). The more poorly differentiated bronchogenic carcinomas have the highest incidence of mediastinal lymph node metastases. Trinkle et al. report a 60 percent incidence of mediastinal lymph node metastases for anaplastic carcinomas.[28] Adenocarcinomas had a slightly lower incidence of mediastinal lymph node metastases (50 percent), and well-differentiated squamous cell carcinomas had the lowest incidence (10 percent). Similar results have been reported by a number of other investigators. The size and location of the primary tumor also influence the incidence of mediastinal lymph node metastases that can be detected by transcervical mediastinoscopy. The larger the lesion, the greater the chance of detecting mediastinal lymph node metastases. Tumors greater than 5 cm in their maximum dimensions have at least a 50 percent incidence of mediastinal lymph node metastases; tumors less than 2 cm in their maximum dimensions are rarely associated with mediastinal lymph node metastases. Lesions of the right upper lobe and right middle lobe have the highest incidence of paratracheal lymph node metastases. The incidence decreases with lesions in the right lower lobe, which are apt to metastasize to the posterior mediastinal lymph nodes. Tumors of the left lung, particularly left upper lobe, left main stem bronchi lesions have a relatively low incidence of paratracheal lymph node metastases. Left lower lobe lesions do metastasize frequently to the contralateral paratracheal areas and, therefore, have a relatively high incident of detection by transcervical mediastinoscopy. Lesions in the lobar bronchi and main stem bronchi have a higher incidence of mediastinal lymph node metastases than do peripheral tumors.

The reported incidence of mediastinal lymph node metastases from peripheral pulmonary nodules has been variable. Stanford et al. report that of 24 of 27 patients with peripheral pulmonary nodules and x-ray evidence of mediastinal lymph node metastases had a positive transcervical mediastinoscopy.[32] In contrast, 15 of 16 patients with peripheral pulmonary nodules without x-ray evidence of mediastinal lymph node metastases had a negative transcervical mediastinoscopy. Our experience at Johns Hopkins demonstrates a 5 percent incidence of mediastinal lymph node metastases in patients with peripheral lesions less than 3 cm in diameter. This is true only if the lesion is distinct from the hilum and is not associated with radiographic evidence of hilar or mediastinal lymphadenopathy. A similar experience has been reported by Hutchinson and Mills[33] and Baggs and Braun.[34] In contrast, Maasen[35] reports a 27 percent incidence of mediastinal lymph node metastases in patients with peripheral lesions, and Mills[36] describes a 17 percent incidence of mediastinal lymph node metastases in patients with peripheral lesions. Neither of these authors defines the precise size of the peripheral lesions, however.

Radiographic evidence of mediastinal lymphadenopathy increases the incidence of positive mediastinoscopy as indicated by the experience of Stanford et al.[32] The absence of x-ray evidence of mediastinal lymphadenopathy, either on plain film or tomograms, should not, however, be considered a contraindication to transcervical mediastinoscopy, since an appreciable number of patients with such x-ray findings have histologic evidence of mediastinal lymph node metastases.[37]

IN PATIENTS WITH BENIGN DISEASE

The results of transcervical mediastinoscopy as a diagnostic procedure in patients with benign disease of the mediastinum and lung are also well established.[28,30,38] If there is evidence of mediastinal widening on the chest x-ray, transcervical mediastinoscopy produces a tissue diagnosis in almost all of the patients with mediastinal sarcoidosis. A histologic diagnosis can be established by transcervical mediastinoscopy in approximately 50 percent of patients with other granulomas of the mediastinum if there is x-ray evidence of mediastinal lymphadenopathy. Transcervical mediastinoscopy is indicated, therefore, in any clinical situation characterized by hilar or mediastinal lymphadenopathy in which a tissue diagnosis is necessary. As previously noted, transcervical mediastinoscopy rarely produces a histologic diagnosis in patients with diffuse parenchymal lesions and no x-ray evidence of mediastinal widening.

TECHNIQUE OF PARASTERNAL EXPLORATION

A parasternal exploration is performed through a vertical incision 2–3 cm lateral to the sternal border. The pectoralis major muscle can be incised in line with the skin incision. The paratracheal exploration is centered over the third intercostal space or through the excised third costal cartilage. The endothoracic fascia is incised, exposing the mediastinal fat medial to the pleura. The internal mammary vessels are either divided or retracted laterally.

Internal mammary nodes are initially looked for and excised for histologic study. In the left parasternal region the mediastinum anterior to the aortic arch is then explored with the finger in an effort to detect lymphadenopathy. If nodes are palpable, the mediastinoscope is introduced and the nodes excised or biopsied for histologic study.

In the absence of lymphadenopathy in the anterior mediastinum, I routinely open the pleura and explore the space between the left pulmonary artery and the arch of the aorta (the aortic pulmonary window). Although this procedure violates the pleural space, I believe it is a useful maneuver for detecting extra-nodal metastases in the aortic pulmonary window, which is a frequent site of metastatic disease from bronchogenic carcinomas arising in the left upper lobe or left main stem bronchus. In selected cases, lesions in the anterior segment of the left upper lobe can also be biopsied by this approach.

Prior to closure of the pleural space a No. 18 French catheter is introduced to evacuate any residual air, and the catheter is removed through a purse-string suture of 4-0 chromic catgut. The remainder of the incision is closed in layers; no effort is made to stabilize the third rib if the costal cartilage has been removed. Right-sided parasternal explorations are performed much less frequently, but the technique is essentially identical except for the different hilar vascular structures confronted during dissection.

Parasternal explorations are associated with a mortality rate of less than 1 percent. Jolly reports a complication rate of 9 percent in 100 consecutive cases.[6] Complications included wound infections (4), pneumothorax (2), bleeding (1), and pneumonitis (2). Parasternal exploration or mediastinotomy is a considerably more extensive procedure than transcervical mediastinoscopy. The risks are slightly higher, and there is more postoperative pain and discomfort than with transcervical mediastinoscopy.

INDICATIONS FOR PARASTERNAL EXPLORATION

Indications in Patients with Bronchogenic Carcinoma

Left parasternal explorations are indicated in any patient with a lesion in the left upper lobe that is greater than 3.0 cm in diameter. Left parasternal explorations are also indicated in any patient who has evidence of hilar lymphadenopathy, regardless of whether the tumor is located in the left upper lobe or left lower lobe. Under most clinical circumstances transcervical mediastinoscopy would precede parasternal exploration because of the very low morbidity of the former procedure. Occasionally both procedures are performed sequentially during the same general anesthesia. If any adenopathy is found during transcervical mediastinoscopy, frozen sections are obtained prior to proceeding with parasternal exploration. In my opinion, parasternal exploration is rarely indicated in patients with lesions of the right lung, since the lymphatic drainage of the right lung is predominantly to the right paratracheal area and exploration of the right hilum is hampered by the presence of the superior vena cava.

Indications for Parasternal Exploration in Benign Disease

Left parasternal explorations are seldom performed in patients with suspected benign disease. When clinically indicated, left hilar nodes can be approached through a left parasternal incision but only after a transcervical mediastinoscopy has ruled out the presence of paratracheal lymph nodes that might provide a histologic diagnosis. I see no indication for parasternal exploration for hilar lymphadenopathy on the right side, since the right paratracheal nodes will usually provide the necessary material for diagnosis. Also, as previously noted, the right hilum is more difficult to expose than the left hilum. Jolly et al. have also employed the parasternal incision to biopsy lesions of the anterior segments of the right upper and left upper lobes.[6] A small anterior thoracotomy in an intercostal space probably provides better access to this type of lesion.

RESULTS OF PARASTERNAL EXPLORATION

In Patients with Suspected or Proven Bronchogenic Carcinoma

In patients with suspected or proven bronchogenic carcinoma, the incidence of anterior mediastinal or subaortic lymph node metastases varies with the histologic type of the primary tumor, the size of the primary tumor, and the degree of hilar lymphadenopathy present on the chest x-ray. As is true with transcervical mediastinoscopy, the more poorly differentiated tumors arising in the left upper lobe or left main stem bronchus such as large cell undifferentiated carcinomas and oat cell carcinomas have a 60–70 percent incidence of metastases to the anterior mediastinal or subaortic lymph nodes. Adenocarcinomas have an approximate 50 percent incidence of metastases if they arise in the left upper lobe or left main stem bronchus, and squamous cancers have a considerably lower incidence of metastases. Peripheral lesions in the left upper lobe that are greater than 3 cm in size and are associated with radiographic evidence of hilar lymphadenopathy have a 50 percent incidence of anterior mediastinal or subaortic lymph node metastases.

In Patients with Benign Disease

As previously noted, parasternal explorations are seldom employed in patients with suspected benign disease. Jolly, however, has reported an experience in 19 patients, all of whom had lung biopsies performed through the parasternal incision.[6] He detected such lesions as interstitial pneumonitis and fibrosis, alveolar proteinosis, histiocytosis, Wegener's granulomatosis, miliary tuberculosis, sarcoidosis, hamartoma, pulmonary infarction, and emphysema. Parasternal exploration is therefore an alternative to open-lung biopsy for diffuse lung disease.

REFERENCES

1. Rouviere H: Anatomie des lymphatiques de l'homme. Paris, Masson et Cie, 1932
2. Vanderhoft: Discussion of, Paulson DL and Urschel HC: Selectivity in the surgical treatment of bronchogenic carcinoma. J Thorac Cardiovasc Surg 62:554–567, 1971
3. Nohl-Oser HC: The lymphatic spread of carcinoma of the bronchus, in Jepsen

O and Sorensen HR (ed): Mediastinoscopy, Proceedings of an International Symposium. Odense, Odense University Press, 1971

4. Pearson FG, Nelams JM, Henderson RD, et al: The role of mediastinoscopy in the selection of treatment for bronchial carcinoma with involvement of the superior mediastinal lymph nodes. J Thorac Cardiovasc Surg 65:382–390, 1972
5. Carlens E, Jepson O: Mediastinoscopy. Otolaryngol Clin North Am 171–192, 1968
6. Jolly PC, Hill LD, Lawles PA, et al: Parasternal mediastinotomy and mediastinoscopy. J Thorac Cardiovasc Surg 66:549–556, 1973.
7. Shah HA, Lambert CJ, Paulson DA, et al: Cervical mediastinal lymph node exploration for diagnosis and determination of operability. Ann Thorac Surg 5:15–22, 1968
8. Stemmer EA, Calvin JW, Steidman RA, et al: Parasternal mediastinal exploration to evaluate resectability of thoracic neoplasms. Ann Thorac Surg 12:375–384, 1971
9. Carlens E: Mediastinoscopy: A method for inspection and tissue biopsy in the superior mediastinum. Dis Chest 36:343–352, 1959
10. Coldberg EM and Radner DB: Mediastinoscopy. Chicago Med Sch Quart 25:60–62, 1962
11. Duvall AJ, Johnson AF, Koop SH, et al: Mediastinoscopy: An evaluation of 100 consecutive cases. Ann Otol 77:843–849, 1968
12. Jepsen O: Mediastinoscopy. Copenhagen, Munksgaard, 1966
13. Foster ED, Munro DD, Dobell ARC: Mediastinoscopy. Ann Thorac Surg 13:273–286, 1972
14. Sealy WC: Mediastinoscopy—Does it have a place in the management of carcinoma of the lung? Ann Thorac Surg 18:433–435, 1974
15. Boyd DP: Discussion of, Jolly PC, Hill LD, Lawless PA, et al: Parasternal mediastinotomy and mediastinoscopy. J Thorac Cardiovasc Surg 66:549–556, 1973
16. Overholt RH: Discussion of, Pearson FG: An evaluation of mediastinoscopy in the management of presumably operable bronchial carcinoma. J Thorac Cardiovasc Surg 55:617–625, 1968
17. Paulson DL, Urschel HC, Jr: Selectivity in the surgical treatment of bronchogenic carcinoma. J Thorac Cardiovasc Surg 62:554–562, 1971
18. Lacquet LK, Mertens A, Kleef JV, et al: Mediastinoscopy and bronchial carcinoma: Experience with 600 mediastinoscopies. Thorax 30:141–145, 1975
19. Kirsh MM, Kahn DR, Gago O, et al: Treatment of bronchogenic carcinoma with mediastinal metastases. Ann Thorac Surg 12:11–21, 1971
20. Bergh NP, Larsson S: The significance of various types of mediastinal lymph node metastases in lung cancer, in Jepsen O and Sorensen HR (ed): Mediastinoscopy, Proceedings of an International Symposium. Odense, Denmark, Odense University Press, 1971
21. Bjork VO: Discussion of, Fishman NH and Bronstein MH: Is mediastinoscopy necessary in the evaluation of lung cancer? Ann Thorac Surg 20:678–685, 1975
22. Ramsey HE, Cahan WG, Beattie EJ, et al: The importance of radical lobectomy in lung cancer. J Thorac Cardiovasc Surg 58:225–230, 1969
23. Konrad RM, Schulte HD: Mediastinoscopy in assessing the operability of carcinoma of the bronchus. German Med Monthly 14:547–551, 1969
24. Bell JW: On the significance of mediastinoscopy. Am J Surg 118:1–2, 1969

25. Elbronal O, Jensen KB, Jepsen O: Mediastinoscopy in Hodgkin's disease, in Jepsen O and Sorensen HR (ed): Mediastinoscopy, Proceedings of an International Symposium. Odense, Denmark, Odense University Press, 1971
26. Akovbiantz A: Mediastinoscopy in carcinoma of the esophagus, in Jepsen O and Sorensen HR (ed): Mediastinoscopy, Proceedings of an International Symposium. Odense, Denmark, Odense University Press, 1971
27. Goldberg EM, Glicksman AS, Khan FR, et al: Mediastinoscopy for assessing mediastinal spread in clinical staging of carcinoma of the lung. Cancer 25:317–353, 1970
28. Trinkle JK, Bryant LR, Hiller AJ, et al: Mediastinoscopy—Experience with 300 consecutive cases. J Thorac Cadiovasc Surg 60:297–300, 1970
29. Reynders H: Mediastinoscopy in bronchogenic cancer. Dis Chest 45:606–611, 1964
30. Tucker JA: Mediastinoscopy: 300 cases reported and literature reviewed. Laryngoscope 82:2226–2248, 1972
31. Inberg MV, Klossner J, Linnmi MI: The role of mediastinoscopy in the treatment of lung carcinoma. Scand J Thorac Cardiovasc Surg 6:293–296, 1972
32. Stanford W, Steele S, Armstrong RG, et al: Mediastinoscopy: its application in central versus peripheral thoracic lesions. Ann Thorac Surg 19:121–126, 1975
33. Hutchinson CM, Mills NL: The selection of patients with bronchogenic carcinoma from mediastinoscopy. J Thorac Cardiovasc Surg 71:768–773, 1976
34. Baggs JK, Braun RA: An evaluation of mediastinoscopy as a guide to diagnosis and therapy. Arch Surg 111:703–706, 1976
35. Maasen W: Results of routine mediastinoscopy in bronchial carcinoma, in Jepsen O and Sorensen HR (ed): Mediastinoscopy, Proceedings of an International Symposium. Odense, Denmark, Odense University Press, 1971
36. Mills NL: Discussion of, Fishman NH and Bronstein MH: Is mediastinoscopy necessary in the evaluation of lung cancer? Ann Thorac Surg 20:678–685, 1975
37. Ginsberg RJ: Discussion of, Fishman NH and Bronstein MH: Is mediastinoscopy necessary in the evaluation of lung cancer? Ann Thorac Surg 20:678–685, 1975
38. Fishman NH, Bronstein MH: Is mediastinoscopy necessary in the evaluation of lung cancer? Ann Thorac Surg 20:678–685, 1975

William R. Bell, M.D.
Toby L. Simon, M.D.

11

Efficacy of Various Techniques for Diagnosing Pulmonary Emboli

Pulmonary embolism remains one of the most common causes of death in hospitalized patients. In no disease of the lung is diagnosis such a critical issue, for pulmonary embolism is diagnosed antemortem in less than 50 percent of cases.[1] Over-diagnosis is also a problem. The answer to this dilemma lies in a high index of suspicion by clinicians, better diagnostic methods and, whenever possible, timely prophylaxis.

This chapter reviews the efficacy of various methods for the diagnosis of pulmonary embolic disease. Most of the best recent data are from the two national studies of thrombolytic agents, The Urokinase Pulmonary Embolism Trial (UPET)[2] and the Urokinase Streptokinase Pulmonary Embolism Trial (USPET).[3] These two studies, in addition to evaluating new treatment, obtained clinical information prior to therapy on 160 and 167 patients, respectively. Thus, the utility of various diagnostic measures can be evaluated in as many as 327 patients whose diagnosis of embolism was confirmed by angiography. These data will be referred to often in this chapter; some are presented here for the first time.

The screening of patients for these trials provides some insight into the difficulties that clinicians face in diagnosing an embolic event. Of 3819 patients in USPET suspected of having an acute pulmonary embolus, 1961 were excluded by a normal lung scan. Moreover, more than 900 patients came to arteriography with the diagnosis confirmed in only 167. Thus, noninvasive tests often fail to determine which patient has actually sustained a pulmonary embolism.

Supported in part by Research Grant Number HL-01601 and Contract Number PH-43-68-1398 from the National Heart, Lung, and Blood Institute. Supported in part by Blood Research and Demonstration Center Grant HL-17265.

Clinical signs and symptoms, although unable to confirm the diagnosis, are important in guiding physicians to the appropriate diagnostic tests. The symptoms seen in over one-half of the USPET and UPET patients[2–4] were chest pain (74 percent pleuritic, 14 percent nonpleuritic), dyspnea, apprehension, and cough. Fever, diaphoresis, and hemoptysis were seen in one-fourth to one-half of the patients. Leg cramps, palpitations, syncope, nausea and vomiting, chills, and angina were examples of less common symptoms. Almost all patients had at least one component of the symptom complex of hemoptysis—chest pain, dyspnea, or apprehension—but there were no magic combinations seen in the majority of patients. A respiratory rate greater than 16 per minute was found in 92 percent of patients, but this is obviously not very specific. Tachycardia (pulse 100, respiratory rate 16 per minute), fever, râles, and increased pulmonic component of the second heart sound each were found in more than 40 percent of the patients. Underlying medical conditions that frequently predisposed to pulmonary embolism included immobilization for any reason (especially postoperative and post-injury states), known thrombophlebitis or other venous disease, congestive heart failure, and malignancy.

ARTERIAL BLOOD GAS DETERMINATION

Clinical findings are not definitive in establishing the diagnosis; therefore, special tests are needed in patients in whom pulmonary embolism is suspected. Arterial blood gases (normal Po_2 80–100 mm Hg; Pco_2 35–45 mm Hg, pH 7.35–7.45) represent one of the most readily available tests. Since significant perfusion abnormalities of the lung secondary to pulmonary embolism would be expected to result in arterial hypoxemia, the arterial Po_2 (measured while breathing room air) should be decreased. Because of other causes for arterial hypoxemia, however, it is nonspecific and other blood gas and clinical data are needed for objective interpretation of the Po_2 value. A normal Po_2 (on room air) has been reported to be rare in the presence of recent pulmonary embolism. In one series of 29 patients, there was only one Po_2 value greater than 80 mm Hg;[5] in a series of 36 patients, there were none.[6] In the USPET-UPET trials, Po_2 (on room air) values greater than 80 mm Hg were uncommon,[2,4] but not as rare as expected from previous reports. In both series, 9 percent of the patients had Po_2 values greater than 80 mm Hg. In USPET, three patients actually had Po_2 values greater than 90 mm Hg. Obviously, the degree of hyperventilation and the oxygen concentration in the inspired air must also be considered when assessing the degree of hypoxemia. Table 11-1 shows the distribution of arterial Po_2 in the combined series. The mean Po_2 values among these patients was 62 mm Hg. The series of Kafer[7] showed a slightly higher mean value of 72.4 mm Hg.

Arterial Pco_2 is less useful. Of the 34 patients in whom this was mea-

Table 11-1
Arterial pO_2 in Pulmonary Embolism

>80– 9%
70–79–13%
60–69–31%
50–59–27%
40–49–15%
<40– 5%

Data obtained from 327 patients[2,3] on room air.

sured in the series of Szucs et al. 28 had values below 40 mm Hg.[6] Three of the six patients with Pco_2 greater than 40 mm Hg had chronic obstructive pulmonary disease. Thirty-three of 36 patients had pH values greater than 7.4. In Kafer's series, arterial Pco_2 ranged from 27 to 53 mm Hg, with a mean value of 37.5 mm Hg.[7] In our experience, hypoxemia in pulmonary embolism is usually accompanied by low Pco_2.

Thus, about one in ten patients that have had a proven pulmonary embolism within the preceding five days may have an arterial Po_2 value greater than 90 mm Hg. It is, therefore, hazardous to exclude the diagnosis of pulmonary embolism on the basis of normal arterial blood gas determinations, although the test is still of some diagnostic use.

ENZYMES AND ISOENZYMES

By contrast, the enzyme determinations, LDH and SGOT, and bilirubin, reported in 1961 by Wacker and associates[8] to be useful in the diagnosis of pulmonary embolism, have ultimately proved to be of minimal value. In the original report, LDH was elevated in virtually all cases (97 percent), usually within 8 to 24 hours after the episode, whereas it was normal in myocardial infarction. The enzyme tests were not of help when renal failure, hemolytic anemia, pernicious anemia, liver disease, myocardial necrosis, other tissue necrosis, or malignancy were present. Nevertheless, in the absence of obvious complicating conditions, elevated LDH with normal SGOT was found helpful in diagnosing pulmonary embolism.

A subsequent study by Szucs et al. in 1971,[6] although it was less enthusiastic, reported LDH increased in 83 percent of patients with angiographically proven pulmonary embolism; with prior heart disease it was 92 percent, whereas without prior heart disease it was 73 percent. The elevation occurred within 24 hours in 87 percent of patients. Bilirubin was increased above normal in only 7 of 34 patients in whom it was tested, whereas SGOT was normal in 60 percent (44 percent within 24 hours; 56 percent after 24 hours). Thus, the triad of increased LDH, normal SGOT, and increased bilirubin was present in only 12 percent, and the combination of increased LDH and normal SGOT was present in only 44 percent.

The increase in LDH in pulmonary embolism, however, has been shown to depend upon release from extrapulmonary sources,[9] as the lung isomer was less elevated following pulmonary embolism than those from liver. In the series of 33 patients with proven pulmonary emboli reported by Konttinen et al., LDH was elevated in 22.[9]

Light and Bell have reported that the incidence of LDH elevation with pulmonary embolism is similar to congestive heart failure and pneumonia and thus is of little use in diagnosing pulmonary embolism.[10] In the UPET trials, 50 percent of patients actually had normal LDH.[2] The lower percentage than in previous studies may relate to the time of diagnosis. Increased LDH and bilirubin with normal SGOT were seen in only 4 percent of the patients, whereas increased LDH with normal SGOT was seen in 20 percent. These enzymes (LDH, SGOT) and bilirubin, therefore, are of little, if any, use in making the diagnosis of pulmonary embolism.

HEMATOLOGIC DETERMINATIONS

The usual hematologic tests are also of limited use. In Szucs' series, 42 percent of the patients had white blood cell counts that were less than 10,000/mm^3, whereas 93 percent were less than 15,000/mm^3. In the UPET-USPET studies[2,3] the average white blood cell count was 11,000/mm^3.

The platelet count was normal in 23 of 26 patients in whom it was measured in Szucs' series. In the UPET-USPET studies, the mean platelet count was 270,000/mm^3. Ten percent of the patients had platelet count determinations of less than 150,000/mm^3, 36 percent were between 150,000 and 249,000/mm^3, 33 percent were between 250,000 and 349,000/mm^3, and 21 percent were greater than 350,000/mm^3 (normal range, 150,000–350,000/mm^3). The data show a tendency toward slightly higher than normal platelet and white blood cell counts, but neither is of diagnostic specificity.

COAGULATION DETERMINATIONS

Clotting time determinations of either the intrinsic or extrinsic system have not been useful. In the UPET-USPET studies, the prothrombin time averaged about 14.4 seconds, compared to a control of 12.5 seconds. Thus, the mean prolongation was only 2 seconds. Gallus et al. have found that shorter partial thromboplastin times and lower antiplasmin levels correlated with a greater mean incidence of thrombosis in surgical patients when measured pre-operatively or on the first postoperative day.[11] The overlap was considerable, however, and no predictive level could be established. In the

UPET-USPET studies, the mean fibrinogen level was 561 mg/100 ml plasma (normal range, 250–400 mg/100 ml plasma). Three percent of the patients had values of less than 250 mg/100 plasma (11 percent had levels between 250 and 349 mg/100 ml plasma, 22 percent had levels between 350 and 449 mg/100 ml plasma) and 64 percent had levels greater than 450 mg/100 ml plasma. The mean plasminogen level was 2.2 caseinolytic units/ml (normal range, 1.75–2.75 units/ml). Twenty-four percent were less than 1.75 units/ml, (29 percent were between 1.75 and 2.24 units/ml, 32 percent were between 2.25 and 2.74 units/ml) and 15 percent were greater than 2.75 units/ml. Although determinations of fibrinogen and plasminogen are of little specificity in diagnosis, an increase in fibrinogen, as an acute-phase reactant, and a slight decrease in plasminogen, probably related to acceleration of in vivo fibrinolysis, result from pulmonary embolism.

The degradation products of fibrinogen-fibrin (FDP-fdp) have also been proposed as laboratory tools for diagnosing pulmonary embolism. One group[12] reported that 12 of 37 postoperative patients with normal lung scans, who were followed with ^{125}I leg scans, showed no elevation in FDP-fdp levels, whereas 25 patients with lung scans suggestive of pulmonary embolism had FDP-fdp elevations. By angiography, 23 of the 25 patients were demonstrated to have pulmonary emboli.[13] In the absence of pulmonary embolism, but with the diagnosis of deep venous thrombosis alone, there was no elevation. The authors were unable to document a relationship to the duration of symptoms.

In 1973 a report by Rickman et al.[14] stated that of 19 patients with angiographically proven pulmonary embolism, the mean level of FDP-fdp (by the staphylococcal clumping test) was 158 $\pm$ 180 μg/ml, with a range of 10–640 μg/ml. Only one of the patients fell into the normal range (less than 20 μg/ml). This was contrasted with 22 patients without pulmonary embolism in whom the range was 1.25–2.0 μg/ml (8.0 $\pm$ 6.0 μg/ml). Only three of these patients had levels greater than 10 μg/ml. Of five patients with equivocal angiograms for pulmonary embolism, two had levels less than 10 μg/ml and three had levels greater than 10 μg/ml. Two patients with proven deep venous thrombosis but no pulmonary embolism had normal FDP-fdp levels. The authors claimed that elevated FDP-fdp levels had a false-negative rate of 2.4 percent, and a false-positive rate of 7.3 percent in this disease. Because two of the three false-positive patients had liver disease, the authors suggested that hepatic dysfunction may interfere with the specificity of the test. The highest levels were in the first three days after embolism was diagnosed. They concluded that FDP-fdp levels are a useful test for diagnosing pulmonary embolism, particularly in the absence of liver disease.

A subsequent study from Great Britain documented an early rise in FDP-fdp levels in dogs, in 8 of 11 cases.[15] Similarly in dogs, Cade et al. have shown that embolism leads to marked increases in FDP-fdp levels at 1, 4, and 24 hours.[16] Heparin therapy lowered the levels successfully. They also showed that elevated FDP-fdp levels were derived mainly from sources other than the original embolus. This was taken as evidence that the amount of fibrin accretion accompanying untreated experimental pulmonary embolism is considerably greater than the fibrin mass of the original embolus itself. Thus, there is experimental documentation of the usefulness of this assay.

Gurewich et al. showed that the staphylococcal clumping test and the serial dilution protamine sulfate tests tended to confirm thromboembolism.[17] They found a protamine sulfate test to be more specific. In their series there was overlap between the normal patients and those with thromboembolism and no evidence that the increase in FDP-fdp levels was specific for pulmonary embolism as opposed to deep venous thrombosis.

Other findings have been reported by Light and Bell[10] and Wood et al.[18] Of 35 patients with angiographically proven pulmonary emboli prospectively studied by Light and Bell elevated levels of FDP-fdp were found in only two, borderline levels in five, and normal levels in 28.[10] They explained the discrepancy between their results and previous results by the time of measurement with respect to the onset of symptoms and the technique used, particularly the amount of thrombin. In Wood's study 27 patients were followed with ^{125}I fibrinogen scans after surgery for fractured neck of the femur.[18] Although the patients with thrombosis had higher FDP-fdp levels than those without, the correlation was better with sepsis, congestive heart failure, or malignancy than with thrombosis alone.

Thus, the usefulness of clinical tests of fibrinogen-fibrin degradation products for pulmonary embolism is in doubt, in part because of lack of specificity, and in part because of technical questions regarding the methodology of measurement. Therefore, such tests cannot be considered a reliable means of diagnosing pulmonary emboli.

Nossel[19] has reported that fibrinopeptide A is elevated in all patients with either thrombophlebitis or pulmonary embolism, with more recent onset of symptoms associated with higher levels. There were, however, elevations in cellulitis with normal venography. This method cannot distinguish between thrombophlebitis alone and pulmonary embolism, and there is overlap with other conditions. At present, it is not a useful clinical test for pulmonary embolism, although it is suggestive that some type of assay for activated coagulation and increased thrombin activity may be useful in diagnosing thrombosis without necessarily distinguishing between deep venous thrombosis and pulmonary embolism.

PLATELET AND FIBRINOGEN SURVIVAL

Platelet and fibrinogen survival measurements have the advantage of being dynamic rather than static tests of the coagulation system.

Steele et al. have shown that platelet survival and increased platelet adhesion were findings of recurrent thrombosis.[20] Harker and Slichter's studies indicate that venous thrombosis leads to parallel decreases in survival of platelets, fibrinogen, and plasminogen.[21] These changes are reversed by anticoagulation. Because these tests take several days to complete, they are not practical in the usual situation. They may, however, be useful in difficult problems of recurrent thromboembolism, particularly with regard to the efficacy of therapy.

The noninvasive studies of β-thromboglobulin,[22,23] anti-fibrin antibody,[24] platelet coagulant activities,[25–28] and activated Factor X (Xa),[29,30] may be helpful in recognizing in vivo thrombus formation, but their ultimate diagnostic value remains to be established.

ELECTROCARDIOGRAM

Although the electrocardiogram may be abnormal in the face of pulmonary embolism, it has been difficult to separate abnormalities due to pre-existing cardiopulmonary disease from those related to pulmonary embolism. In a study of 20 patients with arteriographically proven pulmonary embolism, who were free of pre-existing cardiopulmonary disease, there was one patient with right ventricular strain and three patients with findings suggestive of right ventricular strain that correlated with increased pulmonary artery pressure.[31] In 80 percent of the patients, the ECG was of no specific value. This study suggested that the ECG was unlikely to be of specific value in pulmonary embolism, except where the embolism was massive. The findings of right ventricular strain were confirmed in the report of Spodick.[32] In Szucs' series, 81 percent of the patients had a normal sinus rhythm or a sinus tachycardia.[6] In nine patients, there was atrial fibrillation, but eight of these had heart disease. Fibrillation was new in only three patients (6 percent of the total). Premature atrial or ventricular contractions were found in only two patients. Acute right axis shift was found in seven (15 percent of the series); 57 percent had normal axis; and 28 percent had an axis deviation pre-existing the embolism that did not change. Intraventricular conduction was normal in 75 percent of the series. A pre-existing bundle branch block was found in 17 percent, and a new, incomplete right bundle branch block was found in 8 percent. Nineteen percent of the total series had one electrocardiographic change that was thought to be classical for pulmonary embolism (right axis shift, $S_1Q_3T_3$, or new right bundle branch block). This series also suggested that the ECG was of only limited benefit.

Stein et al.[2,33] have analyzed the electrocardiograms in 90 patients without previous pulmonary or cardiac disease who had angiographically proven pulmonary embolism. Fifty had massive pulmonary embolism and 40 had submassive pulmonary embolism. In submassive embolism, 23 percent of the electrocardiograms were normal, whereas only 6 percent were normal in the massive embolism. The most common abnormality was depressed T-waves, which were found in 42 percent of the patients. The other common abnormalities were: depressed RST segments, found in 26 percent; elevated RST segments, found in 15 percent; and the $S_1Q_3T_3$ finding in 12 percent. Findings in 5–10 percent of the patients were right axis deviation, left axis deviation, incomplete right bundle branch block, complete right bundle branch block, and right ventricular hypertrophy. Premature atrial or ventricular contractions were found in 2 percent and 3 percent of the series, respectively, and atrial ventricular block in 1 percent. Findings more common in massive pulmonary embolism (compared to submassive) were inverted T-waves (46 percent versus 38 percent) and the $S_1Q_3T_3$ (18 percent versus 13 percent). The ECG disturbances were more common in 42 patients with previous cardiopulmonary disease. Twenty-six percent had a rhythm disturbance, 12 percent had an A-V conduction disturbance, 2 percent had cor pulmonale, 76 percent had a QRS change, and 62 percent had an RST segment or T-wave abnormality. The RST segment and T-wave abnormalities were equally common, whether previous cardiopulmonary disease was present or not. It was in rhythm disturbances in particular that patients with previous cardiopulmonary disease were more likely to be abnormal. Stein et al. noted that the $S_1Q_3T_3$ findings all disappeared five or six days after diagnosis, whereas RST segment and T-wave abnormalities were slower to disappear.[33] Their study also showed that a larger perfusion defect and hemodynamic abnormality were associated with more change in the ECG. Electrocardiographic findings remain nonspecific for pulmonary embolism, but in patients with significant pulmonary arterial obstruction they are useful in guiding one toward the diagnosis.

RADIOLOGIC STUDIES

Roentgenograms of the chest usually are abnormal in cases of proven pulmonary embolism.[34] In Szucs' series[6] abnormalities were seen commonly in the lower lobes (51 percent of the patients). In only a minority of cases was the infiltrate or area of consolidation actually wedge-shaped. Pleural effusion was found in 35 percent; elevated diaphragm, in 27 percent. A normal chest x-ray was found in 29 percent of the patients. If one excluded those patients with prior disease, the incidence of infiltrate dropped to 46 percent and pleural effusion to 29 percent, but elevated diaphragm increased to 37 percent.

In another series of angiographically proven cases 93 percent had some abnormality in the chest x-ray.[35] Pleural effusion or infiltrate were each found in more than 50 percent. Forty-four percent had at least two of the following abnormalities: pleural effusion, infiltrate, atelectasis, elevated diaphragm.

Simon[36] has noted that a pleural effusion accompanies 96 percent of pulmonary infarcts and thus is useful when infarction is present in addition to embolism. Elevated diaphragms, found in 62 percent of his series of pulmonary embolism, were due to reduction in lung volume related to focal atelectasis or infarction. In this series of patients some type of pulmonary vascular disease was found in 71 percent, and acute cor pulmonale was seen in 12 percent.

In the analysis of chest x-rays from UPET,[2] 46 percent were found to have an abnormality in lung parenchyma (41 percent consolidation, 20 percent atelectasis, and 2 percent other findings); pleural effusion was found in 28 percent, diaphragmatic elevation in 41 percent, pulmonary vessel changes in 39 percent (distention of proximal pulmonary artery 23 percent, focal arterial findings 15 percent, pulmonary artery increased in size 3 percent, other findings 2 percent), change in the heart shadow 9 percent (right ventricular enlargement 5 percent, left ventricular enlargement 16 percent, right atrial enlargement 2 percent, left atrial enlargement 2 percent).

The findings on chest x-ray are nonspecific, and 7–30 percent of patients with angiographically proven pulmonary embolism may have normal chest x-rays. Similarly, chest x-ray findings in pulmonary embolism can mimic many other pulmonary diseases.

HEMODYNAMIC STUDIES

Hemodynamic and pulmonary function tests have also been used in the diagnosis of pulmonary embolism. In patients free of previous cardiopulmonary disease, pulmonary hypertension is proportional to the amount of obstruction seen on angiography and, in fact, is seen only after 25–30 percent vascular obstruction.[35–37] Cardiac index is infrequently depressed in pulmonary embolism. Increase in mean pulmonary arterial pressure requires obstruction of greater than 25 percent, although with previous cardiopulmonary disease abnormalities are seen with much less obstruction. The mean figures for various hemodynamic measurements in the UPET-USPET trials are shown in Table 11-2. Right heart pressures tend to be higher in patients with previous cardiopulmonary disease, and cardiac index tends to be lower. The hemodynamic data are of importance in planning therapy and predicting prognosis, but since they are usually obtained at the time of angiography, they are rarely critical in diagnosis.

Pulmonary function tests have similarly been found to be of limited use in diagnosing pulmonary embolism.[7] There is a decrease in vital capacity in one-half of the patients, but the findings of obstructive lung disease are infrequent.

Since all the studies discussed to this point tend to be of only limited help in the diagnosis of pulmonary embolism, due to nonspecificity as well as to the absence of abnormalities in a small but significant percentage of patients, emphasis has been on the search for more specific tests. This is of obvious importance, since anticoagulation, the treatment of choice, as well as operative procedures (such as vena caval ligation and pulmonary embo-

Table 11-2
Hemodynamic Variables in Proven Pulmonary Embolism

	Mean Value	Mean Value in Patients with Previous Cardiopulmonary Disease	Mean Value in Patients w/o Previous Cardiopulmonary Disease
Pressures (mm Hg)			
Right arterial mean	6.2	6.9	5.7
Right ventricular end-diastolic	9.0	9.5	8.4
Right ventricular systolic	45.6	49.7	42.3
Pulmonary artery mean	26.6	29.9	25.0
Cardiac index L/min/m^2	2.9	2.7	3.2
Ln total pulmonary vascular resistance[a] (dynes/sec/cm^{-5})	6.1	6.2	5.9
A-V difference	5.3	5.6	5.0

[a] These data were obtained from UPET and USPET patients (2,3), except for "Ln total pulmonary vascular," which were from USPET only.[3]
Ln = natural logarithm.
A-V = arterial-venous blood.

lectomy) pose major hazards and should not be used in patients who have some other explanation for their signs and symptoms. Recent investigation has centered on perfusion and ventilation lung scans and angiographic techniques.

PERFUSION PULMONARY SCAN

During the past 15 years lung perfusion scanning frequently has been utilized to evaluate patients suspected of having pulmonary emboli.[38–44] This procedure provides a simple, safe, sensitive, and precise method to define the status of pulmonary blood flow. Blood flow is determined by imaging the movement of radioactive particles (20–50 μ in diameter), injected into a peripheral vein, as their passage is retarded in precapillary arterioles and capillaries of the lung. This procedure can be performed by technical personnel in seriously compromised patients in 30 minutes.

Although the perfusion lung scan is exquisitely sensitive, providing information about blood flow in vessels as small as 20 μ in diameter, it completely lacks specificity. Anything that will alter blood flow will cause an abnormal perfusion lung scan. The list of pathologic entities that can interfere with pulmonary blood flow is lengthy,[34,45–51] and pulmonary emboli do not occupy a unique position in this list.

Shortly after the introduction and subsequent widespread use of the perfusion scan, a number of reports indicated the merits of this procedure in diagnosis of pulmonary emboli.[39,44,52,53] Despite continued universal use, however, the number of prospective, properly controlled studies in which the findings on perfusion scan have been verified by angiography are very few. In the USPET study, where lung perfusion scanning was used as a screening procedure, 906 patients had scans suggestive of embolism and all had angiography. In 754 of these patients (83 percent), pulmonary angiography (in all patients, selective studies were performed to define abnormal defects seen on scan) was normal. In this study,[3] correlations between perfusion scan and angiogram were carefully evaluated.[54] Lung perfusion scans and pulmonary arteriograms performed within 1 to 2 hours of each other were carried out in 162 patients. They were interpreted separately and independently by experts on perfusion scan and angiogram panels. The expert members on each panel were unaware of the age, sex, clinical history, physical examination, or laboratory findings on the patients.

Among the angiogram panel members there was disagreement about the diagnosis of pulmonary emboli in 6 percent of the patients. Readings by the perfusion scan panel members were in the categories of high, medium, or low probability of embolism, or no evidence of embolism. High probability meant a normal chest x-ray, with characteristic perfusion defects on scan. Low probability meant that, although there were perfusion defects present, their size or shape were not characteristic of embolism, or other explanations were present on chest x-ray. In 22 percent of cases, more than one of the panelists disagreed, and the variation in readings ranged from two or more diagnostic categories (e.g., high to low probability).

When angiographic classification of emboli according to massive, submassive, and nondiagnostic was compared with the scan diagnostic classification of high, medium, and low probability, the correlation was imperfect.[54] There was no instance of a normal scan and a positive angiogram, but of seven cases with nondiagnostic angiograms, two scans were read as high probability; four, as medium probability. Of the 13 scans read as low probability, 3 showed massive embolism on angiogram.

In this study, a comparison was made between the anatomic localization of abnormalities seen on angiogram and those seen on lung perfusion scan (Table 11-3). The right lung was more frequently involved than the left. The two techniques were in agreement most often in patients in whom abnormalities were present in the lower lobe areas. Disagreement was most common in the middle lobes.

Estimation of the extent of perfusion defects by an index lung scan reader is compared with the index angiogram reader,[54] according to the technique described by Walsh et al.[55] (Table 11-4). In 43 percent of the patients analyzed, the estimate by the lung scan technique was within 10 percent of the size of the defect, as demonstrated angiographically. There was a tendency for the scan reader to estimate a larger defect than that reported by

Table 11-3
Localization of Defects of Lobes of the Lungs

	LUL	LING	LLL	RUL	RML	RLL
Angiogram—Pos. scan —Pos.	49	46	96	70	55	112
Angiogram—Neg. scan —Neg.	56	50	19	40	40	7
Angiogram—Pos. scan —Neg.	20	31	8	29	29	16
Angiogram—Neg. scan —Pos.	20	22	23	16	23	11

NOTE: Pulmonary anatomic localization according to lobe of defect or no defect comparing index angiographer and index lung scan reader. LUL = left upper lobe; LING = lingular lobe left lung; LLL = left lower lobe; RUL = right upper lobe; RML = right middle lobe; RLL = right lower lobe. The numerical value indicated in the various anatomic sites is the number of defects tabulated (or no defect) in 162 patients.

the angiogram reader. A relationship was present between more extensive emboli, as estimated by angiography, and the larger perfusion defects estimated by scan.

The size of the perfusion defects, estimated by the index scan reader, was compared to the severity score[2] reported from the angiograms in Table 11-5.

These data point out that there is a general correlation between extent of perfusion defect on scan and severity of lesion and estimated perfusion defect on angiogram. The scan defects, however, are subject to a variety of opinions that related not only to their lack of specificity but also to variations in observer interpretation. There is a need for additional prospective simultaneous studies with perfusion scanning and angiography.

In summary, available data suggest:

1. If all six views (antero-posterior, postero-anterior, right and left laterals and obliques) of a lung perfusion scan are uniformly normal and without defects, the diagnosis of pulmonary emboli is excluded.[56]
2. The lung perfusion scan is a precise, sensitive indicator of pulmonary blood flow and correlates with the extent and location of lesions seen on angiography.
3. The lung perfusion scan completely lacks specificity with respect to the etiology of alteration in blood flow that may be detected.
4. Interpretation of defects observed on lung perfusion scan is extremely difficult and is a significant obstacle to making the correct diagnosis.
5. Abnormalities detected by the lung perfusion scan should serve as a guide for the angiographer to identify potential emboli, with high-quality selective studies resulting in better diagnostic accuracy and reduced patient morbidity (see Chapter 4).

Table 11-4
Comparison of Embolus Size by Angiograph with Size of Perfusion Defect on Lung Scan (Index readers)

Angiogram	Perfusion Defect on Scan (%)	N	%
Massive (100)	0–10	1	1
	11–20	11	11
	21–30	11	11
	31–40	23	23
	41–50	20	20
	51–60	23	23
	61–70	9	9
	71–100	2	2
Submassive (54)	0–10	4	7.4
	11–20	17	31.0
	21–30	15	27.8
	31–40	10	18.5
	41–50	6	11.1
	51–60	1	1.8
	61–70	1	1.8
	71–100	0	0
Nondiagnostic (8)	0–10	4	50.0
	11–20	2	25.0
	21–30	0	0
	31–40	1	12.5
	41–50	0	0
	51–60	0	0
	61–70	1	12.5
	70–100	0	0

NOTE: This table compares the size of the embolus estimated by the index angiographer with the size of the perfusion defect reported by the index scan reader. N = number of patients with the corresponding perfusion defect who had that size emboli or no emboli by angiography. % = the percent of the total number of patients in that angiographic size category with the corresponding scan defect indicated. The number in parentheses is the total number of patients in that angiographic (size) category.

6. A positive diagnosis of pulmonary emboli cannot be definitively established by the lung perfusion scan alone.
7. The scan is a noninvasive test, useful for following perfusion defects during subsequent weeks-months.

PERFUSION–VENTILATION PULMONARY SCANNING

The increasing recognition of the severe limitations of the lung perfusion scan with respect to the diagnosis of pulmonary emboli has demanded additional amplification of this technique. Numerous investigators have indicated that the diagnostic dilemmas that surround patients suspected of

Table 11-5
Comparison of Angiographic Severity Rating with Size of Scan Perfusion Defect (Index readers)

Angiographic Severity Score	Perfusion Defect (%)	N	%
Severe (65)	0–10	1	1.5
	11–20	3	4.6
	21–30	4	6.1
	31–40	12	18
	41–50	16	24
	51–60	21	32
	61–70	6	9
	71–100	2	3
Moderately severe (64)	0–10	1	1
	11–20	15	23
	21–30	15	23
	31–40	14	21
	41–50	12	18
	51–60	2	3.0
	61–70	5	7
	71–100	0	0
Not severe (25)	0–10	4	16
	11–20	9	36
	21–30	6	24
	31–40	6	24
	41–50	0	0
	51–60	0	0
	61–70	0	0
	71–100	0	0

NOTE: This table compares the index angiographers severity rating with the size of the defect on scan reported by the index scan reader. N = number of patients who had the corresponding perfusion defect as indicated. % = the percent of the total number of patients in that severity category who had that size of perfusion defect indicated. The number in parentheses is the total number of patients in that severity category.

having pulmonary emboli arise from many different types of pulmonary pathology.[34,42,45–51,57,58] Any condition that alters intrapulmonary blood flow, be it extrapulmonic or intrapulmonic, may create defects on the perfusion scan that are indistinguishable from the defect of intraluminal blood clots. The major problem emanates from the complete lack of specificity of the perfusion technique. To overcome this problem, the use of radiolabeled gas to examine the ventilatory compartments of the lung has been suggested.[59–63] The perfusion and ventilation compartments can be examined separately. The defects observed in these scans can be attributed to lesions that exist either in the perfusing blood vessels or in the ventilating compartments, or in both. The utility of combining these two techniques is based on the premise that a reduction or alteration in lung perfusion (blood flow) does not cause a corresponding alteration in ventilation. Thus, in the presence of pulmonary emboli, a defect will be visible on perfusion scan, but a corresponding defect on ventilation scan will be lacking. In the presence of normal blood flow, disturbances within the ventilation compartments should not cause defects on the perfusion scan. The vascular and ventilatory compartments, however are in close proximity; in pathologic situations such as infectious infiltrative pulmonary parenchymal disease (bacterial, fungal, neoplastic cells), ventilatory architecture and vascular compartments will both be altered. Likewise, pathologic lesions, similar in type, that begin primarily in the vascular compartment can change the pattern of ventilation.[57,58] Even those pathologic processes that primarily involve the ventilatory areas, such as emphysema, or chronic bronchitis, anatomically or physiologically impinge on the vascular network and alter blood flow. Atelectasis, frequently observed in both embolic and parenchymal lung disease, causes defects on both ventilation and perfusion scans. Peripheral thrombotic lesions that embolize to and totally occlude pulmonic vessels cause vascular damage, loss of vessel integrity, hemorrhage, and infarction. This process results in destruction of the ventilatory saccules of the lung. It is obvious that these pathologic processes result in disturbance to both the perfusion and ventilation systems of the lung. Thus, a single process can cause concomitant defects in both the perfusion and ventilation scans. In actuality, it is difficult to conceive of a pathologic process that always limits itself to only one of these pulmonary systems.

The early studies, combining perfusion and ventilation scans in evaluating patients suspected of having pulmonary emboli reported a significant improvement in diagnostic accuracy.[46,58,63–66] Certain patterns of "diagnostic significance" (abnormal perfusion scan with a normal ventilation scan; a mismatched pattern) emerged that provided an interpretive framework for conclusions about the diagnosis that were not possible with perfusion studies alone.[63–68] Some investigators reported that the concomitant use of these techniques allows documentation of pulmonary emboli.[69–71] Pulmonary angiography, however, was not employed in these studies to substantiate the findings reported in perfusion–ventilation studies.

More recently, it has been demonstrated that pulmonary emboli can be the source of matched perfusion and ventilation defects without radiologically demonstrable infiltrates.[72] Two studies evaluating combined perfusion–ventilation scans in patients suspected of having pulmonary emboli also employed angiography.[73,74] Although both studies were retrospective, the selected data are helpful in evaluating these two techniques used in combination. In the study of 40 patients with pre-existing chronic obstructive pulmonary disease who were suspected of having pulmonary emboli[73] the diagnostic accuracy of emboli was statistically significantly improved when xenon ventilation studies were combined with the perfusion studies. In the second study of more than 100 patients,[74] when the ventilation study was added to the perfusion study the diagnostic accuracy in those patients with multiple large perfusion defects was increased from 80 percent to nearly 100 percent. In those patients with smaller defects and normal ventilation, however, the diagnostic accuracy was only 50 percent.

At present, it is reasonably clear that additional studies employing angiography to verify the results of the combined scanning techniques need to be performed. From the available data, the addition of ventilation scanning may provide some additional help in more accurately making the diagnosis of pulmonary emboli. At present, however, one must conclude that combined perfusion–ventilation studies cannot be substituted for pulmonary angiography to establish the diagnosis of pulmonary emboli in a significant proportion of patients.

PULMONARY ANGIOGRAPHY

Pulmonary angiography continues to be the most precise and specific test available for the detection of pulmonary emboli.[75–78] In a properly staffed and equipped laboratory it can be performed quickly, with minimal discomfort to the patient, and can provide an accurate answer within 30 to 45 minutes. Simultaneously, the hemodynamics of pulmonary and cardiac function can be measured directly. Immediate and long-term management plans can be instituted promptly. In a recent study of patients with pulmonary emboli, over 800 pulmonary angiograms were performed.[2,3,54] The morbidity was less than 1 percent and the mortality was less than 0.01 percent. Special attention is needed to avoid perforation in patients with ventricular aneurysm or myocardiopathy and arrhythmias in patients with irritable ventricles. The other undesirable features are:

1. The procedure is invasive.
2. It requires professional medical and paramedical personnel.
3. It requires sophisticated equipment.
4. It is expensive.

The use of selective arteriography, accompanied by geometric magnification and oblique techniques, significantly enhances the diagnostic sensitivity of this test. Since optimal selective and magnification techniques allow visualization of vessels as small as 0.5 mm in diameter,[34,50] significant emboli should not be missed. Available angiographic–pathologic correlations support this contention[75]. Although two false-negatives were reported in the USPET study, presumably due to the rigid criteria required for the diagnosis,[54] false-positive diagnoses should not occur and false-negative diagnoses should be exceedingly rare when intraluminal filling defects are the criteria. Pulmonary angiography remains the standard test with which all new tests[79] must be compared to evaluate their potential efficacy in making the diagnosis of pulmonary emboli.[80,81]

In a patient suspected of having pulmonary emboli, the decision to perform arteriography must be made by thoughtfully considering the clinical history, physical examination, age, associated diseases, past history of smoking, the findings on chest x-ray, perfusion–ventilation scan, therapeutic considerations, and certain risk factors. At present it is impossible to make all-inclusive statements regarding when angiography should be performed. If any type of surgical procedure (interruption of inferior vena cava, placement of an umbrella, thrombectomy, vein ligation, pulmonary embolectomy) is contemplated, the diagnosis of pulmonary emboli must be established by arteriography. If the patient has a past history of allergy to heparin or coumadin, bleeding while being treated with anticoagulants, contraindications to anticoagulant therapy, resistance to conventional anticoagulants, or recurring emboli while being treated with heparin, angiography must be performed to establish the diagnosis. If the lung perfusion scan in a suspected case of pulmonary emboli is of adequate quality (all four views, and preferably six views) and is interpreted as normal, the diagnosis is not pulmonary emboli and angiography is not indicated.

Venography of the lower extremities is not a substitute for pulmonary arteriography in making the diagnosis of pulmonary emboli. Positive findings on lower extremity venograms, particularly in the presence of an abnormal lung scan, strengthen the suspicion of emboli and provide an indication for institution of anticoagulant therapy but do not make the diagnosis of pulmonary emboli. Venograms of the lower extremities may be normal or without intraluminal thrombi because all thrombi have embolized to the lungs. Similarly, all patients with thrombophlebitis of the lower extremities do not have pulmonary emboli. Thrombi within venous vasculature of the pelvis, abdomen, inferior vena cava, right heart, and upper extremities (structures that cannot be visualized by lower extremity venography) may embolize to the lungs.

SUMMARY: APPROACH TO DIAGNOSIS

Definite diagnosis of pulmonary embolism will require a combination of the techniques described. When clinical suspicion has been aroused, the immediate test of electrocardiogram, chest x-ray, and arterial blood gases should be obtained. Although these tests are primarily useful for diagnosis of associated or alternative conditions, they often provide additional supportive information for diagnosing pulmonary embolism. If normal, they do not exclude the diagnosis. Arterial punctures do carry the risk of serious bleeding if the patient is subsequently anticoagulated; thus, femoral punctures should be avoided and maximal pressure applied to puncture points. A routine blood count is appropriate, but an effort to get coagulation or enzyme data is not worthwhile for diagnosis.

The following are the options for further evaluation when another explanation for the patient's signs and symptoms is not found from the tests:

1. If the patient does *not* have significant pulmonary pathology, a lung scan should be obtained.

a. If the lung perfusion scan is normal, the diagnosis of embolism is excluded.
b. If the lung perfusion scan is interpreted by several experienced observers as "high probability of pulmonary embolism" and the clinical picture strongly supports that diagnosis, angiography need not be obtained and treatment should begin.
c. If the lung perfusion scan is read as medium or high probability of pulmonary embolism or it is read as high probability, but the clinical picture is confusing, angiography should be obtained. Alternatively, if there are signs of deep venous thrombosis, venography can be used and anticoagulation instituted on the basis of a positive study. If the venogram is negative, pulmonary angiography is necessary to establish a diagnosis.

2. If the patient has significant pulmonary pathology (infiltrate, congestive heart failure, atelectasis, emphysema), angiography need not be preceded by a pefusion lung scan in all cases. (Again, venography may substitute for either lung scan or pulmonary angiography if positive). Our angiographers prefer to have a perfusion scan available, if only as a road map for selective angiography and thereby reduce the morbidity of scan angiography. In some institutions, experience with ventilation–perfusion scans may make it reasonable to get that test where objective evidence of underlying lung disease is present. Only one area of clear ventilation–perfusion mismatch is necessary to suggest a high probability of pulmonary embolism. (See Chapters 3 and 4.)
3. Some patients with suspected emboli should have angiography immediately, as previously described (emergency procedure contemplated, contraindication to anticoagulation).

When angiography is done, if possible, right heart pressures should be obtained for prognostic information.

REFERENCES

1. Gorham LW: A study of pulmonary embolism. Arch Intern Med 108:8–90; 189–207; 418–426, 1961
2. The urokinase pulmonary embolism trial. Circulation 47:(Suppl II):1–108, 1973
3. Urokinase-streptokinase embolism trial phase 2 results. JAMA 229:1606–1613, 1974
4. Bell WR, Simon TL, DeMets DL: The clinical features of submassive and massive pulmonary emboli. Am J Med 62:355–360, 1977
5. McIntyre KM, Sasahara A: Determinants of cardio-vascular response to pulmonary embolism, in Moser KM and Stein M (eds): Pulmonary Thromboembolism. Chicago, Yearbook Medical Publishers, 1973, 144–159
6. Szucs MM, Brooks HL, Grossman W, et al: Diagnostic sensitivity of laboratory findings in acute pulmonary embolism. Ann Intern Med 74:161–166, 1971

7. Kafer FR: Respiratory function in pulmonary thromboembolic disease. Am J Med 47:904–915, 1969
8. Wacker WEC, Rosenthal M, Snodgrass PJ, et al: Diagnosis of pulmonary embolism and infarction. JAMA 178:8–13, 1961
9. Konttinen A, Somer H, Auvinen S: Serum enzymes and isoenzymes. Arch Intern Med 133:243–246, 1974
10. Light RW, Bell WR: LDH and fibrinogen-fibrin degradation products in pulmonary embolism. Arch Intern Med 133:372–375, 1974
11. Gallus AS, Hirsh J, Gent M: Relevance of preoperative and postoperative blood test to postoperative leg vein thrombosis. Lancet 2:805–809, 1973
12. Ruckley CV, Dan PC, Leitch AG, et al: Serum fibrin-fibrinogen degradation products associated with post-operative pulmonary embolism and venous thrombosis. Br Med J 4:395–398, 1970
13. Wilson JE, Frankel EP, Pierce AK, et al: Spontaneous fibrinolysis in pulmonary embolism. J Clin Invest 50:474–480, 1971
14. Rickman FD, Handin R, Howe JP, et al: Fibrin split products in acute pulmonary embolism. J Clin Invest 50:474–480, 1971
15. Jones DRB, Ruckley CV, Owens R, et al: Serum fibrin-fibrinogen degradation products after experimental pulmonary embolism. Br J Surg 61:811–813, 1974
16. Cade J, Hirsh J, Regoeczi E: Mechanisms for elevated fibrin-fibrinogen degradation products in acute experimental pulmonary embolism. Blood 45:563–568, 1975
17. Gurewich V, Hume M, Patrick M: The laboratory diagnosis of venous thromboembolic disease by measurement of fibrinogen-fibrin degradation products and fibrin monomer. Chest 64:585–590, 1973
18. Wood EH, Prentice CRM, and McNicol GP: Association of fibrinogen-fibrin related antigen with post-operative deep vein thrombosis and systemic complications. Lancet 1:166–169, 1972
19. Nossel HL: Radioimmunoassay of fibrinopeptides in relation to intravascular coagulation and thrombosis. N Engl J Med 295:428–432, 1976
20. Steele P, Weily HS, Genton E: Platelet survival and adhesiveness in recurrent venous thrombosis. N Engl J Med 288:1148–1152, 1972
21. Harker LA, Slichter SJ: Arterial and venous thromboembolism: Kinetic characterization and evaluation of therapy. Thromb Diath Haemorrh 31:188–203, 1974
22. Moore S, Pepper DS, Cash JD: The isolation and characterization of a platelet-specific β-globulin (β-thromboglobulin) and the detection of antiurokinase and antiplasmin released from thrombin aggregated washed human platelets. Biochem Biophys Acta 379:360–369, 1975
23. Ludlam CA, Moore S, Bolton AE, et al: The release of a human platelet specific protein measured by a radioimmunoassay. Thromb Res 6:543–548, 1975
24. Bosnjakovic VB, Jankovic BD, Horvat J, et al: Radio-labelled antihuman fibrin antibody: A new thrombus-detecting agent. Lancet 1:452–454, 1977
25. Walsh PN: The effect of dilution of plasma on coagulation. The significance of the dilution-activation phenomenon for the study of platelet coagulant activities. Br J Haematol 22:219–236, 1972
26. Walsh PN: The role of platelets in the contact phase of blood coagulation. Br J Haematol 22:237–254, 1972

27. Walsh PN: Platelet coagulant activities and hemostasis: A hypothesis. Blood 43:597–605, 1974
28. King JB, Joffe SN: The prediction of post-operative deep vein thrombosis, using a newly described test of platelet function. Thromb Diath Haemorrh 32:502–509, 1974
29. Yin ET, Wessler S, Stoll PJ: Biological properties of the naturally occurring plasma inhibitor to activated factor X. J Biol Chem 246:3703–3711, 1971
30. Yin ET, Wessler S, Stoll PJ: Identity of plasma-activated factor X inhibitor with antithrombin III and heparin cofactor. J Biol Chem 246:3712–3719, 1971
31. McIntyre KM, Sasahara AA, Littman D: Relation of the electrocardiogram to hemodynamic alterations in pulmonary embolism. Am J Cardiol 30:205–210, 1972
32. Spodick DH: Electrocardiographic response to pulmonary embolism. Am J Cardiol 30:695–699, 1972
33. Stein PD, Dalen JE, McIntyre KM, et al: The electrocardiogram in acute pulmonary embolism. Prog Cardiovasc Dis 17:247–257, 1975
34. Kelly MJ, Elliot LP: The radiologic evaluation of the patient with suspected pulmonary thromboembolic disease. Med Clin North Am 59:3–36, 1974
35. Moses DC, Silver TM, Bookstein JT: The complementary roles of chest radiography lung scanning and selective pulmonary angiography in the diagnosis of pulmonary embolism. Circulation 49:179–188, 1974
36. Simon M: Plain film and angiographic aspects of pulmonary embolism, in Moser KM and Stein M (eds): Pulmonary Thromboembolism. Chicago, Yearbook Medical Publishers, 1973, 197–215
37. McIntyre KM, Sasahara AA: The hemodynamic response to pulmonary embolism in patients without prior cardiopulmonary disease. Am J Cardiol 28:285–294, 1971
38. Quinn JC, Head LR: Radioisotope photoscanning in pulmonary disease. J Nucl Med 7:1–22, 1966
39. Wagner HN Jr: Lung scanning in pulmonary embolism. Bull Physiopathol Respir (Nancy) 6:65–98, 1970
40. Secker-Walker RH, Siegel BA: The use of nuclear medicine in the diagnosis of lung disease. Radiol Clin North Am 11:215–241, 1973
41. Mishkin FS, Johnson PM: The role of lung imaging in pulmonary embolism. Postgrad Med J 49:487–502, 1973
42. Seriff NS, Khan F, Lazo BJ: Acute respiratory failure. Current concepts of pathophysiology and management. Med Clin North Am 57:1539–1550, 1973
43. Schorn D: Aids in the diagnosis of pulmonary embolism. S Afr Med J 47:1951–1952, 1973
44. Anderson TMcD Jr, Mall JC, Hoffer PB et al: Efficacy of emergency radionuclide perfusion lung studies. Radiology 120:125–130, 1976
45. Friedman WF, Braunwald E: Alterations in regional pulmonary blood flow in mitral valve disease by radioisotope scanning. Circulation 34:363–376, 1966
46. Gluck MC, Moser KM: Pulmonary artery agenesis. Diagnosis with ventilation and perfusion scintiphotography. Circulation 41:859–867, 1970
47. Poulose KP, Reba RC, Gilday DL, et al: Diagnosis of pulmonary embolism. A correlative study of the clinical, scan, and angiographic findings. Br Med J 3:67–71, 1970

48. James AE Jr, Cooper M, White RI, et al: Perfusion changes on lung scans in patients with congestive heart failure. Radiology 100:99–106, 1971
49. Moser KM, Longo AM, Ashburn WL, et al: Spurious scintiphotographic recurrence of pulmonary emboli. Am J Med 55:434–443, 1973
50. Haynie TP, Hendrick CK, Schreiber MH: Diagnosis of pulmonary embolism and infarction by photoscanning. J Nucl Med 6:613–631, 1965
51. Shoop JD: Why do a lung scan? JAMA 229:567–570, 1974
52. Wagner HN, Sabiston DC, McAfee JG, et al: Diagnosis of massive pulmonary embolism in man by radioisotopic scanning. N Engl J Med 271:377–384, 1964
53. Tow DE, Wagner HN: Recovery of pulmonary arterial blood flow in patients with pulmonary embolism. N Engl J Med 276:1053–1059, 1967
54. Bell WR, Simon TL: A comparative analysis of pulmonary perfusion scans with pulmonary angiograms. Am Heart J 92:700–706, 1976
55. Walsh PN, Greenspan RH, Simon M, et al: An angiographic severity index for pulmonary embolism. Circulation (Suppl II): 101–108, 1973
56. Greenspan RH: Does a normal isotope perfusion scan exclude pulmonary embolism? Invest Radiol 8:97–99, 1973
57. Griner PF: Blood pleural effusion following pulmonary infarction. JAMA 202:947–949, 1967
58. Stjernholm MR, Landis GA, Marcus FI, et al: Perfusion and ventilation radioisotope lung scans in stenosis of the pulmonary artery and its branches. Am Heart J 78:37–42, 1969
59. Loken MK, Westgate HD: Evaluation of pulmonary function using Xenon-133 and the scintillation camera. Am J Roentgenol Radium Ther Nucl Med 4:835–843, 1967
60. Haddon RWT, Wood DE, Woolf CR: The measurement of ventilation/perfusion relationships using multiple crystal rectilinear scanner. Can Med Assoc J 99:1111–1119, 1968
61. Marks A, Chervony I, Lankford R, et al: Ventilation-perfusion relationships in humans measured by scintillation scanning. J Nucl Med 9:450–456, 1968
62. Newhouse MT, Wright FJ, Ingham GK, et al: Use of scintillation camera and ^{135}Xenon for study of topographic pulmonary function. Respir Physiol 4:141–153, 1968
63. Moser KM, Guisan M, Cuomo A, et al: Differentiation of pulmonary vascular from parenchymal diseases by ventilation/perfusion scintiphotography. Ann Intern Med 75:597–605, 1971
64. Wagner HN JR, Lopes-Majano V, Langan JK, et al: Radioactive Xenon in the differential diagnosis of pulmonary embolism. Radiology 91:1168–1174, 1968
65. Medina JR, Lillehei JP, Loken MK, et al: Use of the scintillation anger camera and Xenon (Xe 133) in the study of chronic obstructive lung disease. JAMA 208:985–991, 1969
66. DeNardo GL, Goodwin DA, Rarasini R, et al: The ventilatory lung scan in the diagnosis of pulmonary embolism. N Engl J Med 282:1334–1336, 1970
67. Jacobstein JG: ^{133}Xe ventilation scanning immediately following the ^{99m}TC perfusion scan. J Nucl Med 15:964–968, 1974
68. Epstein J, Taylor A, Alasraki N, et al: Acute pulmonary embolus associated with transient ventilatory defect: case report. J Nucl Med 16:1017–1020, 1975
69. Yao JST, Henkin RE, Conn J Jr, et al: Combined isotope venography and lung scanning. Arch Surg 107:146–151, 1973

70. Williams O, Lyall J, Vernon M, et al: Ventilation-perfusion lung scanning for pulmonary emboli. Br Med J 1:600–602, 1974
71. Browse NL, Clemenson G, Croft DN: Fibrinogen-detectable thrombosis in the legs and pulmonary embolism. Br Med J 1:603–604, 1974
72. Kessler RM, McNeil BJ: Impaired ventilation in a patient with angiographically demonstrated pulmonary emboli. Radiology 114:111–112, 1975
73. Anderson PO, Rujanavech N, Secker-Walker RH, et al: The role of ^{133}Xe ventilation studies in the scintigraphic detection of pulmonary embolism. Radiology 120:633–640, 1976
74. McNeil BJ: A diagnostic strategy using ventilation-perfusion studies in patients suspect for pulmonary embolism. J Nucl Med 17:613–616, 1976
75. Bookstein JJ: Segmental arteriography in pulmonary embolism. Radiology 93:1007–1012, 1969
76. Bookstein JJ: Pulmonary thromboembolism with emphasis on angiographic-pathologic correlation. Semin Roentgenol 5:291–305, 1970
77. Dalen JE, Brooks HL, Johnson LW et al: Pulmonary angiography in acute pulmonary embolism: Indications, techniques, and results in 367 patients. Am Heart J 81:175–185, 1971
78. Brookstein JJ, Silver TM: The angiographic differential diagnosis of acute pulmonary embolism. Radiology 110:25–33, 1974
79. Tow DE: Thrombus detection: here and now. J Nucl Med 18:90–92, 1977
80. Gilday DL, Poulose KP, DeLand FH: Accuracy of detection of pulmonary embolism by lung scanning correlated with pulmonary angiography. Am J Roentgenol 115:732–738, 1972
81. Moser KM: Pulmonary embolism. Am Rev Respir Dis 115:829–852, 1977

EDITORS' NOTE

The diagnostic approach to the patient with diffuse pulmonary disease varies from physician to physician and from institution to institution, and rightfully so.

At The Johns Hopkins Hospital we have been fortunate in having a team of physicians practicing clinical chest medicine and a long tradition in believing that the secret of success in the care of the patient is in caring for the patient.

Chapters 12 and 13 are designed to be used together to aid the physician engaged in the clinical practice of medicine by providing a practical guide for the investigation of patients with undiagnosed diffuse pulmonary diseases. They are not intended to replace a manual of roentgenological interpretation or a textbook of internal medicine; the emphasis is on adult patients.

The logical starting point in the differential diagnosis of diffuse pulmonary disease is a careful clinical analysis of the whole patient. In arriving at an organized approach, the clinical setting must be used to illuminate the shadows of the chest roentgenogram. Only under these circumstances can we hope to correlate the roentgenographic appearance with the pathophysiology underlying such patterns.

Under most practical circumstances individual patients with diffuse pulmonary disease can be broadly divided into two large categories: the relatively "normal" host and the host who is significantly compromised by an underlying disease or medication. The first category is further conveniently divided by the duration of symptoms. These may be relatively acute or chronic. The duration of these symptoms clearly dictates the speed and need for the physician to determine the appropriate diagnosis. The second major category of patients with diffuse lung disease consists of individuals whose host defenses are grossly altered by some underlying disease or therapy. The compromised host not only is subject to unusual diseases, but he or she often presents with a common disease in an uncommon fashion. Such patients may quickly deteriorate following any minor insult. Therefore a rapid diagnosis is always indicated. Chapter 12 deals with diagnosing diffuse lung disease in the unaltered host, i.e., all patients except those with hematological malignancies or marked immunologic suppression. The chapter is subdivided into the approach to the patient with diffuse pulmonary disease of relatively short duration and the approach to the patient with signs and symptoms present for over 6 weeks. Chapter 13 deals with diagnosis in the patient who has altered host defense mechanisms. The differential diagnosis under these circumstances is as unique as the patient and can be examined separately.

Warren R. Summer, M.D.
Peter B. Terry, M.D.

12

Approach to the Patient with Diffuse Lung Disease

APPROACH TO ACUTE DIFFUSE LUNG DISEASE IN THE PREVIOUSLY "WELL" HOST

Introduction

The patient with acute respiratory symptoms and a chest roentgenogram demonstrating diffuse increased radiodensity is one of the most alarming and intriguing occurrences in all clinical medicine. The designation of diffuse pulmonary disease implies a widespread alteration in the morphology of the lung. By convention this also implies a chest roentgenogram with relatively uniform involvement of both lungs, although several areas may demonstrate slightly more or less involvement. This definition excludes multiple segmental and lobar pneumonias and multiple discrete nodular lesions.

The approach to patients with diffuse lung disease depends on a number of value judgments. Unfortunately, the information necessary for precise decision analysis is almost always lacking.[1] The initial approach is dictated by the physician's clinical diagnostic impression. Does he have a good idea what is producing the pathophysiologic alterations, or is he completely confused? The clinical history most frequently produces the important diagnostic clues. The radiologic characteristics of the pulmonary infiltrates often provide considerable diagnostic assistance, and in some instances the chest roentgenogram, with a compatible clinical history and/or laboratory support, may be essentially diagnostic.

One of the most important considerations in approaching the diagnosis is the time course of the disease. Is it evolving over hours or days? Has the process stabilized, or is it relentlessly progressive? Another factor, almost as important in the diagnostic processes as the time course, is the condition of the patient. Does the patient appear too ill to undergo a potentially complicated procedure, or is he relatively stable? Will therapy differ substantially with different specific etiologies, or is a therapeutic modality likely to help regardless of the differential diagnosis? A further important consideration is the expected gain that the patient may receive by having his condition diagnosed. These considerations may be therapeutic or in some situations even economic. The last consideration in the approach to the patient with diffuse lung disease is the diagnostic modalities available at a particular institution. Some facilities have bronchoscopists expert at transbronchial lung biopsy, whereas others have individuals with extensive experience using transthoracic needle techniques. The choice of the best procedure ultimately hinges on what is available at the time the patient needs the diagnostic study.

The clinical characteristics of a patient with diffuse lung disease may be extremely variable. Since the diagnostic approach interrelates with the patient's signs and symptoms, we will describe a number of representative pictures that illustrate most aspects leading to appropriate diagnosis and therapy.

Clinical Portrait of Patients with Acute Respiratory Distress Syndrome

The most common characteristic of acute diffuse lung disease is the sudden onset of tachypnea following some seemingly unrelated event. Most of these cases can be grouped under the heading of "adult respiratory distress syndrome" (ARDS).[2,3] Where a particular etiologic event can be identified as the most likely cause of the respiratory insufficiency, it should be incorporated in the diagnosis[4]—for example, ARDS associated with acute gastric acid aspiration. Several reviews on this subject have appeared in the literature.[5,6] We see 25 to 30 patients each year with the clinical and/or morphological characteristics of ARDS at The Johns Hopkins Hospital.

Table 12-1 lists the disorders commonly associated with this syndrome. Some of these conditions, such as a fractured femur, drug overdose, or acute pancreatitis, brought the patient to the hospital, whereas others suddenly developed as an untoward complication of hospitalization for some other reason (aspiration following normal delivery of a healthy child, septicemia after a seemingly uneventful transurethral resection). The patient's respiratory status is usually initially stable following the clinical conditions listed in Table 12-1. If respiratory symptoms are noted, the patient often responds to minor supportive respiratory therapy such as suctioning or supplementing oxygen. Several hours up to two days later the patient is noticed to be tachypneic. Within hours this rapidly proceeds to marked respiratory distress. Cyanosis is usually obvious unless the patient is anemic. Frothy, pink to burgundy colored sputum may be observed. The

Table 12-1
Disorders Associated with Adult Respiratory Distress Syndrome

Aspiration
Gastric contents
Freshwater and saltwater
Hydrocarbons
Central Nervous System
Trauma
Anoxia
Increased intracranial pressure
Drug Overdose
Acetylsalicylic acid
Heroin
Methadone
Propoxyphene
Barbiturate
Hematologic Alterations
Disseminated intravascular coagulation
Massive blood transfusion
Postcardiopulmonary bypass
Infection
Sepsis (gram positive or negative)
Viral pneumonia
TB
Peritonitis
Inhalation of Toxins
Oxygen
Smoke
Corrosive chemicals (NO_2, CL_2, NI_3, phosgene, cadmium)
Metabolic Disorders
Pancreatitis
Uremia
Shock
Any etiology (rare in cardiogenic)
Trauma
Fat emboli
Lung contusion (after cardiopulmonary resuscitation)
Nonthoracic

chest roentgenogram reveals a nonspecific diffuse "alveolar" filling process (Fig. 12-1).[7-10]

Staub has demonstrated that the first place edema accumulates in the lungs is in the interstitial space round vessels and bronchi.[5] This is because during lung inflation the pressure is lowest within the interstitium of the lung. Peribronchial cuffing and perivascular haze are therefore early roentgenographic findings in pulmonary edema, whatever the cause of the

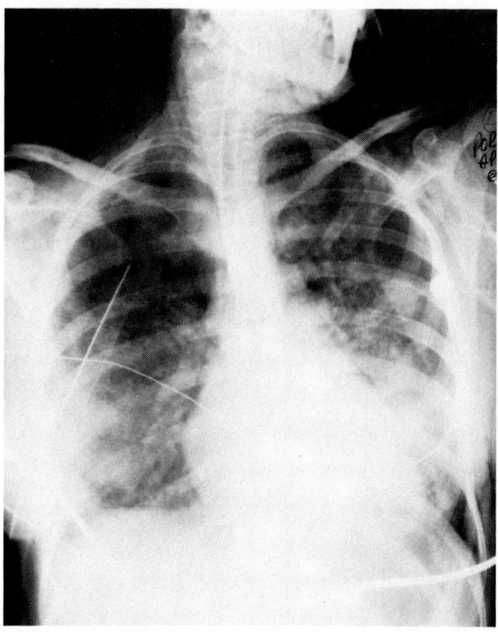

Fig. 12-1. Twenty-nine-year-old white female, with massive aspiration of gastric contents following normal spontaneous delivery of a term pregnancy. Patient developed classic adult respiratory distress syndrome with typical complications of pneumothorax (corrected by chest tube) in right side of chest and subcutaneous emphysema.

fluid accumulation.[11] Obviously, the presence of an enlarged heart should always suggest pulmonary edema of cardiac origin. If the heart is grossly enlarged there is rarely any problem in differential diagnosis. However, up to 20 percent of patients with acute cardiogenic pulmonary edema and the majority of patients with acute fluid overload have a normal-sized heart.[12,13] Pulmonary edema of cardiac origin frequently spares the apices and the costophrenic angles. The densities also tend to fade out (become less radiodense) as they approach the periphery. Intraseptal edema with the production of Kerley's lines and pleural effusions is common.

In the majority of patients with ARDS, the pulmonary capillary endothelium is diffusely injured.[4] The radiographic densities appear uniformly distributed throughout the lung and are monotonously homogeneous. Fissures are not displaced and scattered ill-defined radiolucencies are not observed. In acute diffuse lung disease, therefore, any inhomogeneity in the alveolar densities should suggest an etiology other than ARDS. Intraseptal edema has not, in our experience, been seen in the adult respiratory distress syndrome. That is probably because the diffuse alveolar disease obscures interstitial lines. In spite of the lack of a study evaluating the presence or absence of Kerley's lines in ARDS, our prejudices suggest that when gross septal lines can be observed on x-ray the patient probably has congestive heart failure, lymphangitic spread of carcinoma, or rarely, viral pneumonia. Pleural effusions are also infrequent in patients with ARDS.

The arterial blood gases demonstrate severe hypoxemia with a moderately lowered Pco_2. The vital capacity is markedly reduced as are all lung volumes. The severe hypoxemia must be corrected as soon as possible. Once the hypoxia is improved and the patient is stabilized it is appropriate to proceed with other diagnostic tests. The need for other specific laboratory studies should depend on the circumstances associated with the development of acute respiratory failure such as disseminated intravascular coagulation[14] (See Table 12-1) and the need to rule out congestive heart failure or possible infection.

Heart failure is the predominant problem mistaken for the adult respiratory distress syndrome. This is especially true under circumstances where the patient is very ill and it is technically impossible to obtain a good P-A chest roentgenogram. Fluid overload is a common contributing factor. If the cardiac silhouette is thought to be enlarged or the patient is elderly, it is often wise to determine the pulmonary capillary wedge pressure with a Swan-Ganz catheter.[15] Hypoalbuminemia should be ruled out as a factor contributing to diffuse lung disease and, when present, should be corrected as soon as possible.[13] The need for albumin may be determined through measurements of serum oncotic pressure. Further invasive diagnostic evaluation is rarely indicated unless the patient appears septic and material from potential sites of infection has not been examined. In the presence of fever and no obvious systemic cause, a sputum, or preferably transtracheal, aspiration should be carefully examined and cultured for routine aerobic and anaerobic bacteria.[16] Patients with aspiration pneumonia are often febrile without evidence of infection.[17] Concomitant pleural effusion should be examined if easily obtainable without substantial risk of producing a pneumothorax. When 400–600 cc of pleural fluid is present, it can usually be aspirated without difficulty. In the absence of fever, pleural effusions may be initially observed without aspiration. Frequently, other body fluids (cerebral spinal, peritoneal) should also be examined if there is evidence of altered consciousness, nuchal rigidity, or peritonitis. A determination of the hematocrit, red blood morphology, white blood cell count and differential, as well as the number of platelets is helpful in both diagnosis and therapy. Under most circumstances, electrolytes, blood urea nitrogen, glucose, calcium, and prothrombin time are also measured. Frequently, serial chest films are necessary since pneumothorax and bacterial superinfection are common during the hospital course and often are difficult to assess clinically.[18] Vigorous therapy is indicated, since the mortality in the adult respiratory distress syndrome is approximately 50 percent.

Therapy revolves around physical or physiological recruitment of lung units for gas exchange. This is accomplished by increasing lung volume through the use of some form of positive end-expiratory pressure (PEEP).[19] Immediately following the institution of this type of therapy the chest film often looks substantially improved. The improvement results from the increased lung volume associated with therapy rather than clearing of the pulmonary edema. Depending on the etiology and extent of injury, the chest film may clear gradually over several hours to days or it may remain relatively unchanged until the patient expires. (For example, we have seen heroin pulmonary edema completely clear roentgenographically in less than six hours). Any worsening in the chest film after initial clearing taken at the same level of end-expiratory pressure suggests fluid overload or superimposed infection.

Several acute lung diseases resulting in pulmonary edema are associated with the inhalation of noxious gases.[20] No diagnostic approach other than an understanding of the precipitating events and assessment of extent of injury is necessary. In the unconscious patient found at the scene of a fire, it is often impossible to distinguish the contributing effects of gastric acid aspiration from inhalation injury.

Clinical Portrait of Patients with Acute Diffuse Lung Disease Other Than the Adult Respiratory Distress Syndrome

PRESENTATION

The patient with acute diffuse lung disease which does not fit into the categories of ARDS presents a much more difficult and challenging diagnostic problem. These are usually patients with a more protracted course. The patient often reports a variety of mild to moderate respiratory symptoms for days to weeks preceding the onset of significant dyspnea. Cough, a frequent complaint, is often nonproductive and occasionally is associated with symptoms compatible with upper respiratory infection. Low-grade fever may have been noted. In some patients generalized malaise has been experienced for days to weeks. Weight loss is occasionally noted. Once dyspnea is present, it is usually progressive and severe. Some individuals have small amounts of hemoptysis, and others report pleuritic pain or retrosternal burning.

The chest film reveals diffuse "alveolar" or interstitial lung disease.[7,21,22] Often the roentgenographic pattern is that of a mixed alveolar and interstitial infiltrate. On a number of occasions the same disease may produce either a predominant alveolar or interstitial pattern, depending on the stage of morphologic change at the time of presentation.[7] The diagnostic possibilities are enormous and are listed in Tables 12-2 and 12-3. Some of these conditions can be considered an adult respiratory distress syndrome (viral pneumonia), whereas others, distinctly different, are mistakenly as-

Table 12-2
Differential Diagnosis of "Alveolar" or Acinar Filling Diffuse Lung Disease on the Basis of Predominant Substances Filling the Air Spaces (Modified from Goodman[a])

PUS	
Bacterial	
Pseudomonas	Hospital-acquired, usually during artificial ventilation.
Tuberculosis	Acinar-nodose or miliary. Has been mistaken for ARDS.
H. Influenza	Underlying chronic bronchitis in all
Strep. pneumonia	Saw on case
Viral	
Influenza	Seasonal community or family association, onset usually abrupt.
Adeno	Sporadic, not seasonal
Varicella zoster	Usually have skin lesions
Herpes simplex	Often have lesion of skin or mucous membrane
Measles	Measles
Cytomegalovirus	Almost always in compromised host
Mycoplasma	Young adults; little seasonal predominance, onset usually insidious.
Rickettsial	With Rocky Mountain Spotted Fever & DIC
Fungal	
Histoplasma	Exposure to pigeon, bat, chicken, construction entailing large earth-moving projects.
Aspergilla	Recovery from respiratory failure. Usually still on ventilation or recently removed.
Nocardia	Diffuse disease always in compromised host.
Parasitic disease	Malaria
Protozoan	Pneumocystis carinii
BLOOD	
Contusions	Trauma may be relatively slight without fractured ribs, rarely extreme enough to give diffuse picture. Common after cardiac resuscitation
Multiple infarction	Pleuritic pain common
Goodpasture's syndrome	Renal involvement frequent at onset. Anemia present
Idiopathic pulmonary hemosiderosis	Significant renal involvement absent. Anemia present
Blood dyscrasis-anticoagulants	Hemoptysis may be absent
EDEMA	
Transudate	
Congestive heart failure or left atrial hypertension	Many etiologies

Table 12-2 *(continued)*

Exudate	
ARDS	Seen in Table 12-1
Aspiration pneumonia	Altered consciousness; nasogastric tube in place, frequently mixed alveolar interstitial pattern
Heroin pneumonia	Often delayed in onset, may clear in 24 hours
Near drowning	History; must be differentiated from aspiration of gastric contents
Extrinsic allergic alveolitis	Recurrent problems without previous diagnosis. Exposure not always clear. Air conditioning, humidifier systems may be source
Drug reaction	See Table 12-4. Only these drugs causing acute reactions
Transfusion reaction	WBC antigen and antibody probable cause of pulmonary infiltrate
CELLS	
Sarcoidosis	Relatively well for extent of infiltration
Bronchioalveolar cell CA	Sputum may be copious
Loeffler's	Asymptomatic or minor respiratory and constitutional symptoms. Limited duration of illness. Eosinophilia
Chronic eosinophilic pneumonia	Usually febrile and dyspnic. Eosinophilia absent in 20–30%
Lymphoma	Rare presentation, usually disease obvious elsewhere
Idiopathic pulmonary interstitial pneumonia	Uncommon presentation for this entity Often febrile WBC normal
Histiocytosis	
Metastatic carcinoma	History of previous cancer may be remote and thought to be cured
MUCOPOLYSACCHARIDE	
Alveolar proteinosis	Sputum may be characteristic often only slightly symptomatic. Thought to have recurrent pneumonia
CALCIUM	
Alveolar microlithiosis	Rare—familial—asymptomatic
FOREIGN MATERIAL	
Contrast media	
Lipoid pneumonia	Exogenous—chronic constipation Endogenous—recent history of clinical pneumonia

Table 12-3
Differential Diagnosis of Diffuse Interstitial Lung Disease on the Basis of Localization and Pattern of Morphological Changes in Structures Other Than Air (Modified from Johnson, et al.,[21])

Common	Uncommon	Rare
CONNECTIVE TISSUE PATTERN [Reticular, reticulo-nodular, linear]		
Idiopathic interstitial fibrosis	SLE	Amyloid
Rheumatoid arthritis	Mixed connective tissue	Lymphangiomyomatosis
Scleroderma	Polyarteritis	Tuberous sclerosis
Pneumoconoiosis (asbestosis, silicosis, etc.)	Polymyositis	Neurofibromatosis
Sarcoid	Hemotologic lymphoma	Hemolytic uremic syndrome
Pneumocystis (in altered host)	Hodgkins	Angioimmunoblastic lymphadenopathy
	Waldenstrom macroglobulinemia	IPH
	Alveolar proteinosis	Multiple pulmonary emboli
	Extrinsic allergic alveolitis	
	Viral & Mycoplasma	
	Histiocytosis X	
	Hypersensitivity drugs	
LYMPHATIC PATTERN [Septal lines (b predominantly, a & c occasionally)]		
Interstitial pulmonary edema	Viral	
Lymphangitic carcinoma	Idiopathic fibrosis	
BRONCHIAL PATTERN [Parallel lines, ring shadows]		
	Bronchiectasis	
	Chronic bronchitis	
VASCULAR PATTERN [Prominent vessels w/2° increased flow or distention]		
Mitral stenosis	Polycythemia 1° or 2°	R-L cardiac shunting without severe pulmonary hypertension
DEPOSITION PATTERN: ABNORMAL MATERIAL AND GRANULOMATOUS INFLAMMATION [Miliary, nodular, reticulonodular (late)]		
Tuberculosis	Hemosiderosis	Hematogenous spread of

Table 12-3 (*continued*)

Histoplasmosis	(Mitral stenosis or are welding)	Staphylococcus
Carcinoma (melanoma, Hodgkins, thyroid, renal)	Extrinsic alveolitis (early)	Salmonella
Pneumoconiosis (siderosis, Beryl-liosis)	Bronchoalveolar carcinoma	Coccidiomycosis
Sarcoidosis		Blastomycosis
		Cryptococcus
		Nocardiosis
		Histiocytosis
		Amyloid
		Rheumatoid arthritis
		Idiopathic interstitial fibrosis (early)

sumed to be of similar pathogenesis because of the roentgenographic picture of extensive diffuse lung disease.[23]

The reader will note that the adult respiratory distress syndrome is a condition of sudden onset in which the precipitous nature of the event is common. It is a disorder of various background which is not diagnosed on the basis of the roentgenogram alone, however. Rather, it is a syndrome of diffuse x-ray changes married with a clinical picture of dyspnea and severe hypoxemia not corrected by supplemental oxygen.

The majority of patients with acute diffuse lung disease other than ARDS are suffering from a distinct entity requiring relatively specific therapy. The diseases in Tables 12-2 and 12-3 also include a number of common conditions that may have an extremely atypical roentgenographic pattern and are not commonly considered with acute diffuse lung disease. The diagnosis of these diseases, for example, multiple pulmonary emboli, can result in major therapeutic changes with potentially excellent results.

We see approximately 20 patients a year who fall into this category of acute to subacute diffuse lung disease. Although there are no symptoms that are in themselves diagnostic, the approach to this group of patients can be greatly aided by a more careful scrutiny of the general historical picture just previously outlined. Complete evaluation should begin as soon as the patient is stabilized and adequately oxygenated. The most important diagnostic step is to seek carefully for historical evidence of infection. A history of recent fever and especially shaking chills (true rigors) suggests bacterial infections, although influenza and psittacosis-like organisms may produce overt chills. The patient may report a nonspecific upper respiratory infection or recent contact at work or at home with people experiencing upper respiratory complaints. Community and seasonally associated illnesses may also be suggestive of infection. Most diffuse pulmonary diseases that begin outside of the hospital and are rapidly progressive over a few days are infectious. Purulent or rusty sputum suggest bacterial infection, but may be occasionally associated with viral and mycoplasma infection.[24] However, high fever and shaking chills may be associated with exposure to a variety of organic antigens. On most occasions an avocational or occupational history suggests the possibility of an extrinsic allergic alveolitis. Exposures to antigenic thermophilic actinomycetes in office and home air conditioning or humidification systems have been reported as the source of acute pulmonary hypersensitivity reactions.[25,26] Diagnosis under these circumstances is rarely made during the first attack. Diffuse pulmonary infiltrates may be very unimpressive and only appreciated in retrospect after subsequent chest films are examined. Fever and dyspnea in these latter patients gradually subsides over 24–48 hours. When antibiotic therapy is prescribed, the cessation of symptoms is always attributed to this regimen. The diagnosis of an extrinsic alveolitis should be considered during the first relapse associated with the typical uncomplicated course characteristic of the hypersensitivity pneumonitis. It should be remembered that absence of blood eosinophilia is the rule in most hypersensitivity pneumonias. Epidemiologic evidence is helpful when a number of closely associated individuals have been known to suffer from similar symptoms.

In this group of patients with diffuse disease, gross hemoptysis may be seen with pulmonary vasculitis, Goodpasture's syndrome, and idiopathic pulmonary hemosiderosis (IPH). On a number of occasions we have observed hemoptysis secondary to pulmonary infarction which acutely precipitates severe respiratory symptoms in patients with chronic but relatively asymptomatic diffuse disease. This has occurred recently in our experience in two patients with moderate diffuse rheumatoid lung disease, one patient with metastatic pulmonary carcinoma, and one with diffuse idiopathic pulmonary fibrosis. Without access to a recent baseline chest roentgenogram, the sudden onset of hemoptysis and dyspnea in the patient with diffuse pulmonary densities is usually assumed to be an acute primary pulmonary process. Acute pulmonary emboli or infarction complicating more chronic diffuse lung disease should always be considered a diagnostic possibility.

Retrosternal discomfort or burning aggravated by cough is typical of severe Influenzae pneumonia. Actual precordial pain suggests myocardial infarction and possible cardiogenic pulmonary edema. A previous history of ASHD is a helpful historical clue and is recorded in two-third of patients with cardiogenic pulmonary edema. A history of orthopnea, paroxysmal nocturnal dyspnea, or pedal edema is also frequently reported. We have seen a number of patients with minor precordial pain or recent myocardial infarction who suddenly develop severe shortness of breath and have an x-ray of diffuse pulmonary disease. These patients often have a normal-sized heart on x-ray examination. As a result the pulmonary edema produced by acute papillary muscle dysfunction or rupture (Fig. 12-2) is often mistakenly diagnosed as aspiration or viral pneumonia.

Pleuritic pain is generally uncommon in acute diffuse lung disease. It can be associated with bacterial or viral infection, collagen vascular disease, pulmonary infarction, or, rarely, carcinoma and idiopathic interstitial fibrosis. A history of unilateral leg edema or calf tenderness should always

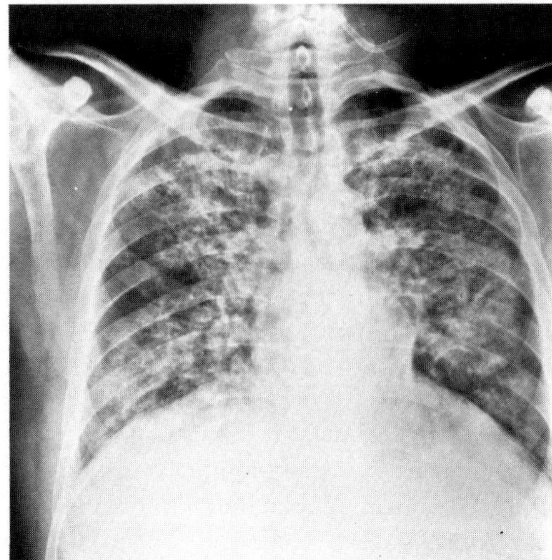

Fig. 12-2. Patient is a 45-year-old white male with acute inferior myocardial infarction who was transferred to The Johns Hopkins Hospital. Chest film showed diffused pulmonary densities. Mean pulmonary capillary wedge pressure was 16 mm Hg. Patient had an uneventful recovery, but the chest film failed to resolve over a five-week period without change in heart size. Subsequent complete cardiac catheterization showed papillary muscle dysfunction with severe mitral incompetence with "v" waves of 40 mm Hg and a mean wedge of 20 mm Hg. Replacement of the mitral valve results in prompt improvement in pulmonary infiltrates.

suggest pulmonary emboli as either the primary or a complicating condition causing pleuritic pain.

Severe headache is characteristic of acute mycoplasma infection and psittacosis, but can be associated with any high degree of fever.

A brief history of polyuria may be seen with secondary diabetes insipidus due to granulomatous involvement of the hypothalamus in eosinophilic granuloma or sarcoidosis. Polyuria may rarely result from hypercalcemia associated with sarcoidosis. We have seen oliguria at the presentation of diffuse Wegener's granulomatosis, but rarely at the onset of Goodpasture's syndrome.

A history of easy bruising, ecchymosis or petechiae over the lower extremities may be noticed prior to the shortness of breath seen with a number of diseases associated with thrombocytopenia or other disorders of coagulation. Alveolar proteinosis has an increased association with acute leukemia, whereas systemic lupus erythematosus may present with an immune thrombocytopenia. In patients with known thrombocytopenia, viral pneumonia may progress to extensive hemorrhagic pneumonitis.

A history of tender skin lesions (erythema nodosum) usually in the anterior aspect of the lower legs is reported most often in sarcoidosis.[27] These lesions may also present in histoplasmosis, coccidiodomycosis, and primary tuberculosis. Other subtle skin changes may be early manifestations of scleroderma and dermatomyositis. Polyarthralgia may be a nonspecific complaint associated with early collagen vascular disease or idiopathic interstitial fibrosis.

Significant weight loss may be reported with tuberculosis, metastatic carcinoma, and, occasionally, idiopathic interstitial fibrosis. The marked lack of symptoms in the presence of impressive diffuse pulmonary involvement is almost diagnostic of sarcoidosis. Alveolar proteinosis, Leoffler's pneumonia, and eosinophilic granuloma of the lung may also be associated with a paucity of clinical symptoms despite impressive roentgenographic abnormality.

A past history of cancer should always suggest metastatic or lymphangitic spread to the lung. Cancer may cause the rapid development of dyspnea with diffuse lung infiltrate. We have seen rapid progression of dyspnea due to metastasis months to years after the primary diagnosis of a variety of apparent ''localized'' malignancies. This is especially true with melanomas (Fig. 12-3) and sarcomas, but also carcinoma of the stomach, cervix, endometrium, prostate, and pancreas. A history of radiation therapy should always raise the possibility of radiation pneumonitis or fibrosis, even when the roentgenographic changes are diffuse.[28] Occasionally, latent radiation injury can be activated by steroid withdrawal.[29]

A variety of medications has been reported to cause acute pulmonary disease (Table 12-4). Although an allergic history is suggestive of this type of hypersensitivity lung disease, a clear-cut documentation of prior hypersensitivity reactions usually is not obtained. In addition, the patient should be questioned for unintentional or intentional aspirin overdosage, since this medication has been associated with acute noncardiogenic pulmonary edema.[30]

A family history of pulmonary disease may be an early clue to the diagnosis of sarcoidosis, idiopathic interstitial fibrosis, or hypersensitivity pneumonitis.[31,32]

Knowledge of the list of organic antigens and means of exposure associated with extrinsic allergic alveolitis is helpful in acute diffuse lung disease.[33] Activities such as caving, picnicking, cleaning chicken coops, or heavy construction work are often linked to acute histoplasmosis. A past history of tuberculosis or exposure should be sought in all patients with acute respiratory disease. Recent travel to tropical climates might aid the physician in suspecting diffuse pulmonary eosinophilia. These patients usually have only minor respiratory symptoms. Patients with underlying abnormalities such as sickle cell anemia or SC anemia have a tendency to develop overwhelming diffuse mycoplasma pneumonia.

Patients already in the hospital under assisted ventilation are prime candidates to develop acute diffuse lung disease secondary to Klebsiella or

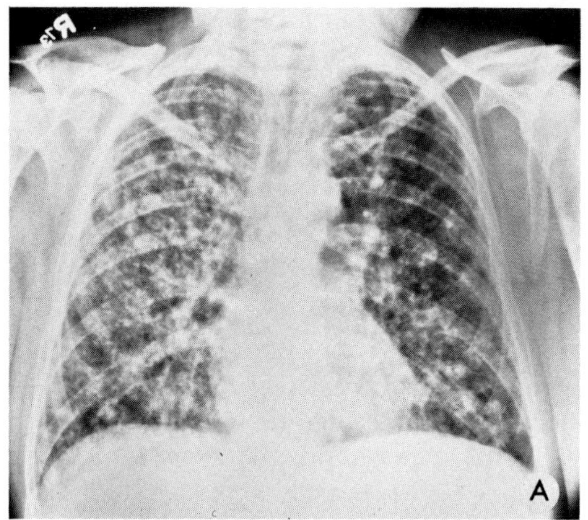

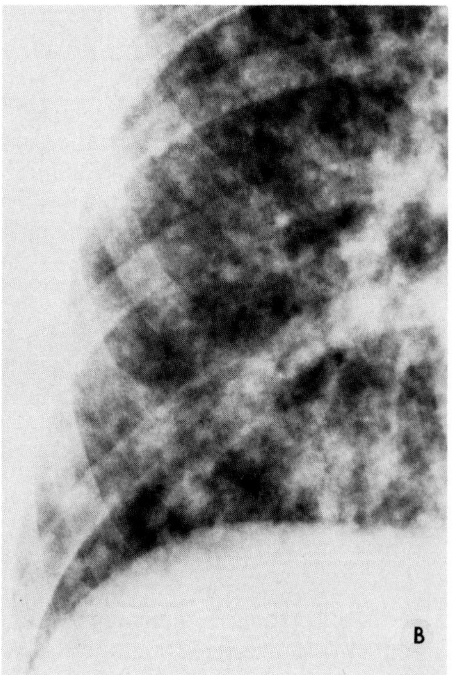

Fig. 12-3. (A) Thirty-two-year-old male with a malignant melanoma removed from his lower back three months prior to admission. Chest film was normal at that time. The patient presents with increasing shortness of breath and nonproductive cough. Chest film shows diffuse pulmonary nodules. (B) Metastatic nodules are usually of various size, but may be miliary in appearance.

Table 12-4
Pulmonary Hypersensitivity Reactions Secondary to Prescribed Drug Administration (Nonchemotherapeutic Agents)

Drug	Acute	Chronic
Nitrofuradantoin	x	x
Sulfonamide	x	
Para-aminosalicylate	x	
Pronestyl*	x	
Hydralazine		
Penicillin-Ampicillin	x	
Haxamathonium-Pentolinium		x
Methylsergide		x
Hydrochlorathiazide	x	
Gold		x
Dilantin	x	?

* A large number of medications have been associated with a lupus like pleural pulmonary disease.[113]

Pseudomonas pneumonia.[34] We have seen two cases of *Aspergilla fumigatus* develop in patients recovering from respiratory failure secondary to severe COPD.

PHYSICAL EXAMINATION

The physical examination is occasionally helpful in the differential diagnosis of acute diffuse pulmonary disease. The presence of elevated neck veins or dependent edema is more often seen with cardiogenic pulmonary edema than with acute cor pulmonale. Skin changes compatible with scleroderma (loss of hair over dorsal aspect of fingers), lupus erythematosus (peringuinal erythema, butterfly rash), erythema nodosum, or generalized vasculitis are of great assistance when present.

Anemia with resulting conjunctival and mucosal pallor is usually present with Goodpasture's syndrome, IPH, or other pulmonary-renal syndromes. Opacified maxillary sinuses or nasal lesions are present in 90 percent of patients with generalized Wegener's granulomatosis, but a limited form of this disease with predominately lower respiratory lesions occurs.[35] The presence of hepatomegaly and/or splenomegaly should suggest disseminated tuberculosis, sarcoidosis, or some hematologic disorder. Hepatomegaly alone may be present in metastatic carcinoma.

Neurologic manifestations such as peripheral neuropathy are commonly reported in lymphomatoid granulomatosis and polyarteritis but may be present in Wegener's granulomatosis.

The presence of muscular weakness is uncommon in acute diffuse pulmonary diseases, but tenderness strongly suggests sarcoidosis or vasculitis and is relatively unheard of in disseminated tuberculosis.[36] Diffuse lymphadenopathy would be most likely in sarcoidosis, whereas regional enlargements can be seen with hematologic diseases, metastatic carcinoma, and SLE.

Clubbing is generally uncommon in the patients currently under discussion. The association of hypotension or acute vascular collapse is rare in diffuse lung disease except during septicemia or far-advanced miliary tuberculosis and disseminated histoplasmosis. A small focus of skin infection may be found as the only cause of acute staphylococcal septicemia.

LABORATORY EXAMINATION

Laboratory tests in patients with acute diffuse pulmonary disease are of limited value and rarely provide the definitive answer. If some systemic disease is discovered, such as leukemia or lymphoma, the diffuse pulmonary disease is still more likely to be infectious.

White blood cell counts above 20,000 suggest bacterial infection, whereas normal or low white counts are most frequently seen in sarcoidosis or tuberculosis. Severe leukopenia (WBC 1000) may be seen with diffuse bacterial pneumonia. This occurs more commonly in alcoholics. Anemia is expected in Goodpasture's, hemolytic uremic syndromes, idiopathic pulmonary hemosiderosis, and pulmonary hemorrhage, but may be found in SLE, metastatic carcinoma, leukemia, lymphoma, Waldenstrom's macroglubulinemia, mycoplasma pneumonia, or miliary tuberculosis.

Many chemical abnormalities can lead to early suspicion of the appropriate diagnosis. Slightly elevated liver enzymes and alkaline phosphatase levels are common in miliary tuberculosis, whereas an isolated alkaline phosphatase abnormality is most frequently seen with sarcoidosis and metastatic disease. Bilirubin is uncommonly elevated, except with severe hemolysis and common duct obstruction from tumor. Hyponatremia secondary to an inappropriate serum antidiuretic hormone level is relatively common in disseminated tuberculosis. Elevated gamma globulins in the serum are too nonspecific to help initial decisions, and immunoelectrophoresis is rarely available for several days. The erythrocyte sedimentation rate is completely nonspecific under these circumstances. The intermediate skin test for tuberculosis can be expected to be positive with tuberculosis and should be placed intradermally during the initial examination. Positive reactions are seen in 60–80 percent of patients with miliary tuberculosis. A negative second-strength skin test essentially rules out tuberculosis except in the most severely debilitated individuals. Other delayed skins tests are usually positive in specific acute fungal disease,[37] but are of questionable significance since they may reflect previous infection.

Serologic tests for acute fungal disease are elevated 80 percent of the time in histoplasmosis and coccidiodomycosis.[38A] Immunologic demonstrations of cryptococcal polysaccharide capsular antigen in serum is simple, rapid, and conclusive proof of pulmonary cryptococsis.[38B] Antinuclear antibodies are elevated in high titer with SLE and mixed collagen vascular disease, but are present in a few patients with idiopathic fibrosis. The presence of overt LE cells in the blood or pleural effusion is essentially diagnostic of SLE. Complement-fixing antibodies to mycoplasma pneumonia are positive in half the patients with acute disease but may also be elevated in sarcoidosis and other disease.[24] A test to determine circulating antiglomerular basement membrane antibodies has recently been described for the diagnosis of Goodpasture's disease.[39]

Arterial blood gases should always be measured in these patients since severe hypoxemia should be expected. The severity of the hypoxemia has little direct relationship to any specific etiology but helps to determine the timing for diagnosis and probably correlates inversely with the initial prognosis. The P_{CO_2} is usually below 40 mm Hg, since some degree of hyperventilation is almost always present. The pH is moderately alkaline due to acute or only partially compensated respiratory alkalosis. If the pH is compensated, it suggests that the underlying process has been present for some days. An acid pH has an ominous connotation being most commonly found in superimposed lactic acidosis secondary to septicemia or cardiovascular collapse. Pulmonary edema following acute heart failure is commonly associated with a metabolic acidosis.[40]

Pulmonary function tests add little to differential diagnosis in acute diffuse pulmonary disease but are valuable in assessing prognosis and response to treatment. These patients are often too ill to cooperate for complete studies. A simple spirogram should reveal a moderate to marked restrictive defect with only occasional trivial airway obstruction.

In IPH the diffusing capacity has recently been reported to be more normal than expected for the degree of restrictive disease. It was postulated that the blood in the alveoli takes up carbon monoxide giving false high values of gas exchange. Radioactively labeled iron may be injected into patients and the rate of disappearance may be followed over several weeks to diagnose IPH. In this diagnostic study, the hematocrit is found to fall while labeled total body iron remains unchanged because it is sequestered in the lung.

ROENTGENOGRAPHIC PATTERNS

The chest roentgenogram is necessary to distinguish diffuse pulmonary disease, as defined in this chapter, from many causes of acute shortness of breath such as lobar pneumonia, pulmonary emphysema, or asthma. Yet the pattern of parenchymal densities in the chest film rarely distinguishes one specific abnormality from another. The diagnostic possibilities listed in Tables 12-2 and 12-3 allow the physician to consider the majority of etiologies. The separation of "alveolar" and interstitial disease where possible may occasionally allow a more focused approach. Diffuse disease that fades or decreases in radiodensity at the periphery of the lung is typical of the pulmonary edema secondary to congestive heart failure, whereas the reverse, a diffuse density that is diminished in opacity toward the hilum, has been described in chronic eosinophilic pneumonia.[41] Idiopathic interstitial fibrosis, lymphomatoid granulomatosis,[42] and collagen vascular disease may appear as acute diffuse disease with a tendency toward basilar involvement, whereas miliary tuberculosis (nodular or mixed alveolar-nodular), and eosinophilic granuloma often show a predilection for upper lobe involvement. On occasion a typical roentgenographic pattern associated with knowledge of patient's age, race, system complex, and physical examination may be essentially diagnostic. An example of such an extremely typical, but unusual pattern is nodular alveolar sarcoid[43] (see Chapter 8, Case 3, Figs. 8-10, 8-11).

Concomitant pleural effusions are commonly observed when diffuse pulmonary disease is associated with CHF, SLE, drug hypersensitivity, and malignancy. Effusions may be present in a host of other diffuse disease such as tuberculosis, bacterial, viral or mycoplasma pneumonia, pulmonary infarction, lymphoma, idiopathic fibrosis, and even sarcoidosis.[44–46] Small effusions are often overlooked. In addition, pleural effusions are frequently infrapulmonary in these patients. Therefore, lateral decubitus films are often helpful in establishing the presence of fluid and should be obtained if there is any suspicion of effusion. Nodular pleural involvement is very suggestive of primary or metastatic neoplasms (Fig. 12-4), lymphomas, or mesotheliomas, which can also produce diffuse parenchymal infiltration.

With diffuse disease it is often difficult to evaluate the hilum. Tomography may be helpful to determine if adenopathy is actually present. Hilar adenopathy suggests sarcoid or lymphoma but has been reported in diffuse pneumonia due to viral, fungal, or tuberculous infection as well as primary and metastatic tumors. In addition, tomography may demonstrate a cavity that would otherwise be overlooked. Such information may help in the diagnosis of diseases such as tuberculosis and Wegener's granulomatosis. Tomography is often not practical in acutely ill patients with marked hypoxemia.

A number of patients with diffuse lung disease experience acute onset of symptoms in the presence of a relatively coarse reticular nodular roentgenographic pattern typical of longstanding interstitial disease (idiopathic fibrosis, rheumatoid arthritis, scleroderma, etc). Old films are often not immediately available to document the duration of the pulmonary infiltrate and should be obtained as soon as possible. Symptoms may have been unimpressive until a few days or hours before admission. In our experience, pneumonia, pneumothorax, or pulmonary emboli are the major precipitating causes of sudden dyspnea in these patients. Purulent sputum, high fever, leukocytosis, or an area of dense consolidation generally points to acute infection. Hemoptysis is rare with thromboemboli, since a major infarct probably would have resulted in death of the patient with chronic interstitial disease. Since lung scans are difficult to interpret with diffuse parenchymal disease, venography or impedence phlebography is very helpful in determin-

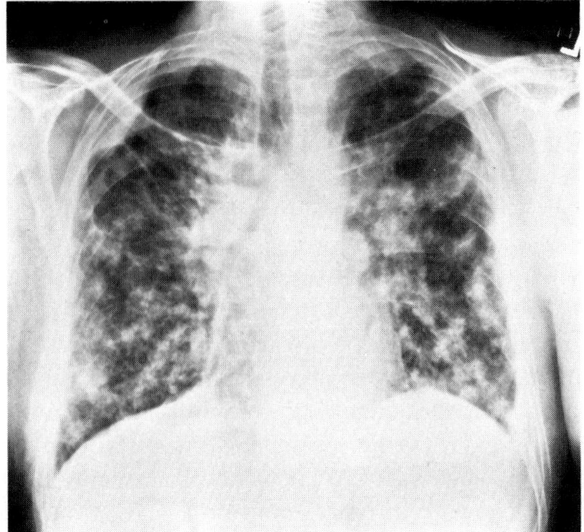

Fig. 12-4. Thirty-five-year-old male, 10 years post-radiotherapy for Stage I Hodgkin's disease discovered in a cervical node. Patient presents with one-month history of progressive shortness of breath and fatigue with 24 hours history of left pleuritic pain. Chest film shows patchy infiltrates, bilateral small pleural effusions, hilar adenopathy and multiple pleural based densities. Patient developed ostenogenic-sarcoma in the sternum following radiation therapy. The tumor metastasized to produce diffuse mediastinal, parenchymal and pleural masses.

ing the need for anticoagulation.[47] If positive, appropriate therapy should be instituted as long as there is no relative or absolute contraindication for anticoagulation. With negative or unavailable venography, a lung scan is still of considerable value. The lung scan is often surprisingly normal in the presence of uncomplicated interstitial fibrosis and, with the exception of sarcoidosis, should not show large or segmental perfusion defects.[48] The concomitant ventilation scan is extremely helpful under these circumstances. If a reasonable possibility of pulmonary emboli still exists after interpretation of the ventilation–perfusion scan, pulmonary angiogram should be performed with selective injection in an area of decreased perfusion most likely to demonstrate a pulmonary embolus. We have recently seen two patients with relatively asymptomatic rheumatoid disease who had a history of acute shortness of breath caused by superimposed thromboembolism. In addition, tumor embolism from a variety of glandular carcinomas may precipitate the admission of a patient with diffuse parenchymal roentgenographic densities secondary to unsuspected lymphangitic spread of carcinoma.

DIAGNOSTIC APPROACH

The initial approach to a patient with acute diffuse lung disease is to narrow the clinical possibilities through all the routine methods previously outlined. The process of elimination, however, often falls short of a precise answer. Some authorities would suggest immediately following Sutton's law.[49] This law was originally popularized in medicine by Dr. William Dock. Dr. Dock, a distinguished professor of Medicine at the State University of New York, observed that, on occasion, every test would be performed except the most obvious. He would quote Willie Sutton, the bank robber, who, when asked why he always robbed banks replied, "Because that's where the money is." Many physicians have interpreted that to mean that if the disease is in a particular area, go right to that area for diagnosis.[50,51] In the case of acute diffuse lung disease, this often implies lung biopsy. However, diagnostic shortcuts are not always practical or rewarding when viewed in conjunction with a risk–benefit ratio. Diagnostic shortcuts may often be harmful. In a number of instances even lung tissue, the "heart" of the problem, may return without specific information. For example, viral pneumonias often yield only compatible tissue and may be confused with idiopathic fibrosis, radiation pneumonitis, extrinsic allergic alveolitis, or drug hypersensitivity reactions. Upon examination of the lung containing alveolar hemorrhage, the pathologist may be unable to distinguish between contusion, aspiration of blood, infarction, or idiopathic pulmonary hemosiderosis. A stepwise diagnostic approach is often safer for the patient and is more likely ultimately to yield an adequate diagnosis. This is not to imply that all noninvasive studies should be performed before lung biopsy or to suggest that financial factors should not be considered. It should be stressed, however that the best care of the patient may result from the caring for the patient.

Our approach is first to rule out the possibility of a treatable infection. Evaluation primarily includes obtaining material for appropriate stain and culture from multiple easily accessible sites, such as sputum, blood, urine, and skin. Appropriate evaluation of sputum is not easily acquired.[52] The quality of gram stain as performed on the wards of most hospitals is often less than adequate to make a decision whether to treat with antibiotics or which specific antibiotic should be used. If the patient has a history of bronchitis, recent antibiotic treatment, or is not bringing up sputum, a transtracheal aspiration may be very helpful. It is an extremely low-risk procedure that can yield definitive bacteriologic information.[53,54] False-positive results may occur with this procedure, but false-negative studies are rare.[55] Transtracheal brushing for culture as described by Aisner in the leukopenic patient is rarely necessary, since adequate material is usually obtained by transtracheal aspiration in the presence of suppuration.[56] A small amount of nonbacteriostatic saline may be lavaged through the transtracheal catheter if a good specimen is not obtained by simple aspiration. Material for bacterial culture obtained by bronchoscopy is frequently contaminated by normal mouth flora.[57] In addition, topical anesthetics may be inhibitory to pathogen.[58] Bronchoscopy may also result in transient bacteremia or frank septicemia when vigorously used in suppurative disease.[59] Sputum should be examined for cellular detail. This may be initially performed by the physician with a fresh wet smear to determine if there are large numbers of neutrophils or eosinophils. In viral respiratory infections, one can often find desquamated ciliated bronchial epithelial cells which have extensive cytoplasmic degeneration. This phenomenon is known as ciliocytophthoria and can usually be rapidly recognized on a fresh smear because of the cells' extremely motile cilia.[52] If tumor or fungus is a possibility, sputum should be sent to the cytopathology laboratory (see Chapter 6). A sputum should also be smeared for acid-fast bacilli and a fresh early-morning preparation subsequently sent to the mycobacteriology laboratory. Serology for cold agglutinins and mycoplasma complement-fixing titers are most rewarding in young adults or patients with sickle cell anemia. Acute viral serology is rarely helpful, but nasal washing, and throat cultures or smears for indirect fluorescent antibody studies may be helpful where available.[60]

If a pleural effusion is present it should be aspirated. Careful analysis may determine the etiology of the diffuse lung disease or lead to appropriate further diagnostic or therapeutic trials. Our experience with pleural effusions at The Johns Hopkins Hospital has recently been reviewed extensively by Light et al.[44] Occasionally, the fluid may be a transudate suggesting for the first time that the patient is in CHF. In the absence of trauma, a bloody effusion is almost always due to cancer or pulmonary embolus. Pleural fluid cytology yields diagnostically abnormal cells in 70 percent of malignant effusions. A bloody, clear, or cloudy exudative effusion often requires a subsequent pleural biopsy. This low-risk study should be performed before any further invasive procedures. Palpable lymph nodes or suspicious skin lesions should also be biopsied early.

The gradual pursuit of invasive tests must be chosen with care in an attempt to obtain the most information with the least risk. Transbronchial lung biopsy or brushing techniques will yield the appropriate diagnosis in up to 80 percent of cases of diffuse lung disease[61] (see Chapter 8). These techniques should be used with caution if the patient is severely hypoxic. Clotting and bleeding parameters should be checked and corrected if abnormal. Thrombocytopenia is very uncommon in such patients. Prolonged prothrombin time is the most commonly seen abnormality and when below 60 percent clearly increases the risk of significant hemorrhagic complication.[62] Transbronchial techniques with the fiberoptic bronchoscope are relatively safe and effective for a variety of diagnostic possibilities.[63] Mycobacterium and fungi can be retrieved by simple brush biopsy in most cases.[64] Transbronchial biopsy has a very high yield in the diagnosis of

Stage II and III sarcoidosis,[65] bronchoalveolar carcinoma, and lymphangitic carcinoma. Transbronchial biopsies are also very useful in the diagnosis of acute lymphomatous involvement of the lung.[66]

Acute idiopathic interstitial fibrosis is a relatively rare disease.[67] Although transbronchial biopsy in appropriate hands usually correlates very well with open lung biopsy,[61,68] its role in this condition has only recently been evaluated. If all sputum cultures and stains for pathogenic bacteria are negative, making infections very unlikely, an adequate tissue specimen compatible with idiopathic interstitial fibrosis is sufficient to allow a trial of steroid therapy. Failure to respond should place the diagnosis of acute fibrosing alveolitis in some doubt. We have made the diagnosis of acute fibrosing alveolitis on the basis of "adequate" tissue from transbronchial and needle biopsy only to find out at a later time that the patient had metastatic carcinoma. Review of the necropsy slides in these cases revealed considerable fibrosis surrounding malignant lesions, which explains the sampling error. Because of this experience, rebiopsy or open-lung biopsy should be considered if the patient continues to deteriorate on steroid therapy.

When collagen vascular disease is considered as a likely possibility in the differential diagnosis of diffuse lung disease, lung biopsy (even open) rarely gives definitive information. Renal or skin biopsies with special staining techniques are certainly more specific for a variety of collagen vascular diseases.

The use of transthoracic percutaneous biopsy or needle aspiration techniques has waxed and waned in popularity for diffuse lung disease.[69] Most groups have shifted to the transbronchial biopsy approach for diffuse disease because of the lower morbidity. Needle aspiration, a relatively safe procedure, is excellent for bacteriologic culture and plays a greater role in the compromised host where diffuse disease is more often of bacterial etiology.[62] Transthoracic needle biopsy certainly has a role in the hands of skilled operators. Greater safety is often ensured by performing the procedure under fluoroscopic guidance to avoid large pulmonary vessels. Several pieces of tissue should be obtained and distributed among the bacteriology, mycology, cytology, and pathology laboratories.

Open-lung biopsy is the ultimate procedure in the diagnosis of acute diffuse lung disease.[70,71] This can be performed through a limited thoractomy with excellent results and relatively low risk.[72] Overall morbidity and mortality may be higher than other invasive diagnostic procedures; however, there are no randomized studies comparing clinical risks between open and closed procedures in similar patients. The more confusing and atypical the case presentation, the more tissue is needed to allow a confident diagnostic impression by the clinician and pathologist. Under certain circumstances a relatively large piece of tissue is needed to obtain special studies. This is particularly true where Goodpasture's syndrome and extrinsic allergic alveolitis are considered likely possibilities. Specific immunofluorescent staining has been reported in the lung in these conditions.[73,74] The more urgent the clinical condition, the more necessary to determine the diagnosis at the earliest moment. Open-lung biopsy usually supplies this information before the incision is closed.

The optimum method of diagnosis must be individualized for each patient. The relative merits and risks of these procedures are often difficult to assess. A definitive diagnosis is not always necessary, and the physician must often resist his intellectual curiosity and fastidious training to always "know" the answer. Cautious diagnostic neglect after a best guess has been made may often be the best approach. We have seen a number of patients with acute diffuse lung disease progressively improve on their own without a diagnosis or specific therapy. This may leave the physician puzzled, but he certainly should be happy for the patient. The disease may recur, and the physician may even be eventually embarrassed by missing an uncommon disease such as extrinsic allergic alveolitis. Certainly, only a minority of cases should lack a definitive diagnosis. When the whole clinical picture is analyzed with the patient's well being as the primary concern, however, the physician will rarely if ever be embarrassed, and all parties may be better off not being able to file the chest film in a teaching collection.

APPROACH TO CHRONIC DIFFUSE LUNG DISEASE IN THE PREVIOUSLY "WELL" HOST

Introduction

The patient with diffuse pulmonary disease which has been present for some uncertain length of time always presents a difficult diagnostic problem. This is not surprising since the history of dyspnea and cough is nonspecific, the physical findings are often limited to the lung, and the chest x-ray is rarely unique. Of the large number of etiological conditions listed by Buechner capable of producing diffuse lung disease,[75] only about half produce characteristic bronchial secretions, physical findings, detectable extrapulmonary manifestations, or laboratory derangements. Gaensler has stated that only 10 percent of patients with diffuse pulmonary disease are diagnosed after history and physical examination alone, and one-third of the patients remain undiagnosed after prolonged investigation, including a variety of nonpulmonary biopsies.[70] It is a medical axiom that a specific diagnosis allows more intelligent treatment and humane planning for the patient's future. However, a specific diagnosis is too often the only concern of the physician. The exact diagnosis may not be possible in a variety of symptomatic complaints that a patient acquires, and specific answers often relieve the physician's anxieties more than they help to remove the patient's symptoms. The mature clinician strives to ensure an accurate diagnosis, but on occasion is willing to try to maintain his patient in optimum health based only on a firm clinical impression.

With regard to the dilemma of chronic pulmonary disease, most authorities subscribe to some preconceived stepwise diagnostic approach, whereas a few champions of Sutton's law would proceed to open-lung biopsy after initial history; physical, and laboratory results return without specific diagnostic leads. We are proponents of a limited but thorough diagnostic search prior to proceeding with any invasive procedures. We have no set format except for a complete history and physical examination. All other diagnostic studies are individualized. Subsequent procedures are determined by their potential yield in relation to the patient's needs. Because socioeconomic factors are increasingly more important in medicine today, hospital work-up should not be unnecessarily long or utilize all associated hospital facilities simply because they are available. On the other hand, financial factors should not be considered the major motivating force to proceed rapidly to open lung biopsy.[50] Chronic diffuse disease usually progresses relatively slowly, so that the entire work-up may proceed without haste—with intermissions for careful observation, depending on the severity of symptoms.

Clinical Portrait of Patients with Chronic Diffuse Lung Disease

PRESENTATION

Essentially all patients with chronic diffuse lung disease have dyspnea. Often it is first noted with moderate exercise, but eventually shortness of breath is present during activities of daily living. Dyspnea may be the only symptom in approximately 25 percent of patients. Cough is the next most frequent complaint. It is usually associated with dyspnea but may be the most troublesome or primary symptom in 10 percent of cases. The cough is characteristically nonproductive, but, may be associated with nonpurulent phlegm and even hemoptysis.

Nonspecific symptoms of weight loss, fatigue, and night sweats are not infrequent, but are usually unimpressive except when the diffuse pulmonary disease is secondary to neoplastic disease or tuberculosis. Vague chest discomfort is often present, but significant pleuritic pain is rare.[76] Mild joint pains are common in a number of conditions, but true arthritis is only present with collagen vascular disease. Specific destructive joint abnormalities are characteristic of rheumatoid arthritis. Other symptoms suggesting collagen vascular disease include erythematous eruptions, dysphagia, Raynaud's phenomenon, lymphadenopathy, CNS abnormalities, and muscle weakness. Patients with collagen vascular disease are more often female and are younger on the average than patients with idiopathic fibrosis. Sudden SOB from a spontaneous pneumothorax is a well-reported presentation of sarcoidosis and eosinophilic granuloma, but it can occur with any diffuse lung disease. Repeated pneumothorax and hemoptysis in women of child-bearing age should suggest lymphangioleiomyomatosis. An acute unrelated upper respiratory illness prompts a modest number of patients to seek a physician. Fever, usually not present, suggests infection, malignancy, or collagen vascular disease. Fever is also seen in sarcoidosis and radiation pneumonitis. Superimposed acute events necessitating clinical attention such as thrombotic or tumor emboli in patients with lymphagitic pulmonary carcinoma or a superimposed nocardia infection with alveolar proteinosis have been reported in the literature.[77,78] Approximately 10 percent of the patients will have no respiratory symptoms but are referred after a routine chest film is interpreted as being abnormal.

A history of industrial exposure is extremely important in the ultimate diagnosis of chronic diffuse pulmonary disease. Frequently, individuals do not appreciate that in their occupations there are many inorganic substances that are present in high enough concentrations to produce pulmonary injury. The physician should clarify all industrial contacts. The patient may have limited knowledge of exposure to metal fumes or "toxic dusts." The patient's union representative, plant physician, or pulmonary specialist may be a useful source of specific information on injurious environmental exposure. It is often helpful to consult an industrial hygienist if the patient's occupation is unfamiliar to the physician. Often a particular occupation has an exposure related to the work environment rather than the job activity. For example, industrial plumbers often come into an environment that is contaminated with asbestos from the removal of insulation just prior to their arrival. Careful detective work may be helpful, but often lung biopsy must be performed to determine industrial lung injury. A number of inorganic dusts are known to result in chronic pulmonary fibrosis.[74]

What is less well appreciated is that family members are also at risk from low-dose, long-term exposure to toxic or sensitizing foreign materials. This is because the foreign material may be brought into the house by a person who never develops pulmonary symptoms. Such an association has been suggested to occur between the pigeon breeder and the person who cleans his clothes.[79]

The family history may be of some value in suggesting idiopathic interstitial fibrosis,[80] sarcoidosis[81] or hypersensitivity pneumonitis.[33]

PHYSICAL EXAMINATION

Tachypnea is the only physical finding that is common to the majority of these patients. Clubbing is reported in up to 70 percent of patients with idiopathic pulmonary fibrosis (IPF) while hypertrophic osteoarthropathy is rare.[67,76] Auscultation usually reveals râles or rhonchi in these patients. The presence of pan-inspiratory "crackling" râles and clubbing in a patient with radiographic chronic diffuse lung disease is so characteristic of idiopathic interstitial fibrosis that Scadding feels further biopsy confirmation is probably unnecessary in these patients.[82] Cyanosis is commonly reported. The extent of the hypoxemia is usually underestimated on clinical grounds, but occasionally cyanosis is clinically suspected in patients with measured arterial oxygen saturation above 88 percent due to a mild erythrocytosis. Cardiac examination is usually normal. A number of patients with idiopathic pulmonary fibrosis will have evidence of an increased pulmonic valve closure sound which suggests the presence of pulmonary hypertension.[67,76] Signs of congestive failure such as elevated neck veins, hepatic congestion, and pedal edema are very late manifestations of an "end-stage lung." Other physical abnormalities can be observed when the pulmonary process is a manifestation of a systemic disease. Hepatomegaly is usually present in the patient with pulmonary lymphangitic carcinomatosis. Hepatosplenomegaly has frequently been described in sarcoidosis, Wegener's granulomatosis, lymphoma, amyloidosis, and systemic lupus erythematosus. Patients with severe fibrotic sarcoidosis often have chronic skin and bone changes. Evidence of vasculitis or arthritis are not infrequent with collagen vascular disease, whereas peripheral neuropathy would favor Wegener's or lymphomatoid granulomatosis, amyloidosis, and polyarteritis.

LABORATORY EXAMINATION

A number of laboratory tests that frequently are abnormal in these patients are unfortunately completely nonspecific. These include the erythrocyte sedimentation rate, total serum protein and albumin:globulin ratio. The hemoglobin is usually normal, but it may be nonspecifically decreased in any chronic disease. Very low hemoglobin levels suggest blood loss, hemolysis, or marrow replacement. The white blood cell counts may be low in sarcoidosis, tuberculosis, or primary hematologic disease. Absolute lymphopenia has been reported in Hodgkin's lymphoma and other malignancies. Increased eosinophils are not uncommon with periarteritis when it is associated with bronchospasm and other pulmonary manifestations. Moderate eosinophila is common with chronic eosinophilic pneumonia but may be seen with disseminated carcinomatosis, Hodgkin's disease, and sarcoidosis. Elevated eosinophil counts may be present with the diffuse pulmonary infiltrate of drug-related hypersensitivity, but are usually not elevated when pulmonary disease is due to inhalation of organic antigen.

Routine and special laboratory studies will document the most likely etiology in approximately 50 percent of patients with chronic diffuse pulmonary disease. Some of these diseases will require lung biopsy confirmation, whereas others cannot be expected to show specific pulmonary histology even in the presence of specific disease. For example, systemic lupus erythematosus or mixed collagen vascular disease will have high ANA titers. With SLE, however, one usually can document the presence of LE cells on appropriately prepared blood specimens. A lung biopsy will be much less specific than a skin or renal biopsy in these conditions[83] and should not be performed unless some additional information is needed prior to beginning therapy. Abnormal ANA and elevated rheumatoid factor has been described in idiopathic fibrosis. Although some series report a very high incidence of abnormal serologic findings, our experience is in keeping with the recent report of Crystal et al., which found a relatively low incidence of ANA or abnormal latex fixation titers.[76] When present in IPF, the ANA and rheumatoid factors are usually in low titer. A high frequency of circulating cryoimmunoglobulins has recently been reported in idiopathic fibrosis.[76] Elevated muscle enzymes are unique to polymyositis, dermatomyositis, and sarcoidosis. An elevated alkaline phosphatase may represent granulomatosus and metastatic liver disease or metastatic bone disease. An abnormal BSP test or elevated serum 5′ neucleotidase will differentiate liver from bone involvement. A bone or liver scan may help to localize lesions that can subsequently be biopsied for a definitive diagnosis. Without chemical or clinical evidence of liver disease, blind biopsies are no longer recommended for chronic diffuse lung disease.

Sputum should always be examined for acid-fact bacilli, fungal forms, and abnormal cytology. These are generally low-yield procedures in chronic diffuse pulmonary disease, but are without any risk to the patient and may pleasantly surprise the investigator. An intermediate skin test for tuberculosis is of value in excluding tuberculosis as well as deciding on whether INH is indicated in the future if the patient is subsequently placed on steroids. Fungal skin tests and serology may be positive but usually are not helpful subsequently in deciding on the specific diagnosis of active fungal infection. Serologic studies may be helpful in following responses to therapy once a particular fungus has been identified.[84]

Urine beryllium and a beryllium patch test should be obtained if an appropriate exposure can be elicited. If a patient with chronic diffuse lung disease is essentially asymptomatic, it may be advisable to insert a Kveim test for sarcoidosis and temporarily forego other diagnostic work-up. This skin test usually takes six weeks to complete but is extremely safe and operationally specific for sarcoidosis in the presence of a compatible clinical picture.[85] If the patient is ill and the physician is pressed for a therapeutic decision, it is not worthwhile to wait for the diagnostic information supplied by the Kveim test. The concomitant administration of steroids may prevent the development of intradermal noncaseating granuloma, resulting in false-negative results. Recently, biochemical measurements of serum lysozyme and serum angiotension-converting enzyme, which can be rapidly performed, have shown promise in confirming the diagnosis of sarcoidosis.[86]

An evaluation of carcinoembryonic antigen (CEA) may be helpful. Although there are many causes of false-positive tests, there are relatively few false-negative results in the presence of pulmonary carcinomatosis from sites such as the pancreas or other portions of the gastrointestinal tract.[87] We have seen prostatic carcinoma present as diffuse pulmonary disease, and therefore usually obtain an acid-phosphatase level in men over 60 even without other evidence of primary carcinoma (Fig. 12-5). A normal acid-phosphatase is found in 20 percent of cases with metastatic carcinoma of the prostate.[87B]

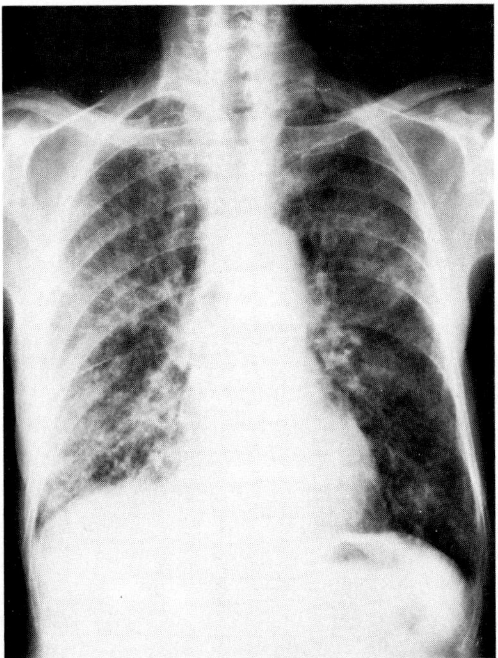

Fig. 12-5. Sixty-three-year-old male with two months' history of progressive cough and shortness of breath. Prostatic exam showed 1 cm hard nodule, acid phosphate was mildly elevated and multiple blastic lesions were observed in the pelvis. Chest film shows diffuse interstitial infiltrates and a small right sided pleural effusion. Pulmonary infiltrates improved dramatically after estrogen therapy.

Patients suspected of having an extrinsic allergic alveolitis, but without an occupational or known antigenic exposure, should have their home and, where possible, their work environment examined for the presence of thermophilic actinomycetes.[88] Serum samples should also be obtained from these patients and examined by the agar gel immunodiffusion method for precipitating antibodies to various antigens known to cause hypersensitivity pneumonitis.[74] Extracts of cultures of micro-organisms from the patient's environment may also be examined for antigen reactivity with the patient's serum.

Pleural effusion should always be diagnostically evaluated. The fluid in patients with chronic diffuse pulmonary disease is almost always an exudate with predominantly mononuclear cells unless there is concomitant heart failure. Bloody and chylos effusions are usually due to cancer. Serous effusions with pH below 7.30 and less than 5 percent mesothelial cells are most likely caused by tuberculosis.[89] A pleural fluid glucose 50 percent lower than a simultaneously drawn blood glucose usually indicates infection. Tuberculous effusions only occasionally produce low pleural fluid glucose, rarely less than 30 mg/ml. Rheumatoid arthritis is often characterized by a very low pleural fluid sugar, which is often less than 10 mg/100 ml in the presence of a normal blood glucose; however, we have seen a number of typical rheumatoid effusions with normal glucose levels. Long-standing malignant effusions may also result in a low pleural fluid glucose. In the presence of a low pleural fluid sugar, malignant effusions almost always have positive cytology, and infected effusions have micro-organisms on routine microscopic examination. The finding of an LE cell or an RA cell ("ragocyte" or polymorphornuclear leukocyte that contains cytoplasmic inclusion bodies thought to represent phagocytose rheumatoid factor) within the effusion is thought to be diagnostic of systemic lupus erythematosus or rheumatoid arthritis, respectively (see Chapter 6). At our institution pleural fluid cytology and pleural biopsy results in a diagnosis of malignancy in 80 percent of malignant effusions.[90] Culture of the biopsy for tuberculosis and histological examination for granuloma produce a positive diagnosis in over 80 percent of the cases of tuberculosis.[91] The yield of pleural biopsy is further increased in both malignant and granulomatous disease by obtaining specimens under direct vision with the use of a small endoscope.[92] Vasculitis may be observed in a rare biopsy specimen and may confirm the presence of angitis from drug or other etiologies.

PULMONARY FUNCTION TESTING

These patients have classical restrictive defects. The lung volumes are reduced, with the vital capacity most affected and the residual volume least altered. In far-advanced disease, there may be some mild obstructive changes caused by general anatomical airway distortion from severe fibrosis. Scleroderma and asbestosis are most likely to produce a significant combined obstructive and restrictive defect. A rare patient may have moderate dyspnea with only trivial reductions in lung volume. Diaphragmatic weakness has recently been reported in SLE and may contribute to the sensation of dyspnea in this condition.

The steady-state diffusing capacity ($DLCO_{SS}$) is almost always reduced in the presence of significant symptoms. However, the single-breath diffusing capacity ($DLCO_{SB}$) may occasionally be normal.[76] The reduced DLCO is caused by loss of alveolar capillary surface area, usually with destruction or obliteration of capillary bed.

The Po_2 may be at the lower limits of normal during the early course of the disease, but the alveolar-arterial oxygen gradient ($A\text{-}aO_2$) is almost always increased. The reduced arterial oxygen tension is due to perfusion of poorly ventilated lung units. In end-stage honeycomb lung, severe refractory hypoxia often develops secondary to fixed right-to-left intrapulmonary shunting. Mild to moderate hyperventilation with a compensated respiratory alkalosis is present in the majority of patients.

It is often difficult to correlate the degree of pulmonary function impair-

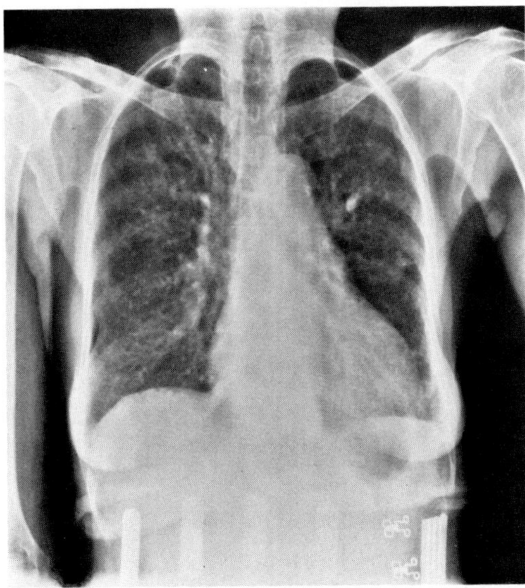

Fig. 12-6. Fifty-two-year-old black female with shortness of breath and cough of six months' duration increasing in severity. Chest film was interpreted as showing prominent pulmonary vascularity (note relative size of left upper lobe bronchus and companion vessel). ECG showed right ventricular hypertrophy. Cardiac catheterization demonstrated severe pulmonary hypertension. Pulmonary function test showed severe restriction and marked reduction in diffusing capacity. Pulmonary compliance was significantly reduced. Open lung biopsy revealed severe idiopathic interstitial fibrosis.

ment with the degree of parenchymal involvement observed morphologically. Crystal et al., have suggested that the elastic recoil of the lung at full inflation and the A-aO_2 gradient with a specified work load correlated best with the degree of underlying fibrosis found in idiopathic interstitial fibrosis.[76] In some cases there is a poor correlation between the extent of disease radiologically and the pulmonary function abnormalities. If the patient has dyspnea and the PFTs are reproducibly abnormal, it is extremely likely that an open-lung biopsy will demonstrate altered morphology despite a normal chest roentgenogram.

The pulmonary function tests are occasionally helpful in differential diagnosis. We and others[93] have seen cases of idiopathic fibrosis in which the chest film resembles primary pulmonary hypertension or multiple pulmonary emboli (Fig. 12-6). Classically, primary pulmonary hypertension has only a slight decrease in lung volume and only mild changes in diffusing capacity. When a chest roentgenogram is suggestive of primary pulmonary

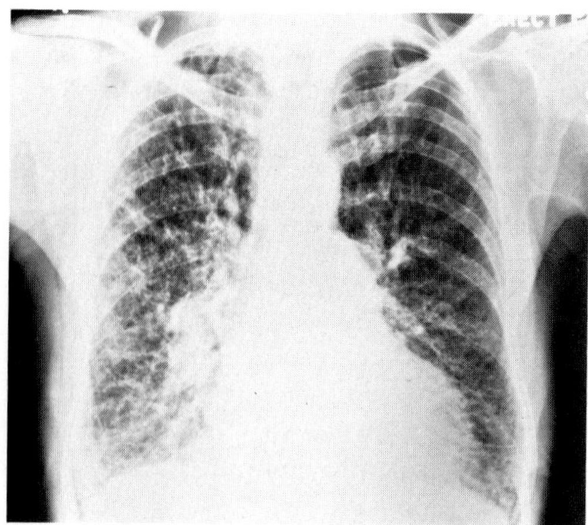

Fig. 12-7. Fifty-two-year-old white female with one-year history of progressive shortness of breath and frequent paroxysm of nonproductive coughing. Chest film shows classical linear interstitial marking with obvious honeycombing seen best in upper lobes.

hypertension and the PFTs demonstrate moderate to marked restriction with a significant decrease in diffusing capacity, the patient most certainly has some form of parenchymal infiltrative disease. This is most often idiopathic interstitial fibrosis, but patients with sarcoidosis and scleroderma have also been reported to have marked pulmonary hypertension and a paucity of roentgenologic evidence of parenchymal lung disease.[93A,93B]

Pulmonary function tests have value in establishing a prognosis and serial testing in following a patient's progression with or without therapeutic intervention. The use of pulmonary function tests to assess operative risk has not been carefully examined in these patients.

ROENTGENOGRAPHIC PATTERNS

The chest film usually shows an interstitial or mixed pattern in these patients. A number of diseases may telescope to a final common appearance the "end-stage lung" which morphologically is nonspecific.[94] If there is coarse reticulation (honeycombing), the morphology is almost always nonspecific fibrosis (Fig. 12-7). A homogeneous hazy, ground-glass pattern with air bronchograms or air alveolograms often correlates with the more active alveolitis morphologically associated with early idiopathic interstitial fibrosis.

Certain chronic diffuse pulmonary diseases tend to demonstrate a predilection for the upper or lower zones. Sarcoidosis, eosinophilic granuloma, and tuberculosis commonly show predominant fibrocystic disease in the upper lungs. Idiopathic interstitial fibrosis, recurrent aspiration, lipoid pneumonia, and scleroderma are predominately basilar in distribution.

In many patients with pneumoconiosis there is a characteristic roentgenographic pattern.[95] The presence of bilateral diaphragmatic calcification with or without pericardial calcification is essentially pathognomonic for asbestosis (Fig. 12-8).

The presence of well demarcated Kerley B lines in the absence of chronic heart failure is extremely suggestive of lymphangitic carcinoma.

A number of associated findings may give a clue to appropriate diagnosis. High diaphragms with trivial parenchymal densities have been described in systemic lupus and idiopathic interstitial fibrosis. Diffuse pulmonary disease with bilateral pleural effusion and a normal-sized cardiac silhouette is usually caused by carcinoma or lymphoma, but miliary tuberculosis, recurrent emboli, drug hypersensitivity, and collagen vascular disease are occasionally responsible. Mild pleural thickening is nonspecific; however, marked thickening or lobulation of the pleura is characteristic of asbestosis and may even indicate the development of a diffuse mesothelioma.[96]

Fissures and mediastinal structures are usually not displaced early in the course of idiopathic interstitial fibrosis due to the general uniform involvement of the lung.[76]

Although hilar nodes have usually regressed in fibrocystic sarcoidosis, there is an occasional case of residual adenopathy. Calcification of these nodes has been reported. A thin layer of calcium in the periphery of the hilar node—i.e., "egg-shell" calcification—is strongly suggestive of sarcoid or coalworks pneumoconiosis. Mediastinal adenopathy does not usually recur in Hodgkin's disease after adequate radiotherapy (Fig. 12-5). Evidence of marked pulmonary hypertension suggests end-stage pulmonary fibrosis or an occasional case of lymphangitic carcinomatosis with recurrent thrombotic and/or tumor emboli.[77] Careful inspection of the bony thorax to detect metastatic or cystic lesions has helped lead to a diagnosis of metastatic disease, eosinophilic granuloma, or lymphoma.

Practical Approach to the Patient with Chronic Diffuse Lung Disease

In the majority of patients with chronic diffuse lung disease it is not possible to make a specific diagnosis without lung biopsy. This was demonstrated in one large series in which the primary preoperative diagnosis was not corroborated by open-lung biopsy in over half the cases. Furthermore, in approximately one-third of the patients, the correct diagnosis was not even suspected preoperatively.[70] On the other hand, in a significant number of patients it is not possible to make a specific diagnosis even with adequate tissue because of the lung's limited morphological response.[94]

The most difficult decision to resolve in the care of patients with chronic diffuse lung disease is whether a lung biopsy could result in some possible gain to the patient. For example, in most patients with pneumoconiosis the diagnosis rests on a history of exposure of adequate intensity and duration—

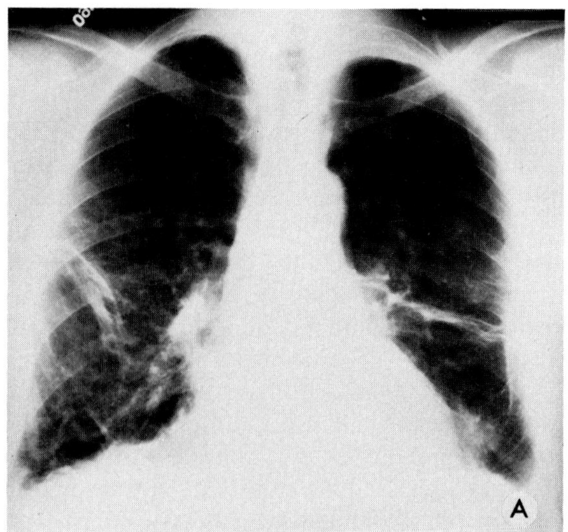

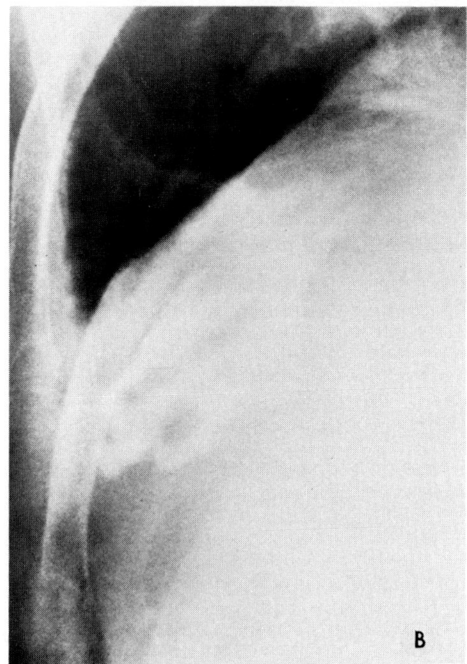

Fig. 12-8. (A) Sixty-two-year-old male ship builder who presented with four-year history of increasing shortness of breath on lessening degrees of activity. Chest film shows bilateral diffused linear densities, predominantly in the lower lung fields, and bilateral pleural disease. (B) Over-penetrated oblique view of right diagram shows large calcified diaphragmatic placque. Bilateral lower lobe fibrosis with pleural thickening and calcification in a ship builder is almost certainly due to pleural pulmonary asbestosis.

a characteristic x-ray and significant impairment in pulmonary function (Fig. 12-8).

Another difficult question facing the physician presented with a case of chronic diffuse lung disease is when to biopsy. Some authors feel a biopsy should be performed in 2–3 days after the routine laboratory data have been evaluated. Others recommend lung biopsy only as a last resort.[50,70,71] We employ an individualized approach that does not invariably lead to lung biopsy. The first step is often an aggressive and sometimes prolonged search for old films when presented with a patient reporting clinically stable symptoms for a number of years. Sometimes, roentgenographic evidence of an abnormal lung may be eventually uncovered following re-examination on an upper gastrointestinal series taken at another hospital several years previously. The relative stability of the infiltrate with definite lower lobe involvement may markedly lessen the possibility of a specific etiological entity being discerned after histological examination of pulmonary tissue. Therapy can then practically and almost certainly safely proceed along nonspecific avenues.

The final major decision is the mode of lung biopsy. Demands for more tissue are increasing for a variety of potentially informative and sophisticated studies.[97] These include electron microscopic, mineralogic, and immunologic investigations. These sophisticated procedures in conjunction with the routine histologic examination and microbial studies require more than the usual large wedge of tissue measuring 4 × 4 × 5 cm obtained by open-lung biopsy. The decision whether special studies requiring larger amounts of tissue are needed often dictates the appropriate method of biopsy for a particular patient with chronic diffuse lung disease. Fortunately, in most of these patients, a small piece of tissue usually produces a histologic picture sufficiently specific or typical to proceed with appropriate clinical management.

We see approximately 25–30 patients each year with diffuse chronic lung disease at The Johns Hopkins Hospital. Over 80 percent of these patients are eventually diagnosed as having idiopathic interstitial fibrosis, sarcoidosis, or carcinoma (primary or secondary).

APPROACH TO THE ASYMPTOMATIC PATIENT WITH CHRONIC DIFFUSE LUNG DISEASE

If the patient is essentially asymptomatic, the majority of the pertinent work-up may be performed prior to hospitalization. Since therapeutic alternatives are questionable in this type of patient, early diagnosis is not indicated except for pressing emotional or other personal reasons. Asymptomatic chronic diffuse lung disease is often discovered on a routine x-ray prior to relocating residence for a new job, obtaining life insurance, leaving the country, or leaving military service. In these individuals, if a reliable Kveim skin test is available, it should be evaluated prior to invasive biopsy procedures. A positive Kveim biopsy site six weeks after administration is satisfactory evidence that the asymptomatic diffuse lung disease is sarcoidosis. In the presence of significant patient anxiety, no available Kveim, or an indication for more rapid diagnosis, transbronchial lung biopsy has been extremely efficient in retrieving sufficient tissue to allow an appropriate diagnosis. The transbronchial lung biopsy with the fibroptic bronchoscope is especially productive in diffuse lung disease resulting from noncaseating granuloma and is the diagnostic procedure of choice at our institution.[62,63,65] If biopsy is initially unsuccessful, it should be repeated. Significant complications are minimal.[68] Where hilar adenopathy is obvious or can be demonstrated by tomography, mediastinoscopy is an almost certain method of diagnosing sarcoidosis (see Chapter 10). The risk of this procedure is minimal.[98] The choice between transbronchial biopsy and mediatinoscopy in diffuse pulmonary sarcoidosis with hilar adenopathy is not clear, but at present the transbronchial approach is favored. The choice, besides depending on what is available and most reliable at a particular institution, may be influenced by the sex and race of the patient. Mediastinoscopy leaves a small, but often conspicuous scar which could be cosmetically unpleasant, especially in a patient prone to develop keloid. In the presence of nonspecific results, the patient with asymptomatic diffuse lung disease can be followed without the physician's manifesting undue anxiety.

APPROACH TO THE SYMPTOMATIC PATIENT WITH CHRONIC DIFFUSE LUNG DISEASE

Fever. The patient with chronic diffuse lung disease and fever represents a specific problem. Routine sputum and blood cultures are usually not helpful. Although infection is unlikely when the symptoms of dyspnea and cough have been present for several months, tuberculosis, fungal, or other unusual infections have been reported to run a relatively chronic course prior to diagnosis.[99]

The fever recorded on presentation to the physician may not have been appreciated by the patient or may be of recent onset, marking a superimposed infection. An intermediate tuberculosis skin test should be inserted in all of these patients on admission to the hospital. If the patient has a known or suspected collagen vascular disease, it should be evaluated by serologic tests and the activity of the disease assessed by measuring the erythrocyte sedimentation rate and complement level. Skin and renal biopsy yield a more specific histologic picture and, therefore, are preferable to pulmonary biopsy. When a patient is receiving high doses of steroids or is immune suppressed, rapid diagnosis is mandatory (see Chapter 13). Patients with diffuse pulmonary disease should be questioned carefully for the possibility of recurrent aspiration pneumonia, especially when the roentgenographic densities are predominately basilar in distribution. We have seen patients with chronic shortness of breath from repeated aspiration who had recurrent fever and slowly progressive symptoms of respiratory insufficiency (Fig. 12-9). If aspiration is suspected on a historical basis, a cine esophagram should be obtained. In the presence of fever, primary hematologic malignancy should be considered a cause of pulmonary infiltration, and a bone marrow biopsy should be performed if there are any abnormalities in the peripheral smear. Occasionally, a buffy coat smear will yield abnormal cellular morphology when a routine smear appears unremarkable. This is especially helpful in Hodgkin's disease. The majority of patients with difuse pulmonary disease associated with untreated lymphoma or leukemia have either obvious peripheral or hilar adenopathy. These lymph nodes should be biopsied before more invasive diagnostic procedures are contemplated. Pleural effusions are also very common in hematologic malignancies and should be examined and biopsied early. Following the return of initial laboratory studies, if a site is not defined for further investigation, it is statistically unlikely that a lung biopsy can be averted in patients with symptomatic chronic diffuse lung disease. In addition, febrile patients may suddenly deteriorate. Transbronchial lung biopsy should be performed within 3–5 days so as not to produce undue anxiety in the patient or incur unnecessary expense. Several specimens should be obtained (Chapter 8). Once adequate tissue is retrieved for pathology, subsequent specimens should be cultured for routine organisms, mycobacteria, and fungal forms. Histologic evaluation is most important, and the biopsied material should be delivered to the surgical pathology laboratory with the appropriate request for routine and special staining to ensure that maximum information is obtained from the small pieces of tissue. Depending on the results and the patient's clinical condition, transbronchial biopsy may be repeated. On a number of occasions the results from this procedure are nonspecific, and the physician must decide if this information is consistent with the condition producing the symptoms in these patients. If the histologic information is unsatisfactory or does not seem to explain all the patient's symptoms, an open biopsy should be performed (see Chapter 7). A lingular biopsy is not recommended because this area of the lung is often a site of chronic nonspecific inflammation.[71]

Afebrile. The majority of patients with symptomatic chronic diffuse lung disease are afebrile and have a history of progressive shortness of breath associated with some degree of chronic cough. A careful history of industrial exposure is very helpful in these cases. The patient should also be extensively questioned concerning drug exposures[100] (see Table 12-4). For example, did the patient have a chronic urinary-tract infection which periodically flared, requiring recurrent or continuous treatment with nitrofuradantoin? Another very important aspect in the work-up of the patient with symptomatic chronic diffuse lung disease, is a careful search for old films. A relatively stable x-ray film for several months is against most infectious or malignant etiologies. Although fever is present at the onset in 85–95 percent of the cases of miliary tuberculosis, some patients are afebrile

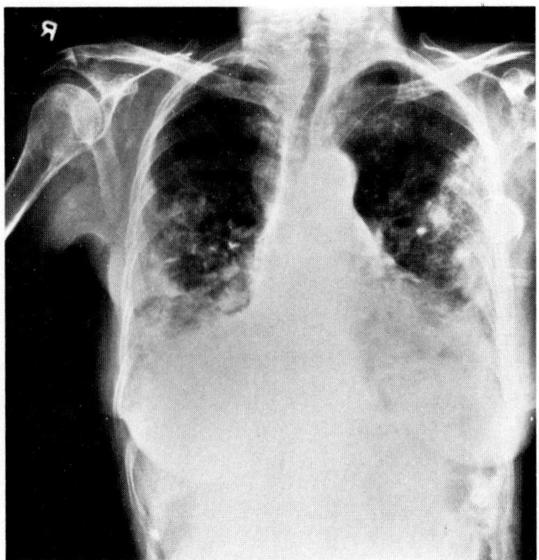

Fig. 12-9. Seventy-two-year-old white female with history of frequent episodes of nocturnal regurgitation (water brash) over five-year period. Presented with six-month history of progressive shortness of breath and episodes of dyspnea. Chest film demonstrates bilateral lower lobe and peripheral infiltrates. Autopsy revealed interstitial pneumonitis most compatible with recurrent aspiration pneumonia.

and remain so for long periods.[99] Sahn et al. have recently demonstrated that miliary tuberculosis can present with a wide variety of roentgenographic and clinical manifestations and is currently most often seen in elderly patients.[101] As previously mentioned, an intermediate tuberculosis skin test should therefore be placed on all these patients even if tuberculosis seems extremely unlikely. Skin anergy to a variety of antigens should always suggest sarcoidosis, but may be present in malignant disease and miliary tuberculosis.

In approximately 10–20 percent of elderly "healthy" patients routine antinuclear antibody tests are positive.[102] However, this is usually in low titer. The erythrocyte sedimentation rate may also be elevated in these individuals. If collagen vascular disease is suspected on the basis of abnormal laboratory data, a full immunologic work-up is indicated. Characteristic skin biopsies and elevated muscle enzymes may suggest a mixed collagen vascular disease as the cause of diffuse symptomatic lung disease. In the elderly patient, systemic lupus often presents predominantly as a pulmonary or cardiopulmonary disease without renal or joint manifestation.[103] Drug-implicated lupus syndromes are less commonly associated with skin abnormalities, and renal disease is usually absent.[104] Serum complement is usually normal in drug-induced lupus. Sjogren's syndrome has recently

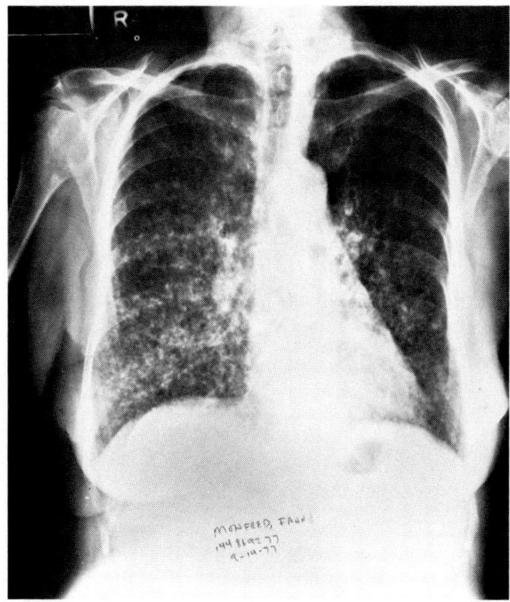

Fig. 12-10. Sixty-five-year-old black female with three-month history of nonproductive cough and 15-pound weight loss. Chest film shows bilateral lower lobe linear densities. Transbronchial biopsy demonstrated tissue compatible with lymphocytic lymphoma.

been reported to have a 10 percent incidence of diffuse pulmonary disease.[105]

The newly described entity of angioimmunoblastic lymphadenopathy has been reported to produce diffuse interstitial pneumonitis.[106] This diagnosis is usually made by biopsy of involved lymph nodes. Primary amyloidosis frequently involves the lungs[107] and may appear predominantly or exclusively as a diffuse pulmonary process. A skin biopsy of a suggestive lesion (especially purpuric lesions around eyelids) or a rectal valve biopsy should be obtained in the presence of nonspecific adenopathy, unexplained splenomegaly, or a variety of monoclonal or polyclonal immunoglobulin abnormalities in order to rule out amyloidosis.

Malignant tumor must always be considered in the group of patients with symptomatic chronic diffuse lung disease. Prominent weight loss is unusual in any of the other diffuse lung diseases, unless associated with obvious systemic symptoms. Lymphoma may be characterized by predominant pulmonary findings, but often it is associated with disturbances in immunoglobulins, pleural effusion, or hilar adenopathy (Fig. 12-10). Alveolar cell carcinoma may present as a diffuse alveolar or nodular alveolar interstitial pattern (Fig. 12-11). Thus, sputum cytology should always be obtained in patients with chronic diffuse lung disease, although it is often not appre-

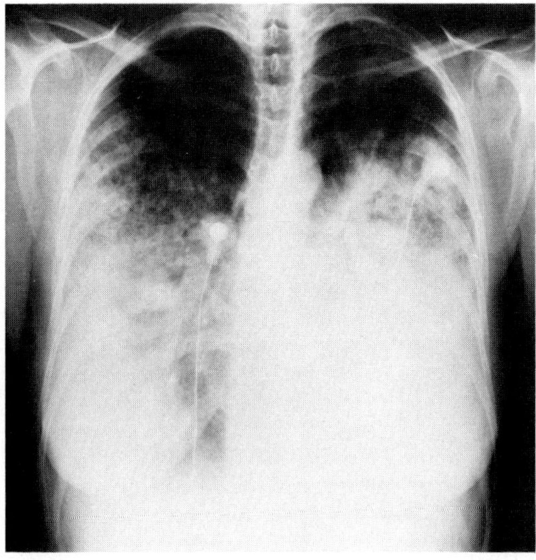

Fig. 12-11. Fifty-six-year-old black female with six-month history of cough productive of copious amounts of foamy mucoid sputum and a one month history of progressive shortness of breath and weight loss. Chest film shows diffuse alveolar filling infiltrates. Transbronchial biopsy demonstrated alveolar cell carcinoma.

ciated as positive in alveolar cell carcinoma because the expectorated cells may be well differentiated.

The possibility of metastatic pulmonary disease always appears to be a concern of physicians taking care of these patients. The doctor often launches into an extensive search for the primary tumor. This is probably unreasonable. It is the least satisfactory diagnosis to make from the patient's point of view and certainly will eventually make itself known to all concerned parties. A tumor search is expensive, and often a number of the procedures are uncomfortable. Occult carcinoma may be suspected by demonstrating elevated alkaline or acid phosphatases or carcinoembryonic antigen.[87] Lymphangitic carcinoma is easily diagnosed by transbronchial brushing and biopsy.

An ever-increasing number of organic antigens has been implicated in causes of diffuse lung disease.[34] Long-term, low-dose exposure to thermophylic actinomycetes from air conditioning or humidifiers may produce a chronic diffuse pulmonary fibrosis.[74,79] Subtle seasonal exacerbations or knowledge of other individuals at home or work with similar symptoms should alert the physican to obtain special studies for serum precipitins.

In patients between 40 and 65 years of age without any extrapulmonary manifestations and relatively slowly progressive dyspnea, the most likely diagnosis is idiopathic interstitial fibrosis. This disease entity has been variously named and divided into a number of subcategories, but is currently felt to be single entity with morphologic changes that vary during the course of the disease.[32,67,76,82] Early in the disease there is predominant cellular interstitial infiltration, whereas with the passage of time increasing amounts of collagen deposition occurs. Crystal et al. have recently reviewed their experiences with idiopathic pulmonary fibrosis.[76] Approximately 40 percent of their patients have circulating cryoimmunoglobulins. Certain radiographically similar conditions termed lymphoid interstitial pneumonia have been reported.[108] These are separate diseases and are characterized by interstitial infiltrations with mature small and large lymphocytes and plasma cells producing diffuse linear and reticular shadows on chest x-rays which tend to become confluent. A number of these cases have been associated with monoclonal gammopathies.

If the chest roentgenogram shows marked honeycombing and the patient has definite clubbing, we agree with Scadding and others who feel that no further biopsy documentation of interstitial fibrosis is necessary.[82] This opinion is based on the observation that biopsy in these patients usually demonstrates a nonspecific, morphologic, end-stage lung. Clubbing is rare in sarcoidosis and generally is not seen in lymphangitic carcinoma of the lung. Patients with advanced interstitial fibrosis often have evidence of significant pulmonary hypertension.[109] The risk of complication following transbronchial lung biopsy is thought to be increased in this group of patients,[110] therefore, it is preferable to observe these patients or attempt therapeutic trials without a tissue diagnosis as long as infectious etiologies can be adequately excluded. Patients with advanced fibrosis, pulmonary hypertension, or cor pulmonale are rarely febrile without an acute superimposed insult, and the duration of their symptoms is usually sufficiently long to exclude chronic infection.

If chronic pulmonary edema associated with silent mitral stenosis, chronic congestive heart failure, or pulmonary veno-occlusive disease cannot be ruled out on clinical grounds, the patient should undergo complete cardiovascular evaluation. This includes echocardiography and subsequent cardiac catheterization where indicated. If primary pulmonary hypertension or chronic pulmonary emboli are suspected, the patient should have a right-heart catheterization and selective pulmonary angiography. Angiography should be obtained only if there is evidence of segmental or subsegmental ventilation–perfusion mismatches following ^{99m}Tc scanning of the lung (see Chapter 4).

If the patient with symptomatic chronic diffuse lung disease is not severely dyspneic, most of the routine and special laboratory studies should be obtained prior to hospitalization. Following thorough evaluation, if a number of etiologies appear possible and a specific diagnosis has not been established, a transbronchial lung biopsy should be performed in the absence of clinical evidence of significant pulmonary hypertension (see Chapter 8).

Several biopsy specimens should be obtained and examined appropriately (see Chapters 7 and 8). If adequate tissue is obtained, the diagnostic yield in granulomatous disease or primary and secondary lymphangitis carcinoma approaches 100 percent in our experience. Transbronchial lung biopsy has been shown to correlate with open-lung biopsy in a number of different diffuse pulmonary diseases.[61] If nonspecific fibrosis is obtained, again from an adequate *alveolar* sample of lung tissue, then idiopathic interstitial fibrosis is the most likely diagnosis in a patient with symptomatic chronic diffuse lung disease and nonspecific diagnostic laboratory results. Although multiple samples are usually taken, only a small portion of the total lung will be available for morphologic examination. This potentially allows for a sampling error and often prevents prognostication based on the extent of cellular inflammation versus irreversible generalized fibrosis. Since all the lung can only be observed at autopsy, however, most clinicians will attempt a therapeutic trial of steroids regardless of the extent of irreversible scarring found even on open-lung biopsy.

Several large studies have demonstrated the effectiveness and reliability of percutaneous lung biopsy with cutting or trephine needles in diffuse lung disease.[61,62,109,111,112] Even groups with the largest experience using needle-biopsy techniques prefer transbronchial biopsy in diffuse lung disease because of the ease and lack of complications from this procedure.[109] At present we prefer to use transbronchial biopsy rather than needle biopsy as the initial technique for diagnosis of diffuse lung disease.

In complicated or confusing cases or when large pieces of tissue are desired for special mineralogic or immunologic studies, an open-lung biopsy through a limited thoracotomy will undoubtedly provide the most information. Cases with suspected vasculitis involving the lung should have an open biopsy, since transbronchial specimens do not usually contain pulmonary vessels larger than capillaries. Various portions of the thorax, including the hilar and mediastinal nodes, may be examined at thoracotomy. The appropriate site for taking the biopsy specimen is usually an area not severely involved but rather representative of the general process as observed directly by the surgeon. Occasionally, more than one specimen must be obtained. Marginal areas that include a transition from mild to moderate involvement frequently result in more specific diagnostic morphology. End-stage fibrosis, or honeycombing, is a result of a number of conditions and always leaves a question as to the etiology. Sometimes open-lung biopsy simply supplies more nonspecific tissue than transbronchial lung biopsy. All specific diseases, however, will be adequately diagnosed by the open-lung biopsy method if tissue is handled properly (see Chapter 7).

Respiratory insufficiency is not a contraindication to open-lung biopsy. The mortality from this procedure in a large number of cases from various series ranges from less than 1 percent to approximately 5 percent.[51,70] Major complications are uncommon. In some cases of idiopathic interstitial fibrosis, adequate lung biopsy allows the physician to determine the degree of inflammation versus fibrosis and encourage more aggressive therapeutic attempts where they might have been assumed to be hopeless.

Patients with chronic diffuse lung disease rarely, if ever, suddenly resolve their clinical symptoms or roentgenographic abnormality. Their problem must be ultimately resolved in some way or another. Appropriate decisions often spare the patient undue anxiety and unnecessary expense.

REFERENCES

1. Schwartz WB, Gorry GA, Kassirer JP, and Esssig A: Decision analysis and clinical judgment. Am J Med 55:459–472, 1973
2. Ashbough DG, Bigelow DG, Petty TL, et al: Acute respiratory distress in adults. Lancet 2:319, 1967
3. Petty TL, Ashbough DG: The adult respiratory distress syndrome: Clinical features, factors influencing prognosis and principle of management. Chest 60:233–239, 1971
4. Murray JF: The adult respiratory distress syndrome (may it rest in peace). Am Rev Respir Dis 111:716, 1975
5. Staub NC: Pulmonary edema. Physiol Rev 54:678, 1974
6. Briscoe WA, Smith JP, Bergofsky E, King TKC: Catastrophic pulmonary failure. Am J Med 60:248, 1976
7. Theros EG: The value of radiologic-pathologic correlation in the education of the radiologist. Am J Roentgenol Radium Ther Nucl Med 107:235, 1969
8. Zishim MM, Weill H, Bnechner HA, Brown M: Recognition of distinctive radiologic patterns in diffuse pulmonary disease. Arch Intern Med 114:108, 1964
9. Goodman W: Differential diagnosis of pulmonary alveolar infiltrates. Am Rev Respir Dis 95:681, 1967
10. Felson B: The roentgen diagnosis of disseminated pulmonary alveolar disease. Semin Roentgenol Vol. II, No. 1 Greene & Shetlon, Inc., New York, 1967
11. Chait A: Interstitial pulmonary edema. Circulation 45:1323, 1972
12. Dodek A, Kassebaum DG, Bristown JD: Pulmonary edema in coronary artery disease without cardiomegaly. N Engl J Med 286:1347, 1972
13. Stein L, Bernard JJ, Morissette M, et al: Pulmonary edema during volume infusion. Circulation 52:483, 1975
14. Bones RC, Francis B, Pierce AK: Intravascular coagulation associated with the adult respiratory distress syndrome. Am J Med 61:585, 1976
15. Swan JHC, Ganz W, Forrester J, et al: Catheterization of the heart in man with the use of a flow-directed balloon typed catheter. N Engl J Med 283:447, 1970
16. Hahn HH, Beaty HN: Transtracheal aspiration in the evaluation of patients with pneumonia. Ann Intern Med 72:183, 1970
17. Bynum LJ, Pierce AK: Pulmonary aspiration of gastric contents. Am Rev Respir Dis 144:1129, 1976

18. Ashbough DG, Petty TL: Sepsis complicating the acute respiratory distress syndrome. Surg Gynecol Obstet 135:865, 1972
19. Ashbough DG, Petty TL: Positive end-expiratory pressure: physiology indications and contraindications. J Thorac Cardioasc Surg 65:165, 1973
20. Summer W: Acute pulmonary disease from noxious gases, vapors and fumes. In Shibel E, Moser K, Mosbey C (eds): Respiratory Emergencies. St. Louis, CV Mosby, 1977
21. Johnson TH, Gajaraj A, Feist JH: Am J Roentgenol Radium Ther Nucl Med 109:516, 1970
22. Fraser RG: Diagnosis of diseases of the chest. Chapter 4 In: J.A.P. Vol. Philadelphia, W.B. Saunders Co., 1977, p. 341
23. Huseby JS, Hudson LD: Miliary tuberculosis and the adult respiratory distress syndrome. Ann Intern Med 85:609, 1976
24. Murry HW, Mason H, Senterfit LB, et al: The protein manifestations of mycoplasma pneumonia infection in adults. Am J Med 58:229, 1975
25. Banaszak EF, Thieds WH, Fink JN: Hypersensitivity pneumonitis due to contamination of an air conditioner. N Engl J Med 283:271, 1970
26. Fink JN, Banaszak EF, Thiede WH, et al: Interstitial pneumonitis due to hypersensitivity to an organism contaminating a heating system. Ann Intern Med 74:80, 1971
27. Kory RC, Smith JR: Medical history: Physical examination in the assessment of pulmonary disease. In Baun, GL (ed): Textbook of Pulmonary Disease, 2nd. ed. Boston: Little Brown, 1974, p. 14
28. Bennett DE, Millian RR, Acherman LV: Bilateral radiation pneumonitis: A complication of the radiotherapy of bronchogenic carcinoma. Cancer 25:1001, 1969
29. Costellino RA, Glalstein E, Turlow MM, et al: Latent radiation injury of lungs or heart activated by steroid withdrawal. Ann Intern Med 80:593, 1973
30. Bowers RE, Brigham KL, Owen PJ: Salicylate pulmonary edema: The mechanism in sleep and review of the clinical literature. Am Rev Respir Dis 115:261, 1977
31. Scadding JG: Diffuse pulmonary alveolar fibrosis. Thorax 29:271, 1974
32. Allen DH, Basten A, William GV, et al: Familial hypersensitivity pneumonitis. Am J Med 59:505, 1975
33. Fink JM: Hypersensitivity pneumonitis. A case of mistaken identity. Hosp Practice, March, 1974
34. Jaffee N: Roentgenologic aspects of primary pseudomonas aeruginosa pneumonia in mechanically ventilated patients. Am J Roentgenol Radium Ther Nucl Med 107:305, 1969
35. Cassan SM, Coles DT, Harrison EG: The concept of limited forms of Wegener's granulomatosis. Am J Med 49:366, 1970
36. Talbot AS: Sarcoid myopathy. Br Med J 4:465, 1967
37. Chick EW, Baum GL, et al: The use of skin tests and serologic tests in histoplasmosic, coccidioidomycosis, and blastomycosis. Am Rev Respir Dis 108:156, 1973
38A. Buechner HH, Seabury JH, Campbell CC, et al: The current status of serologic, immunologic and skin tests in the diagnosis of pulmonary mycosis. Chest 63:259, 1973

38B. Fisher RD, Armstrong D: Cryptococcal interstitial pneumonia: Value of antigen determination. N Engl J Med 297:1440, 1977
39. Schacter EN, Finkelstein FO, Bastel C, et al: Diagnostic problems in pulmonary-renal syndrome. Am Rev Respir Dis 115:155, 1977
40. Fulop, M, Horowitz M, Aberman A, et al: Lactic acidosis in pulmonary edema due to left ventricular failure. Ann Intern Med 70:180, 1973
41. Carrington CB, Addington WW, Groff AH, et al: Chronic eosinophilic pneumonia. N Engl J Med 280:727, 1969
42. Clinical conferences at The Johns Hopkins Hospital. Johns Hopkins Med 139:279, 1976
43. Onal E, Lopata M, Lourence RV: Nodular pulmonary sarcoidosis. Roentgenographic and physiologic courses in five patients. Chest 72:296, 1977
44. Light RW, Mac Gregor MI, Luchsinger PC, et al: Pleural effusions: The diagnostic separation of transditis and exudates. Ann Intern Med 77:507, 1972
45. Weick JK, Kriby JM, Harrison EG, et al: Pleural effusion in lymphoma. Cancer 31:848, 1973
46. Beckman JF, Zimmet SM, Chum, BK, et al: Spectrum of pleural involvement in sarcoidosis. Arch Intern Med 136:323, 1976
47. Hull R, Van Aken WG, Hirsh J, et al: Impedence plethysmography using the occlumin cuff technique in the diagnosis of venous thrombosis. Circulation 53:696, 1977
48. Shibel EM, Tisi GM, Moser KM: Pulmonary photoscan and roentgenographic comparisons in sarcoidosis. Radiology 106:770, 1969
49. Strauss MB: Familiar Medical Quotations. Boston, Little Brown, 1968
50. Case records of the Massachusetts General Hospital. Case 4-1977. N Engl J Med 296:215, 1977
51. Roy JF, Lawton BR, Myers WD: Open lung biopsy: Nineteen-year experiences with 416 consecutive operations. Chest 69:43, 1976
52. Epstein RL: Constituents of sputum: A simple method. Ann Intern Med 77:259, 1972
53. Schreiner A, Digranes A, Myking O: Transtracheal aspiration in the diagnosis of lower respiratory tract infection. Scand J Infect Dis 4:49, 1972
54. Bartless JG, Rosenblatt JE, Finegold SM: Percutaneous transtracheal aspiration in the diagnosis of anaerobic pulmonary infection. Ann Intern Med 79:535, 1973
55. Davidson M, Tempest B, Palmer D: Bacteriologic diagnosis of acute pneumonia: Comparison of sputum, transtracheal aspirates and lung aspirates. JAMA 235:158, 1976
56. Aisner J, Kroles LK, Sickles EA, et al: Transtracheal selective bronchial brushing for pulmonary infiltrates in patients with cancer. Chest 69:367, 1976
57. Bartless JG, Alexander J, Mayhew J: Should fiberoptic bronchoscopy aspirates be cultured? Am Rev Respir Dis 114:73, 1976
58. Conte BA, Laforet EG: The role of the typical anesthetics in modifying bacteriologic data obtained by bronchoscopy. N Engl J Med 267:957, 1962
59. Pereira W, Kornat DM, Khan MA, et al: Fever and pneumonia after flexible fiberoptic bronchoscopy. Am Rev Respir Dis 112:59, 1975
60. Douglas RG: Influenza: The disease and its complications. Hospital Practice, December 1976

61. Ellis JH: Transbronchial lung biopsy via the fiberoptic bronchoscope. Chest 68:524, 1975
62. Greenman RL, Goodall PT, King D: Lung biopsy in immunocompromised host. Am J Med 59:488, 1975
63. Zavala DC: Diagnostic fiberoptic bronchoscopy: Techniques and results: 600 patients. Chest 68:12, 1975
64. Thieds WH, Banaszak EF: Selective bronchial catheterization. N Engl J Med 286, 526, 1972
65. Koontz CH, Joyner LR, Nelson RA: Transbronchial lung biopsy via the fiberoptic bronchoscope in sarcoidosis. Ann Intern Med 85:64, 1976
66. Feldman NT, Pennington JE, Ehrie MJ: Transbronchial lung biopsy in the compromised host. JAMA 238:1377, 1977
67. Livingston JL, Lewis JL, Reid L, et al: Diffuse interstitial pulmonary fibrosis. Q J Med 33:71, 1964
68. Havson RR, Zavola DC, Rhodes ML, et al: Transbronchial biopsy via flexible bronchoscope: Results in 164 patients. Am Rev Respir Dis 114:67, 1976
69. Zavola DC, Bedell GN: Percutaneous lung biopsy with a cutting needle. Am Rev Respir Dis 106:186, 1972
70. Gaensler EA, Moister VB, Hann: Open lung biopsy in diffuse pulmonary disease. N Engl J Med 270:1319, 1964
71. Ray JF, Lawton BR, Myers WO: Open lung biopsy, nineteen year experience with 416 consecutive generations. Chest 69:43, 1976
72. Klassen KP, Andrew NC: Biopsy of diffuse pulmonary lesions: A 17 year experience. Ann Thorac Surg 4:117, 1967
73. Poskitt TR: Immunologic and electron microscopic studies in Goodpasture's syndrome. Ann J Med 49:250, 1970
74. Fink JM, Baraszek EF, Baroriak JJ, et al: Interstitial lung disease due to contamination of forced air system. Ann Intern Med 84:406, 1976
75. Buechner HA, Rabin CB, Schepers GWH, et al: Diffuse pulmonary lesion problems of differential diagnosis. Dis Chest 43:155, 1963
76. Crystal RG, Fulmer JD, Roberts WG, et al: Idiopathic pulmonary fibrosis clinical, histologic, radiologic, physiologic, suntigraphic, cytologic, and biochemical aspects. Ann Intern Med 85:769, 1976
77. Winterbauer RH, Elfenbein IB, Ball WC Jr: The incidence and clinical significance of tumor embolization to the lungs. Am J Med 45:271, 1968
78. Davidson JM, Macleod WM: Pulmonary alveolar proteinosis. Br J Dis Chest 63:13, 1969
79. Riley DJ, Saldane M: Pigeon breeder's lungs: Subacute course and the importance of indirect exposure. Am Rev Respir Dis 107:456, 1973
80. MacMillan JM: Familial pulmonary fibrosis. Dis Chest 1951:18, 330
81. Wiman LG: Familial occurrence of sarcoidosis proceeding to the VI international conference on sarcoidosis.
82. Scadding JG, Kinson KFW: Diffuse fibrosing alveolity (diffuse interstitial fibrosis of the lung). Thorax 22:291, 1967
83. Koffler D, Schur P, Kunkel HG: Immunological studies concerning the nephritis of systemic lupus erythematosus. J Exp Med 126:607, 1967
84. Picardi TL, Kaufman LA, Schwarz J, et al: Detection of precipitating antibodies to histoplasma by counterimmunoelectrophoresis. Am Rev Respir Dis 114:171, 1976

85. Siltzbach LE: Significance and specificity of the Kveim reaction. Acta Scand Med (Suppl 425)176:74, 1964
86. Littner MR, Schachter EN, Putman CE: The clinical assessment of roentgenographically atypical pulmonary sarcoidosis. Am J Med 62:361, 1977
87A. Hansen HJ, Synder JJ, Miller, et al: Carcinoembryonic antigen (CEA) a laboratory adjunct in the diagnosis and management of cancer. Hum Pathol 5:139, 1974
87B. Murphy GP, Reynoso G, Kenny GM, and Gaeta JF: Comparison of total and prostatic fraction serum acid phosphatase levels in patients with differentiated and undifferentiated prostatic carcinoma. Cancer 23: 1309–1314, 1969
88. Barboiak JJ, Fink JN, Scribner G: Immunologic cross-reactions of thermophilic actinomycetes isolated from home environments. J Allergy Clin Immunol 49:81, 1972
89. Light RW, MacGregor MI, Ball WC Jr, et al: Diagnostic significance of pleural fluid pH and Pco_2. Chest 64:591, 1973
90. Salger WR, Eggleston JC, Erozon YS: Efficiency of pleural needle biopsy and pleural fluid cytopathology in the diagnosis of malignant neoplasm involving the pleura. Chest 67:536, 1975
91. Scerbo J, Keltz H, Stove D: A prospective study of closed pleural biopsies. JAMA 218:377, 1971
92. Ash SR, Manfredi F: Directed biopsy using a small endoscope: Thoroscopy and peritoneoscopy simplified. N Engl J Med 291:1398, 1974
93A. Williams MH, Adler JJ, Colp C: Pulmonary function studies as an aid in the differential diagnosis of pulmonary hypertension. Am J Med 47:378, 1969
93B. Salerni R, Rodnan GP, Leon DF, et al: Pulmonary hypertension in the CREST syndrome variant of progressive systemic sclerosis (scleroderma). Ann Intern Med 86:394, 1977
94. Genereuh GP: The end-stage lung. Radiology 116:279, 1975
95. Morgan WKC, Seaton A: Occupational Lung Disease. Philadelphia, W.B. Saunders Co., 1975
96. Seaton A: Asbestosis in Occupational Lung disease. Philadelphia, W.B. Saunders Co., 1975, Ch 9, p 124
97. Ruttner JR, Spycher MA, Sticker H: The detection of etiologic agents in interstitial pulmonary fibrosis. Hum Pathol 4:497, 1973
98. Pearson FG: Mediastinoscopy. A method of biopsy in the superior mediastinum. J Thorac Cardiovasc Surg 49:11, 1965
99. Proudfoot AT, Achtar AJ, Douglas AC, et al: Miliary tuberculosis in adults. Br Med J 2:273, 1969
100. Rosenow EC III: The spectrum of drug induced pulmonary disease. Ann Intern Med 77:979, 1972
101. Sahn SA, Neff TA: Miliary tuberculosis. Am J Med 56:495, 1974
102. Rowley MJ, Buchanan H, Mackey IR: Reciprocal changes with age in antibody to extrinsic and intrinsic antigens. Lancet 2:24, 1968
103. Eisenberg H, Dubous EL, Sherwin RP, et al: Diffuse interstitial lung disease in systemic lupus erythematosus. Ann Intern Med 79:37, 1973
104. Blomgren SE, Condem JH, Vaughan JH: Procainamide-induced lupus erythematosus. Clinical and laboratory observations. Am J Med 52:338, 1972
105. Strimlan CV, Rosenow EC III, Diverte MB, et al: Pulmonary manifestations of Sjögren's syndrome. Chest 70:354, 1976

106. Schwarz MI, Stanford RE: Interstitial pneumonia in angio-immunoblastic lymphadenopathy with dysproteinemia. Ann Intern Med 85:752, 1976
107. Himmelfarb E, Wells S, Rabinowitz JG: The radiologic spectrum of cardiopulmonary amyloidosis. Chest 72:327, 1977
108. Case Records of the Massachusetts General Hospital. Case 38-1977. N Engl J Med 297:652, 1977
109. McLoes B, Fulmer J, Adin N, et al: Correlative studies of pulmonary hypertension in idiopathic pulmonary hypertension. Am Rev. Respir Dis (Suppl) 115:354, 1977
110. Cunningham JH, Zavola DC, Corry RJ, et al: Trephine air drill, bronchial brush and fiberoptic transbronchial lung biopsy in immunosuppressed patients. Am Rev Respir Dis 115:213, 1977
111. Zavola DC, Bedelll GN: Percutaneous lung biopsy with a cutting needle: An analysis of 40 cases and comparisons with other biopsy techniques. Am Rev Respir Dis 106:186, 1972
112. King EG, Bachynski JE, Mielke B: Percutaneous trephine lung biopsy. Evolving role. Chest 70:212, 1976
113. Rosenow EC III: Drug-induced hypersensitivity disease of the lung: Immunologic and infectious reactions in the lung. In Kirkpatrick CH & Reynolds HY (eds) Vol 1 in: Lung Biology in Health & Disease (Exec. Ed. C Leafant) New York, Marcel Pekker Inc., 1976, pp 261–288

Peter B. Terry, M.D.
Warren R. Summer, M.D.

13

Pulmonary Disease in the Immunocompromised Host

INTRODUCTION

The immunocompromised host with pulmonary disease represents one of the most difficult management problems facing physicians. The differential diagnosis is broad and the rate of clinical deterioration unpredictable. Rapid diagnosis and appropriate therapeutic interventions are therefore critical for patient survival. An approach to these patients is outlined in the following pages.

The compromised host with lung disease must first be recognized by the physician as one whose immune system is deficient. This deficiency may be related to the patient's underlying disease, e.g., leukemia, related to drug therapy in an otherwise immunocompetent host, e.g., steroid treatment of giant cell arteritis, or a combination of underlying disease and drug therapy, e.g., chemotherapy for Hodgkin's disease.

The symptoms or signs that bring the compromised host to the physician's attention may be explosive in onset or deceptively subtle. Typically these patients have fever and an abnormal chest roentgenogram. *Infection, progression of underlying disease, and drug-related abnormalities* constitute the three broad diagnostic categories for consideration in these patients. Empitus is to proceed rapidly with evaluation since infection is the most common cause of pulmonary infiltrates, and any delay in delivery of appropriate therapy may be fatal. The diagnostic and therapeutic process requires the close cooperation of a team of physicians.

We here confine our discussion to the most frequently seen immunosuppressed hosts, for they represent the spectrum of disease in which to demonstrate the principles of an orderly diagnostic approach. In most cases these

Table 13-1
Classification of Primary Immunodeficiency Disorders

Type	Suggested Cellular Defect		
	B-cells	*T-cells*	*Stem Cells*
Infantile X-linked agammaglobulinemia	+		
Selective immunoglobulin deficiency (IgA)	+		
X-linked immunodeficiency with hyper-IgM	+	?	
Thymic hypoplasia (pharyngeal pouch syndrome, DiGeorge's syndrome)		+	
Episodic lymphopenia with lymphocytoxin		+	
Immunodeficiency with normal or without hyper-immunoglobulinemia	+	+	
Immunodeficiency with ataxia-telangiectasia	+	+	
Immunodeficiency with thrombocytopenia and eczema (Wiskott-Aldrich syndrome)	+	+	
Immunodeficiency with thymoma	+	+	
Immunodeficiency with short-limbed dwarfism	+	+	
Immunodeficiency with generalized hematopoietic hypoplasia	+	+	+
Severe combined immunodeficiency			
(a) autosomal recessive	+	+	+
(b) X-linked	+	+	+
(c) sporadic	+	+	+
Variable immunodeficiency (common, largely unclassified)	+	+ (sometimes)	
Others	*Nonspecific Defect*		
A. Primary complement deficiency	C-3		
B. Lazy leukocyte syndrome	Neutrophil mobility		
C. Job's syndrome	Neutrophil chemotaxis		
D. Chediak-Higashi	Intracellular killing impairment		
E. Chronic granulomatous disease	Neutrophil hydrogen peroxidase deficiency		
F. Congenital neutropenia	Neutrophil production deficiency		
G. Sickle cell disease	Heat-labile opsonins		
H. Diabetes mellitus	Phagocytosis, others?		

immunodeficiency states are acquired disorders. Table 13-1 is a listing of the numerous inherited immunodeficiency states.

To proceed intelligently with the diagnostic work-up in immunocompromised patients, it is necessary for the physician to understand (1) immunocompetence, (2) drug-related pulmonary disease, (3) the natural progression of the underlying disease as it may present intrathoracically, and (4) common pathogens that infect the immunosuppressed host.

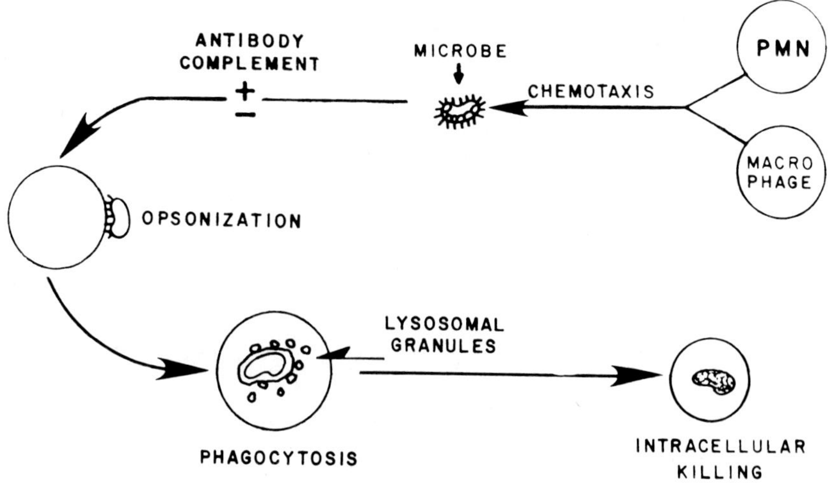

NONSPECIFIC HOST DEFENSE MECHANISMS

Fig. 13-1. Diagram of nonspecific host mechanisms.

IMMUNOCOMPETENCE

The capacity of the patient to defend himself against invasion by microbes depends upon intact host defense mechanisms. These may be broadly categorized as *nonspecific, cellular, and humoral* host defense mechanisms. Although a complete understanding of these mechanisms has not yet been elucidated, we appear to understand the framework of the system.

The nonspecific host defense mechanisms are actually the first line of defense in combating infection (Fig. 13-1). The principal cells involved are the polymorphonuclear leukocyte (PMN) and the mononuclear cell. These cells initially migrate to the site of invading organisms, being drawn to the area by substances released from the damaged tissue (chemotaxis). If the host has previously formed antibodies, these may unite on the surface of the invading microbe (opsonization) with the third component of complement, thereby facilitating ingestion of the organism (phagocytosis) by the PMN, or mononuclear cell turned macrophage. Lysosomal granules containing cidal material are released within the cell and kill the ingested organism.[1] Certain organisms such as *M. tuberculosis, Listeria monocytogenes,* and *Brucella* species resist this intracellular destruction and may persist as chronic intracellular infections. Deficiencies in one or a combination of these steps occur commonly in the immunosuppressed host and thereby predispose to infection.

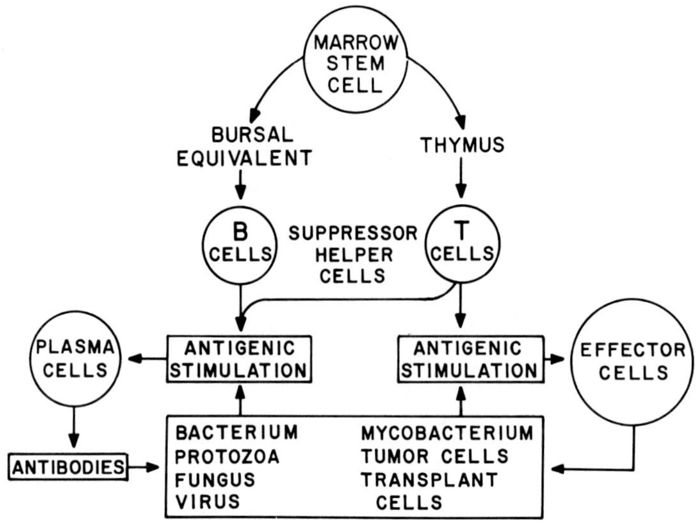

Fig. 13-2. Diagram of specific humoral and cellular host defense mechanisms.

During embryonic life, bone marrow stem cells differentiate into two general classes of lymphocytes—thymus-derived T cells and bursal dependent B cells (Fig. 13-2). Each cell line has a specific anatomical distribution, specific functional characteristics, and can be identified by in vitro stimulatory tests and morphologic features.

T cells, whose maturation is dependent on the thymus, are responsible for the development of delayed-type cellular immune response as exemplified in the host's attempts to control tuberculosis, viral, and fungal diseases. These cells have a long life, recirculate constantly, and demonstrate a memory which allows for a rapid cellular response to previously recognized antigens, as demonstrated by the cellular response to PPD antigen in the skin. T cells may also help or suppress B cell responses to antigens.[2] T cells represent approximately 60–85 percent of the circulating blood and thoracic duct lymphocytes. They are also found in paracortical areas of lymph nodes, the spleen, and in small numbers in bone marrow.[3,4] They can be recognized by scanning electron microscope because of their relatively smooth cell surface.[5] Normal sheep red blood cells will attach themselves to human T cells in a rosette pattern. This does not occur when B cells are mixed with sheep red cells.

B cells represent the principal component of bone marrow lymphocytes. In lymph nodes, they are found in the germinal centers, subcapsular areas, and medullary cords, whereas in the spleen they are found in the germinal centers, red pulp, and peripheral white pulp.[2] In contrast to T cells, they have a variably rough surface with characteristic villous projections.

B cell differentiation in birds is dependent on the bursa of Fabricius. In man a bursal equivalent, possibly fetal liver, is required for B cell maturation to plasma cells, which then generate humoral antibodies in the form of immunoglobulins.[6] Immunoglobulin production is critical in host defense against bacterial invasion. Surface immunoglobulins on B cells have been detected with fluorescent anti-immunoglobulin serum. Receptors for the third component of complement are also present on these cells.

A variable percentage of the circulating lymphocytes cannot be defined as T or B cells and are known as null cells.

Lung defense mechanisms and their relationship to general host defenses are only now being defined. The effects of immunosuppression on the mucociliary clearing mechanism, so necessary for removal of inhaled particles, are unknown. It has been suggested that high concentrations of oxygen, often required in immunosuppressed hosts, will reduce normal ciliary function.[7]

The alveolar macrophage is a mononuclear cell that is responsible for the ingestion and destruction of inhaled foreign particulate matter including bacteria. The supply of pulmonary alveolar macrophages is derived from the bone marrow and the tissue histiocytic pool.[8]

The macrophage system, which comprises the primary defense system of the lung against inhaled bacteria, is suppressed by cytoxic drugs, immunosuppressive agents, and treatment with irradiation.[9] The suppression of phagocytic activity in the immunosuppressed host is multifactoral, with direct interference with the function of resident macrophages as well as depletion of the pool of tissue histiocytes. It has been demonstrated in animal studies that acute viral infections produce a direct suppressive effect on the bactericidal capacity of the lung, presumably mediated by inactivation of the alveolar macrophage population.[10] The state of increased susceptibility to bacteria induced by virus infection is a quantifiable phenomenon; it is observed between the sixth and tenth days of acute virus infections.

The roles of antibody and cell-mediated immune responses within the lungs of immunosuppressed hosts are unknown. In otherwise normal individuals the presence of specific IgA antibody in nasal and upper respiratory tract secretions is better correlated with resistance to infection than specific serum antibiodies.[11] Secretory IgA antibody levels in immunosuppressed hosts have not been measured. Cell-mediated immune responses, localized to the respiratory tract, have recently been described, but their significance is unknown.[12]

DRUG RELATED PULMONARY DISEASES

Corticosteroids

Corticosteroids have been described as the drugs most commonly associated with opportunistic infections, whether in the immunosuppressed or immunincompetent host.[13] This predisposition to infection may relate to inhibition of several steps in the nonspecific host defense mechanisms, including leukocyte migration, and phagocytosis.[14] Corticosteroids combined with antibiotics may alter intestinal flora and promote tissue invasion. Craig has described disseminated visceral fungal infections in patients receiving combined therapy.[15] Experiments in which mice were subject to inhalation of fungal spores demonstrate that control animals can tolerate large doses of inhaled spores, whereas animals maintained on corticosteroid therapy rapidly develop a fatal pneumonitis.[16]

Pneumocystis carinii pneumonia has long been associated with immunosuppressive doses of corticosteroids.[17] Frenkel et al. used corticosteroids to induce *P. carinii* infection in rats.[18]

Tuberculosis reactivation with corticosteroids has been well described, although a recent article suggests that low-dose steroids are not associated with an increased incidence of reactivation.[19,20]

Corticosteroids may confuse the clinician concerned with pulmonary disease by producing mediastinal lipomatosis, with resultant mediastinal widening on the roentgenogram. These individuals have a cushingoid habitus, supraclavicular fullness on physical examination, and prominence of the epicardial fat pad on chest roentgenogram.[21] Discontinuance of steroids results in disappearance of the lipomatosis.

Methotrexate

The incidence of methotrexate-induced pulmonary toxicity is unknown, but it has been associated with the treatment of acute leukemia, skin diseases, and connective tissue disorders.[22,24,99] There appears to be no correlation with sex, underlying disease, or duration of therapy, but it is unusual in patients receiving less than 20 mg per week.[23] Symptoms may occur between 12 days and 5 years after initiation of therapy, with an average of 130 days elapsing before symptoms occur. Pulmonary changes have occurred more frequently in patients taking the drug orally. This may be explained by the excellent absorption and sustained blood levels seen with this mode of intake.

Symptoms, including nonproductive cough, dyspnea, and fever up to 105°F, may precede roentgenographic changes by a week or more.[24] Physical findings are often minimal when pulmonary function tests and chest roentgenograms are markedly abnormal. Eosinophilia is found in approximately 50 percent of patients. The roentgenogram characteristically demonstrates diffuse bilateral infiltrates, which initially appear to be interstitial with a late acinar component. Transient hilar and mediastinal adenopathy have been noted, but pleural effusions are rare.[23] Pulmonary function tests demonstrate restrictive changes. The lung biopsy shows round cell infiltrates, and occasional noncaseating granulomata. Cessation of the drug usually results in rapid clearing of the infiltrates. Corticosteroids are reported to increase the resolution rate when methotrexate is discontinued but may not prevent the abnormalities from occurring when methotrexate is continued.

Bleomycin

This drug, which has a propensity to concentrate in epithelial tissue, has frequently been reported to cause interstitial pulmonary fibrosis. Disease usually is dose related, with total doses greater than 300 mg being associated with a higher incidence of fibrosis. Pulmonary function changes, however, may be seen with lower doses. Clinical symptoms are nonspecific. Changes in pulmonary function may be seen within two weeks of initiation of therapy, with the vital capacity and the diffusing capacity being reduced in 30 percent or more of patients in some series.[25] Radiographically the most common pattern seen is a bilateral basal, interstitial infiltrate, with an occasional patient showing a fine nodular pattern. The changes in many cases are irreversible.

Busulfan

This alkylating agent may cause a chronic intra-alveolar fibrotic reaction characterized clinically by symptoms of progressive cough, dyspnea, and fever 9 months to 8 years after initiation of the drug.[26] The chest roentgenogram shows a combined diffuse interstitial and alveolar process. Pulmonary function tests demonstrate restriction. Unlike methotrexate lung, eosinophilia is uncommon. Sputum cytology, which may be diagnostic, shows bizarre, atypical cells thought to be damaged type II granular pneumocytes. Bronchial epithelial cells may also be characteristically abnormal, but histologic sections of the lungs demonstrate a nonspecific organizing fibrous edema. If the disease is far advanced, cessation of the drug and institution of corticosteroids may be of no benefit.

Cyclophosphamide

Another of the alkylating agents, cyclophosphamide has also been associated with a small number of cases of interstitial fibrotic disease that are quite similar to Busulfan-related fibrosis.[27,28] Clinical symptoms of dyspnea and cough generally have occurred after a minimum of 4 months of therapy. Pathologically a bronchiolo-alveolar lining cell dysplasia is seen. Deterioration of pulmonary function appears to be the rule in spite of cessation of the drug.

Melphalan

A single case of progressive interstitial fibrosis, with roentgenographic changes, similar to that seen with Busulfan fibrosis has been reported.[29]

The patient, being treated for multiple myeloma, developed unrelenting dyspnea, later respiratory decompensation, and finally died with respiratory insufficiency. Histologic evaluation of the lungs revealed a proliferation of alveolar and terminal bronchiole lining cells, fibrinous intra-alveolar exudates, and interstitial fibrosis.

Combination Chemotherapy

Recently combined immunotherapy has been implicated in a reversible interstitial process.[30,31] The combinations have been procarbazine, vincristine, and cyclophosphamide in one patient, and nitrogen mustard, vincristine, procarbazine, and prednisone in another. Symptoms were dyspnea, nonproductive cough, and fever after 1–2 months of therapy, with pulmonary function tests demonstrating restrictive changes and the chest roentgenograms showing interstitial-alveolar processes. A nonspecific alveolitis was found at biopsy in both cases. Cessation of drug therapy resulted in significant resolution of symptoms and improvement of restrictive disease. Of the two drugs common to both regimens, only procarbazine has been suggested as a cause of lung disease.[32] Whether a synergistic effect of drugs occurs is unknown.

IMMUNOSUPPRESSED HOSTS

Leukemia

IMMUNE STATUS

Patients with acute leukemias appear to have neither humoral nor cellular immune deficiencies early in their disease. In contrast, patients with chronic lymphocytic leukemia appear to be deficient in both functions. Both groups, however, have quantitative and qualitative defects in mature granulocytes. The qualitative defects include impaired migration, altered phagocytosis, and reduced ability to kill ingested organisms.[33] Lymphopenia and neutropenia (less than 1,000 PMNs), when present, appear to be correlated with an increased incidence of infection.

The quantitative and qualitative defects do not completely explain the predisposition of these patients to infection, for there is an increased incidence of infection during relapse when compared with remission at similar granulocyte levels.[34] Initiation of chemotherapy further compromises the host by inducing leukopenia, depressing cellular and humoral immunity, and predisposing the gastrointestinal barrier to permit invasion by resident flora.[35]

PROGRESSION OF PRIMARY INTRATHORACIC LEUKEMIA:

Roentgenographically discernible hilar and mediastinal lymphadenopathy are present in 5–35 percent of terminal leukemics, with the incidence being higher in the lymphocytic than myelocytic forms.[36] However the roentgenogram is generally insensitive, as demonstrated by the fact that 50 percent of leukemics may have hilar and mediastinal adenopathy at autopsy. The most common roentgenographic pattern in leukemia is bilateral hilar nodes. The nodes are most commonly discretely lobulated in appearance.

Pulmonary parenchymal infiltrates are frequently evident at autopsy but usually are not seen roentgenographically during life.[37] The most common pattern is a diffuse bilateral reticular pattern resembling lymphangitic spread of carcinoma.[38] Ill-defined nodular lesions may be seen that can represent either interstitial infiltrates or infarcts created by leukemic invasion of small vessels. Because roentgenographic evidence of parenchymal leukemia is so uncommon, evidence of infiltrates and especially localized lesions, should raise the suspicion of infection.

Pleural effusions, usually unilateral, occur in approximately 15 percent of leukemics. These are often associated with mediastinal adenopathy and are thought to be secondary to lymphatic obstruction. Actual leukemic infiltration of the pleurae is uncommon.

INFECTIONS

Bacterial. Approximately 70 percent of febrile episodes in patients with leukemia and lymphoma are ultimately proved to be infectious, the majority being bacterial.[39] The lung is the commonest site of bacterial infection. Symptoms are generally nonspecific, most commonly cough, sputum, and hemoptysis. The increased incidence of gram negative bacilli implicated in hospital-acquired infections is reflected in an increased incidence of these organisms in leukemics. Pneumonias, in most cases resulting from initial upper respiratory tract colonization, reflect this tendency, with *Pseudomonas pneumoniae* being the most common infection in some series.

Other gram negative organisms that have caused severe infection include *Klebsiella, E. Coli, Serratia, Proteus, Salmonella,* and *Bacteroides.*[40] Poor prognostic factors include persistent and profound granulocytopenia, cardiovascular shock, azotemia, and failure to develop fever. Roentgenographically these pneumonias usually show up as bronchopneumonic infiltrates or homogenous consolidations and are initially localized to a single lobe. This point may be helpful in distinguishing pneumonias from the more generalized leukemic infiltrates.

The incidence of *Staphylococus aureus* infections has decreased significantly, being found in only 5 percent of fatal infections in several series.

Other gram positive organisms include *Streptococci, Clostridia* and, rarely, organisms thought to be nonpathogenic, as *Staphylococcus albus*.

The liberal use of antibiotics has led to the emergence of drug-resistant organisms with increasing frequency. Resistance, due to the transfer of Ⓡ factor, occurs most commonly between gram negative organisms. Resistance to groups of antibiotics, e.g., kanamycin, neomycin, streptomycin, is the rule. Compounding this problem is the fact that *Pseudomonas,* one of the most lethal organisms, may be only one of several organisms simultaneously infecting the patient. The development of gentamicin, carbenicillin, and recently amakacin has somewhat improved the prognosis of patients with gram negative pneumonias. In spite of this improvement, the mortality rate of severe pulmonary infections approaches 80 percent in some series. This devastating rate appears due more to failure of host defense mechanisms than to antibiotic failure.

Fungal Infections. Invasive fungal infections are common in leukemic patients. Candidiasis, aspergillosis, and mucormycosis are the most frequently observed infections and appear to be related to the use of chemotherapy. The incidence of histoplasma and cryptococcal pulmonary infections is less common but also increased.

Candidiasis is the most common fungal infection in leukemics and lymphoma patients; *C. albicans* is the most frequently implicated species. The ubiquity of the organism which is found routinely in the intestinal tract, on the skin, and hands of medical personnel, as well as in the oral flora of 50 percent of normals partially explains its frequency.[41,42] It is generally thought that neutropenia contributes to its invasive propensity. Invasion of the gastrointestinal tract appears to be common, as does pulmonary involvement. Other manifestations of candida infection in leukemics are thrush, urinary tract infections, septicemia, meningitis, and endophthalmitis.

When pulmonary involvement with *Candida* occurs, symptoms are nonspecific and the chest roentgenogram is commonly abnormal.[43] Lower lobe pneumonitis, generally a bronchopneumonia, with or without pleural effusions has been reported. Patchy consolidation, and abscesses have been seen less frequently. The pattern is generally nonspecific.

The ubiquity of *Candida* and its tendency to colonize requires that the diagnosis of invasive disease be made only when the organism can be demonstrated pathologically in tissue.

The only exceptions to this criterion are positive cultures from pleural fluid, abscesses, or peritoneal fluid.[44] The value of pseudohyphae formation, previously thought to indicate invasion of tissue, has recently been questioned, as has the value of transtracheal aspiration in patients with thrush.

Candidemia, seen not uncommonly in the presence of intravenous catheters, is not adequate evidence of invasion, for the organism often disappears from the blood spontaneously when the catheter is removed. In the compromised host however, candidemia appears to be of more serious consequence, with one series reporting only 25 percent of its cases as noninvasive candidemia.[45] Recently a counterimmunoelectrophoresis test has been demonstrated to be quite accurate in diagnosing invasive candidiasis.[46] A positive test is not, however, considered adequate evidence for institution of therapy.

Aspergillosis is the second most common fungal infection in leukemia and lymphoma patients, but probably represents the single most common pulmonary fungal infection. *A. fumagatus, A. Flavus,* and *A. glaucus* are the most frequent pathogens. The lung is the usual portal of entry.[47] Transmission of the airborne spores has been implicated in hospital-acquired infections.[102] Immune defenses against aspergillus are not well defined, although there is evidence suggesting that PMNs may be necessary for host defense.

The most common indications are a necrotizing bronchopneumonia and hemorrhagic pulmonary infarction, with lobar consolidation being described less often.[48] Symptoms include tachypnea, fever, dyspnea, and, with infarction, hemoptysis and pleuritic pain. Roentgenographic patterns are nonspecific, showing patchy infiltrates, consolidation, and occasional cavitation and atelectasis.

The value of a positive sputum culture for *Aspergillus* is unclear. A small but significant percentage (5–15 percent) of COPD patients, and normals have positive sputums without evidence of disease.[49] Bodey, however, has demonstrated invasive aspergillosis at autopsy in all patients with positive antemortem sputum, urine, and fecal cultures.[50] Unfortunately sputum cultures are infrequently positive in invasive pulmonary aspergillosis. Serologic tests are not presently considered reliable for the diagnosis of invasive aspergillosis. It is usually necessary to resort to biopsy procedures to establish invasion.

The genera *Rhizopus* and *Mucor* are most commonly implicated in phycomycosis of leukemia patients. Inhalation of the fungus results in the most common expression of disease, pulmonary phycomycosis. Why these patients differ significantly from the diabetic patients who present with rhinocerebral phycomycosis is unknown.[44] Common presenting symptoms are those of fever, cough, hemoptysis, and pleuritic pain resulting from vascular invasion and thrombosis, much as with aspergillosis. Mixed infections with bacteria or other fungi are common.

The roentgenographic findings are nonspecific, generally a patchy infiltrate, consolidation, a cavity, or effusion.[51] It has been suggested that the individual lesions are larger and progress more rapidly than in aspergillosis or nocardiosis. A negative chest roentgenogram does not exclude the diagnosis.

Sputum examination is rarely rewarding, and in some cases even when tissue has been available and appropriate septate hypal forms present, the organism could not be cultured. The diagnosis is usually made by lung biopsy, or occasionally skin biopsy.

Hodgkin's Disease

IMMUNE STATUS

Early studies in patients with Hodgkin's disease demonstrated a significantly lower incidence of PPD reactivity when compared to controls.[52] This observation emphasizes the most significant defect of immunity in these patients, specifically abnormalities in cellular immune responsivity due to an acquired T cell deficiency. This anergic state, as manifest by negative skin testing to common antigens, appears to be infrequent in individuals with well localized disease (Stage I), and in those without evidence of systemic symptoms. Those with the nodular sclerosing and lymphocyte predominant forms of the disease also appear to retain the delayed hypersensitivity reaction. In contrast, anergy is more frequently associated with end stage disease (Stage IV), systemic symptoms and the cell types in which lymphocytes are decreased in number.[53]

Humoral antibody responsivity appears to remain intact until far advanced disease is present, but subtle abnormalities in antibody formation have been manifest by decreased ability to form antibodies to weak antigens, and failure to maintain antibody levels over periods of time when compared with controls.[54]

The staging of Hodgkin's disease with splenectomy has been associated with an increased incidence of bacterial infections.[55] Furthermore, radiotherapy and immunosuppressive chemotherapy soon render incompetent those host defense mechanisms previously only minimally impaired.

These observations suggest that initially the Hodgkin's disease patient has either intact defenses, or T cell deficiencies at most, but with progression of disease, radiation, drug therapy, splenectomy, or a combination of these, immune competence diminishes so that ultimately the patient is subject to virtually any infection.

PROGRESSION OF PRIMARY INTRATHORACIC HODGKIN'S DISEASE

Clinical symptoms of intrathoracic involvement are generally cough, dyspnea, pleuritic pain, or occasionally retrosternal pain signifying mediastinal node involvement.

The most common roentgenographic abnormality, seen in 50 percent of patients, is bilateral asymmetric mediastinal adenopathy with paratracheal nodes being involved as frequently as bronchopulmonary nodes.[56] Anterior mediastinal masses and retrosternal nodes are not uncommon and may signify sternal invasion. Calcification of nodes may occur after radiotherapy.[57,58]

Parenchymal involvement rarely occurs without accompanying mediastinal adenopathy. The rare exceptions to this rule occur after mediastinal radiotherapy or with evidence of concurrent extrathoracic disease.[59] The parenchymal involvement is thought to result from extension of the disease from mediastinal nodes along the lymphatics of the bronchovascular sheaths.

Consolidative lesions of variable size with shaggy borders occur occasionally. These infiltrates usually contain air bronchograms since airways are frequently spared in this form of parenchymal invasion. Other roentgenographic patterns include cavitating lower lobe lesions, diffuse miliary or reticulonodular processes, or, uncommonly, atelectasis due to endobronchial invasion. Pleural effusions are present in about 30 percent of patients. These may be chylous or serosanguinous.[58]

Some patients demonstrate sternal, rib, or thoracic vertebrae erosion, thought due to direct invasion from adjacent nodes. Vertebral invasion may be osteoblastic, giving rise to the "ivory vertebrae," whereas rib involvement may mimic that of multiple myeloma.

INFECTIONS

Bacterial. Patients with localized, or early stages of Hodgkin's disease do not have increased susceptibility to bacterial infections because B cell function is intact. As the disease process spreads or the patient undergoes radiotherapy and/or chemotherapy, the propensity for bacterial infections increases. Splenectomy further increases the tendency to *Streptococcus pneumoniae* and *H. influenzae* infections.

In the end stages of the disease, when immunosuppressive therapy no longer controls the disease, bacterial infections occur frequently. Common infecting organisms are *Pseudomonas aeruginosa, Staphylococcus aureus,* and *Escherichia coli.* Tuberculosis, previously quite common in patients with Hodgkin's disease, now occurs in only approximately 5 percent of these patients.[60,61]

Fungal. The T cell deficiency of Hodgkin's disease had been implicated in the unique association of this disease with cryptococcosis. In one series 8.5 percent of all cryptococcal infections were associated with Hodgkin's disease.[100] The organism is ubiquitous, being found in soil, pigeon and chicken droppings, in fruit juice, and even in milk.[62] The species *Cryptococcus neoformans* is the most common pulmonary pathogen in these patients, with *C. albidus* occasionally implicated in this disease. The usual portal of entry is the lung.

The commonest roentgenographic finding is a circumscribed solitary mass 2 to 8 cm in diameter, with the lesion generally found peripherally in a lower lobe.[63,64] Infrequently, cryptococcosis presents as a segmental consolidation, cavitation, miliary pattern, or even less commonly, as multiple discrete lesions. Hilar or mediastinal adenopathy and pleural effusions are uncommon.[65]

The disease may present with no symptoms, subtle personality changes, headaches, fever, skin lesions, or cough. Although *C. neoformans* may rarely be found in the sputum of some patients with no evidence of cryptococcosis, it is not known whether this lack of correlation holds true for the immunosuppressed host.[66] Demonstration of pulmonary cryptococcosis is an indication for lumbar puncture in the immunosuppressed host regardless of symptoms since CNS involvement is common.[101]

There is no reliable skin test antigen to document cryptococcal infection.[67] Diagnosis of invasive disease is best made by open-lung biopsy, transbronchial biopsy, or transthoracic needle biopsy. Invasion of the central nervous system is correlated with the presence of cryptococcal antigen in the cerebrospinal fluid. Care must be taken in making the diagnosis by this method since false-positive reactions have been reported with one form of the test in patients with rheumatoid arthritis.

Viral. Varicella zoster infections have been observed in up to 25 percent of patients with Hodgkin's disease. These infections often occur before clinical evidence of Hodgkin's disease; they are generally in rash form, and do not often disseminate to the lungs.

Late in disease, Casazza et al. have demonstrated the frequent occurrence of a wide range of bacterial, fungal, viral, and protozal infections.[68]

Non-Hodgkin's Lymphomas

This group includes the lymphosarcomas, reticulum cell sarcomas, and follicular lymphomas.

IMMUNE STATUS

Cellular immune defense mechanisms are impaired in this group in a fashion similar to that of Hodgkin's disease. Humoral antibody generating capacity appears to be intermediate between Hodgkin's disease (normal) and chronic lymphocytic leukemia (markedly abnormal). Approximately 15 percent of patients with lymphosarcoma have decreased serum gamma globulin levels with an even higher incidence in those who are evolving into lymphocytic leukemias.[69] Evidence of decreased antibody formation to viral antigens has also been reported.

PROGRESSION OF PRIMARY INTRATHORACIC DISEASE

This group of patients rarely has primary intrathoracic lesions, but when they do, the initial clinical symptoms are dyspnea, cough, and pain.[70]

As the disease progresses 50 percent of patients will demonstrate secondary pulmonary involvement, most commonly manifested by mediastinal or bronchial lymphadenopathy. Other secondary manifestations include solitary or multiple pulmonary nodules, varying in size from 3 mm to 7 cm in diameter.[71] These lesions are usually found endobronchially in the lower half of the lungs and may result in atelectasis and/or obstructive pneumonitis. Pleural effusions, when present, are most commonly due to mediastinal or hilar obstruction of lymphatics. Autopsy studies reveal a 70 percent incidence of intrathoracic involvement.

Because the immune status of these patients is similar to that of the patients with Hodgkin's disease, similar bacterial, fungal, and protozoal infections occur.

TRANSPLANT RECIPIENTS

This group of patients add yet another factor to the decision-making process. The value of the graft must be weighed against the lethal potential of continued immune suppression in the infected host.

Renal Transplants

IMMUNOLOGY

Renal transplant patients are the prototype of the transplant group. In recent years it has been recognized that uremia alone increases susceptibility to bacterial infections, impairs delayed hypersensitivity reactions, and delays skin homograft and kidney transplant rejections.[72] Post-transplant the immunosuppressive agents used to prevent rejection result in both T and B cell deficiency states as well as suppression of the nonspecific host defenses. In addition the liberal use of steroids during rejection crises may facilitate the invasion of certain organisms.

The elective nature of these surgical patients does allow for the minimization of some potential pathogens. Staphylococcal carriers can be treated preoperatively. INH may be given prophylactically even with a negative PPD because of the aforementioned anergic state. Blood products can be screened for hepatitis B antigen, and indigenous flora regularly monitored.

INFECTIONS

Infections in this group generally occur at least two weeks post-transplant. Males are infected more frequently for unknown reasons. The respiratory tract is the most common portal of microbial entry. Bacteria account for approximately half of all infections, whereas fungi, viruses, protozoa, and mixed infections constitute the remainder.

BACTERIAL

The incidence of gram positive infections has been reduced considerably with the elimination of *Staphylococcus* carriers. Gram negative organisms, specifically *Pseudomonas, E. coli,* and *Klebsiellae* are now more common and often result in death in this group of patients. Mixed infections of bacteria and fungi are not common.

FUNGAL

Fungal infections occur commonly in patients with renal transplants with one series demonstrating twenty fungal infections in 51 transplant patients.[73] The infecting organisms are similar in frequency to those reported in leukemics and lymphoma patients, with *Aspergillae* and *Candida* predominating, and occasional cases of *Cryptococcosis* and *Phycomycosis* being found. It has been suggested that the potential for infection increases with the number of rejection episodes but is not necessarily associated with leukopenia. Because these fungi have been reviewed in a previous section, they will not be further detailed here.

PROTOZOA

Pneumocystis carinii is the single most common cause of diffuse interstitial pneumonitis in immunosuppressed hosts.[74] It is a common accompaniment to the use of chemotherapy, most commonly corticosteroids, and cyclophosphamide. *P. carinii* rarely causes disease in transplant patients not taking medication. It appears that disease caused by *P. carinii* is due more to the immune state of the patient than to the virulence of the organism.[76] Frequently, pneumonitis does not present itself until steroids have been tapered.[75] It has been suggested in animal studies that this observation is due to the return of immunocompetence with inflammation and exudate occurring as the host defenses become more competent and attempt to kill the organisms. This inflammatory state then causes the deterioration of pulmonary function and the typical clinical presentation. Other associated predispositions are hypogammaglobulinemia and protein deficiency states.[76]

Recent studies have suggested that the organism may be transmitted between persons, but invasive disease has not been documented by this route.[77] The clinical syndrome characteristically has a rapid onset of dyspnea and nonproductive cough. Fever is common, but physical findings are often minimal or absent. We have been impressed, as have others, by the discrepancy between the minimal physical and roentgenographic findings and the severity of hypoxemia.

Roentgenographic presentation is most typically a bilateral, perihilar interstitial infiltrate but frequent variations, ranging from a peripheral alveolar presentation to nodular or unilateral infiltrates occur.[78] Minimal radiographic abnormalities may be present weeks before clinical symptoms occur and may remain unimpressive during the initial development of significant respiratory complaints. Pleural effusions are rare. Blood studies are nonspecific with the exception of the poor prognosis associated with leukopenia. Because sputum examination is usually unrewarding, the diagnosis is made most frequently by obtaining lung tissue or via bronchial brushing. Pathologic sections of lung tissue characteristically show a foamy eosinophilic material filling the alveoli and alveolar septal thickening with minimal cellular infiltrates.[79] The organism, best seen with a silver stain, is found within the foamy material. At present the organisms cannot be cultured in the average laboratory, so that the diagnosis rests solely on pathologic demonstration. Approximately 20 percent of patients with *P. carinii* infection have a concurrent infection, typically bacteria or cytomegalovirus.[80]

Toxoplasmosis, with a prevalence rate of 50 percent in some population studies, less commonly manifests clinical symptoms in the immunocompromised host. When it does so, it is often associated with other organisms.[81] The clinical presentation is most commonly a neurologic syndrome, but an interstitial pneumonitis picture has been described. Disease due to toxoplasmosis has been extensively reviewed elsewhere and will not be discussed further because of its infrequency.[82,91]

VIRAL

Cytomegalovirus (CMV) is a member of the herpes virus family which includes *Herpes simplex,* Varicella, and the Epstein-Barr virus. CMV commonly presents as a pneumonitis in the immunosuppressed host.[83] It appears to arise from a latent infection present either in the recipient or donor kidney which proliferates when immunity is significantly depressed.[84,85] Rejection phenomena have also been associated with emergence of the infection.

The clinical presentation is generally that of fever, dyspnea, and nonproductive cough beginning 40 days after transplant. Simultaneous infections with *Candida, Aspergillae,* and *Pneumocystis* are common. Roentgenographic findings are variable, and include a bilateral peripheral infiltrate of 2–4-mm nodules, a reticular pattern, and a normal roentgenogram.[86] The diagnosis is complicated by the fact that the organism is ubiquitous. In one series 65 percent of individuals without clinical evidence of disease had positive urine cultures. Serologic testing commonly shows elevations in the titer post-transplant, even in individuals without clinical evidence of disease. Moreover, CMV has been cultured from lung tissue which did not have the typical haloed "owl-eyed" intranuclear inclusions thought characteristic of infections.[87] Presently the best diagnostic criteria for invasive disease include both characteristic pathologic changes on biopsy and a positive culture of the biopsy tissue.

Bone Marrow Transplants

Bone marrow transplantation is currently being performed in patients with leukemia or aplastic anemia. A nonspecific interstitial pneumonia is the most frequent cause of death in these patients.[88] It is often unassociated with culture or histologic evidence of known pathogens. Possible explanations include the additive effects of drugs plus radiation injury, graft versus host reactions within the lung, or combinations of these insults.

IMMUNOLOGY

Successful engraftment of donor marrow requires total destruction of the pre-existing immune system, with leukopenia and lymphopenia naturally occurring. This suppression is accomplished by total-body irradiation and/or multiple drugs, including cytosine arabinoside, 6 thioguainine, daunorubicin, cyclophosphamide, and procarbazine. Antihuman globulin is used in some aplastic anemia patients.

INFECTIONS

Bacterial. Infections with these organisms are uncommon, perhaps due to the pretransplant sterilization of the intestines and the early institution of broad-spectrum antibiotics at the first sign of infection.

Fungal. Candida infections may occur early in the post-transplant period and are usually fatal.[89] Respiratory infections are rarely seen in the absence of disseminated candidiasis.

Viral. Cytomegalovirus (CMV) is the major lethal pathogen in marrow transplant patients, and occurs in the lung as an interstitial pneumonitis. The presence of the virus can be documented in many individuals who do not develop clinical infections. These patients frequently excrete the virus in the urine, and demonstrate significant complement fixation antibody titer rises. When CMV is associated with a lethal pneumonitis, the virus is less often recovered from the urine, and the serologic response is usually absent or insignificant. In our hospital sputum cytology has been helpful in diagnosing suspect CMV pneumonia. Characteristic changes seen are cellular enlargement, enlarged nuclei showing coarsely granular basophilic chromatin condensed into a ring along the inner surface of the nuclear membrane, and around a central large, single basophilic inclusion.

Cardiac Transplants

This procedure has rarely been performed in recent years. The patients involved have end-stage cardiac disease and chronic pulmonary congestion. This latter point may partially explain the high incidence (50 percent) of pulmonary infections found in this group.

IMMUNOLOGY

Preoperatively these patients differ from the renal transplant patients because they have no immune deficiencies. With surgery and the institution of therapy, including corticosteroids, azothioprine, cyclophosphamide, and antilymphocyte globulin, these individuals develop deficiencies in all three host defense systems—the nonspecific, cellular, and humoral.

INFECTIONS

Bacterial infections occur and gram negative infections predominate. It is not uncommon to have infections with multiple bacterial organisms or mixed bacterial and fungal infections. Remington et al. have reported fungal infections to be common in these patients with *Aspergillae* and *Nocardia* being most prevalent.[90]

CLINICAL APPROACH

Rapid, appropriate decision making in these patients is critical. In one's haste to arrive at the correct diagnosis, definitive procedures should not take precedence over a carefully taken history and meticulous physical examination, for these may obviate the need for invasive procedures with considerable risk. Steroids or antimetabolites should be discontinued if possible, with the hope for rapid return of immunocompetence.

History

The immunocompromised host with pulmonary disease generally presents in one of two ways—with fever or with symptoms referable to pulmonary involvement. Depending on the underlying disease, fever may or may not heighten one's suspicion of an infectious process. In patients with chronic lymphocytic leukemia and multiple myeloma, fever almost always represents infection, whereas approximately 30 percent of acute leukemia, Hodgkin's disease, and lymphoma patients have fever due to their underlying disease. Fever due to transplant rejection is a somewhat uncommon but well-known entity. In the appropriate setting a history of Busulfan or methotrexate therapy should raise the possibility of drug-related fever.

Symptoms are generally nonspecific and tend to underestimate the extent of disease. Unique symptom complexes should, however, arouse suspicion of specific etiologies as exemplified by the pleuritic chest pain and hemoptysis seen with invasive aspergillosis or phycomycosis.

A careful drug history is extremely helpful for it allows one to include or exclude drug-related pulmonary problems. The history of recent steroid withdrawal should raise the suspicion of *P. carinii* infection and also make one consider corticosteroid replacement for possible adrenal insufficiency. A recent history of high-dose immunosuppressive therapy with resultant granulocytopenia should raise one's suspicion of an opportunistic infection. The time-span of leukopenia can often be predicted from knowledge of specific drug effects.

The specific underlying disease and its activity may suggest a diagnosis. Stage I or II Hodgkin's disease with a localized pulmonary lesion and fever suggest cryptococcosis. This may be most quickly and easily diagnosed by lumbar puncture rather than lung biopsy. Alternatively, knowledge of end-stage refractory Hodgkin's disease broadens the differential diagnosis to include virtually any infection or progression of the primary disease.

Physical Examination

A meticulous physical examination is extremely helpful. Particular attention to the eyes, skin, mucous membranes, and rectal area may reward one with the findings of early *Candida endophthalmitis,* disseminated fungal infections to the skin, perianal herpetic lesions, or rectal abscesses.

When the patient is leukopenic and cannot generate a significant inflammatory reaction, signs of pulmonary consolidation may be absent and abscesses may be watery and non-tender. Inspection of all indwelling catheters may reveal an early site of infection. Daily physical exams may be the only reliable method of assessing progression of disease.

Laboratory Evaluation

Blood studies are routinely obtained to measure the total leukocyte count, lymphocyte count, and gamma globulin concentration. These reflect B cell and nonspecific host defenses; skin testing may be used to demonstrate delayed hypersensitivity and, indirectly, T cell function.

Serologic tests for fungal disease may be drawn but, because of their delay in return, will not generally influence decision-making.

Platelet counts and prothrombin times are mandatory in defining procedural risks. Increased risk of bleeding from cutting and aspirating needle biopsy, as well as open-lung biopsy have been reported with prothrombin times less than 60 percent of control regardless of the platelet count.[92] In the same study there was a definite increased risk of bleeding when the platelet count was less than 100,000/mm,^{3} but the risk did not increase progressively as the platelet count decreased, and thrombocytopenia did not preclude performance of a lung biopsy. Successful transbronchial biopsies in patients with platelet counts less than 20,000/mm^3 have been performed after platelet infusion.[93]

On the other hand a hemorrhagic fatality has been reported after bronchial brushing in a patient with a platelet count less than 10,000/mm^3. Azotemia has also been associated with an increased incidence of hemorrhagic complications of biopsy procedures.[95]

Cultures of the oropharynx, sputum, blood, and urine should be obtained, and smears from appropriate body fluids or sites should be stained with acid-fast, KOH, Gram, or methenamine silver stains. Cerebral spinal fluid India ink preparations should be routine when lumbar puncture is indicated.

Assuming an unrewarding routine evaluation to this point, and bearing in mind that clinical diagnoses correlate poorly in these patients with their ultimate diagnoses, the physician now must decide upon a potential sequence of diagnostic procedures.

Diagnostic Sequences

The necessity of an accurate diagnosis cannot be overemphasized. Diagnosis of a treatable disease may be associated with a 70 percent recovery rate.[92] Continued or increased immunosuppressive therapy for presumed progression of underlying disease could prove fatal if the correct diagnosis is infection. Broad-spectrum antibiotic coverage for presumed infection invites resistant organisms, potential toxic reactions, and delay of correct diagnosis. Under very select circumstances the physician may have no alternative but to employ broad-spectrum antimicrobial therapy.

The sequence of procedures and timing will be influenced by the underlying disease, characteristics of the present illness, available diagnostic procedures, their risks, and yields. Examples are given below.

A leukemic or myeloma patient with fever and a localized infiltrate on chest roentgenogram has approximately a 70 percent chance of the infiltrate's representing infection (Fig. 13-3). These are generally bacterial. Mixed infections are not uncommon in these patients. The combination of CMV and *P. carinii* infections in the immune-suppressed host is well known. Less well appreciated is the frequency and multiplicity of gram negative bacillus infections. Valdivieso et al. found 43 episodes of mixed infections in 217 occurrences of gram negative infections.[106] More than two organisms were implicated in some infections, and cure rate appeared to depend on the number of organisms. A transtracheal aspirate, assuming correction of inadequate clotting parameters, would then be most likely to reveal one or more pathogens. If stains are unrewarding, consideration of a transthoracic needle aspiration is then appropriate, for this procedure generally has a high yield in infections and reasonably low morbidity, provided coagulation defects are corrected.[96] Supportive facilities for pneumothorax control and blood replacement must be available. Lacking needle aspiration capabilities, trephine biopsy, or the transtracheal brushing technique described by Aisner may be helpful in defining viral, fungal, or bacterial infections.[97] Transbronchoscopic procedures are not helpful in defining specific etiologies because of the frequent contamination when passing the bronchoscope through the oropharynx or nasopharynx.

If severe clotting deficits preclude biopsy or the procedures mentioned

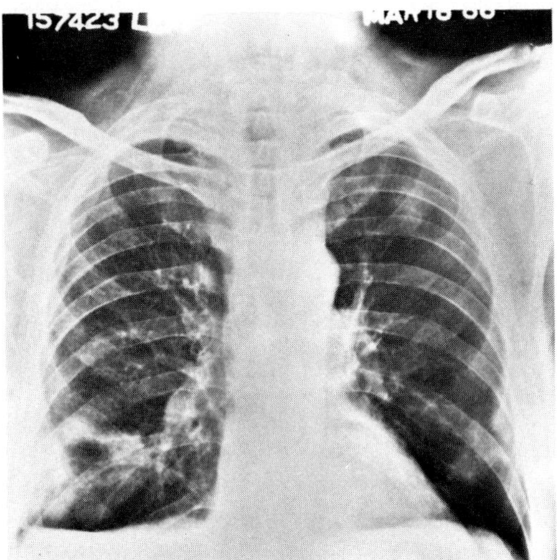

Fig. 13-3. This patient with leukemia presented with fever and a right lower lobe infiltrate. Diagnostic studies revealed a mixed infection of proteus mirabilis, klebsiella species, and pseudomonas species.

above are not available, an alternate course may be that of 48 hours of empiric broad-spectrum antibiotics. If clinical improvement does not occur, and if cultures are still negative, then consideration may be given to open-lung biopsy. The point has been repeatedly made that bleeding tendencies can be more easily controlled during open biopsy, and that control of hypoxemia and extubation are less problematic in these restricted patients than in obstructed patients.

The granulocytopenic patient with fever, pulmonary involvement, and clinical signs of sepsis requires a broad-spectrum antibiotic regimen before a definite diagnosis can be made. Mortality rates approach 60 percent in this situation when antibiotics are withheld for 48 to 72 hours.[105] When broad-spectrum coverage is begun early, approximately 70 percent will respond. Recently granulocyte transfusions in conjunction with antibiotics have been demonstrated to be effective in decreasing the mortality rate, particularly in those with persistent granulocytopenia.[103,104]

The diagnostic sequence may be dictated by the rate of progression of the present illness. In individuals with rapid deterioration of pulmonary reserve, as demonstrated by progressive arterial desaturation and dyspnea, we have elected to go directly to open lung biopsy. The rationale for this approach is the feeling that time would allow but one procedure, and therefore we have chosen the single diagnostic study with the highest acknowledged yield. An alternate approach, which we have used on occasion, is to take the individual to the operating room, intubate him, and while preparing him for thoracotomy, perform a transbronchial biopsy. If frozen sections, touch

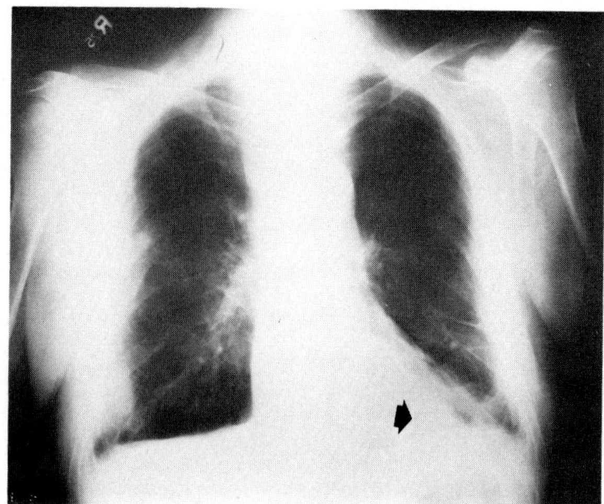

Fig. 13-4. 59-year-old renal transplant patient with retrocardiac aspergillus fumagatus abscess.

preps, and appropriate stains are negative, an open-lung biopsy can be performed immediately.

An occasional patient has respiratory decompensation of such severity that respirator support is immediately required, and all biopsy procedures appear to be contraindicated. This is not always the case. It is possible to brush and do transbronchial biopsies through a small adapter that allows the patient to remain on the respirator. If necessary, positive end-expiratory pressure (PEEP) can be maintained during the procedure. There are no strict criteria to guide the diagnostician through this decision. The facility of the bronchoscopist, presence of underlying obstructive pulmonary disease, pulmonary hypertension, level of PEEP, and a multitude of other factors must be considered.

The individual more prone to develop one of the opportunistic infections is exemplified by the renal transplant patient or one who is in an early stage of Hodgkin's disease. The approach to these patients is dictated somewhat by the roentgenographic presentation. Localized, slowly progressive disease suggests initially a transtracheal aspiration to rule out bacterial, fungal, viral, or the occasional localized *P. carinii* infection (Fig. 13-4). In our institution this would be followed by bronchial brushing and a transbronchial biopsy. An alternative procedure would be transthoracic needle aspiration, although we would prefer the bronchoscopic procedure because the incidence of pneumothorax is generally lower (approximately 5 percent versus 10 percent). If necessary, either of these procedures may be repeated.

A similar patient with a diffuse symmetrical process generally, though not always, suggests a viral, protozoal, mixed infection, or drug-related dis-

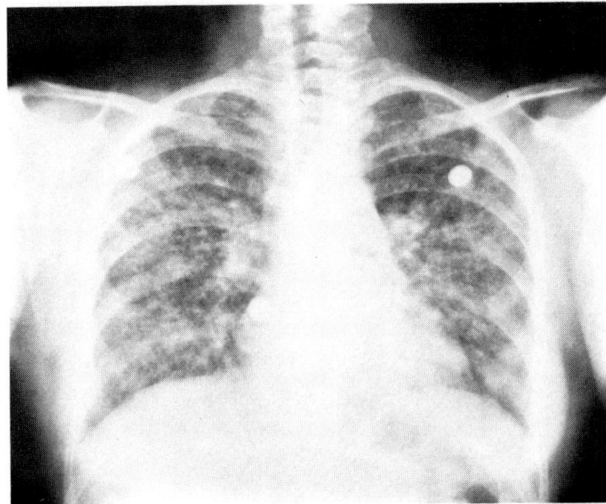

Fig. 13-5. 16-year-old renal transplant patient with Pneumocystis carinii pneumonia proven by open lung biopsy.

ease (Fig. 13-5). Assuming an unrewarding transtracheal aspiration, we then would do a transbronchial brushing and biopsy. *Pneumocystis carinii* can be identified in more than 80 percent of cases using this technique and fungi in approximately 40 percent of proven cases. Occasionally viral cytopathologic changes are diagnostic.[94] Again transthoracic needle aspiration is an acceptable alternative. If no specific diagnosis is obtained by the previous procedures, an open biopsy would follow rather than consideration of repeating either of the less invasive procedures.

Progression of underlying disease as exemplified by end-stage lymphoma patients, immunosuppressed collagen vascular disease patients, or patients with suspect drug-related injury may initially have a transtracheal aspirate to rule out infection (Fig. 13-6). This may then be followed by a transbronchial biopsy and brushing. Needle aspiration is less attractive because we are seriously entertaining diagnoses best evaluated by histologic specimens. Open biopsy is the most helpful procedure in this group, but consideration should be given to biopsying sites other than the lingula because, although its readily accessible, it may demonstrate chronic changes related more to its anatomic configuration and poor drainage than to the underlying process.

The adequacy of biopsy specimens from transbronchial, needle, or trephine biopsy is always questioned when the pathology report returns describing nonspecific inflammatory changes. Although a nonspecific diagnosis is often the final diagnosis at autopsy, we have generally chosen to proceed with open-lung biopsy, being unwilling to assume that the less invasive procedure was totally representative. Although open-lung biopsy is the ultimate diagnostic procedure, even this may be inadequate. Greenman et

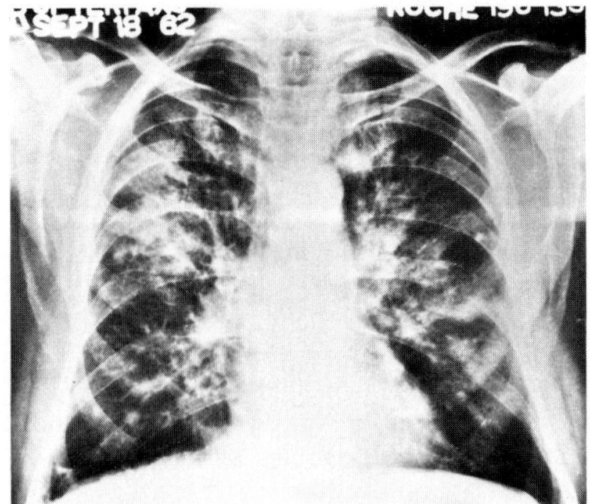

Fig. 13-6. This 67-year-old man died in the hospital while being treated for carcinoma of the vocal cord. Autopsy revealed diffuse Hodgkin's disease involving both lungs.

al. described three patients in whom open-lung biopsy was not representative of the total process found at autopsy, and we have seen similar instances.[92]

Hypoxemia in this group of patients appears to correlate with the length of disease prior to biospy. Not surprisingly, then, hypoxemia has been correlated in general with a poor prognosis.

A thorough, prospective study correlating underlying disease, clinical presentation, and diagnostic procedures of choice has yet to be done in this group of patients. Advances in serologic testing, vaccination against opportunistic organisms, and tissue-specific immunosuppressive agents may minimize the need for invasive procedures in the future.

REFERENCES

1. Carpenter PL: Immunology and Serology. Philadelphia: W. B. Saunders Company, 1975, p. 243
2. Richter M, Algom D: The heterogeneity of lymphocytes, a consideration of future developments and their impact on clinical medicine. Med Clin North Am, 56:305–317, 1972
3. Craddock CG, Longmire R, McMillan R: Lymphocytes and the immune response, N Engl J Med 285:324–331, 1971
4. Borella L, Sen L: The distribution of lymphocytes with T and B cell surface markers in human bone marrow. J Immunol 112:836–843, 1974
5. Polliak A, Lampen N, Clarkson BD, et al: Identification of human B and T lymphocytes by scanning electronmicroscopy, J Exp Med 138:607–624, 1973
6. Gatti RA, Good RA: The immunological deficiency disease, Med Clin North Am 54:281, 1970

7. Sackner MA, Landa J, Hirsch J, et al: Pulmonary effects of oxygen breathing: A 6 hour study in normal man. Ann Intern Med 82:40–43, 1975
8. Godleski JJ, Brain JD: The origin of alveolar macrophages in mouse radiation chimeras. J Exp Med 136:630–643, 1972
9. Green GM, Kass EH: The role of the alveolar macrophage in the clearance of bacteria from the lung. J Exp Med 119:167–176, 1964
10. Jakob GJ, Green GM: The effect of Sendai virus infection on bacteriacidal and transport mechanisms of the murine lung. J Clin Invest 51:1989–1998, 1972
11. Perkins JC, Tucker DN, Knapf HLS, et al: Comparison of protective effect of neutralizing antibody in serum, and nasal secretions in experimental rhinovirus type 13 illness. Am J Epidemiol 90:519–526, 1969
12. Waldman RH, Henney CS: Cell-mediated immunity and antibody responses in the respiratory tract after local and systemic immunization. J Exp Med 134:482–494, 1971
13. Rosenow EC: The spectrum of drug-induced pulmonary disease. Ann Intern Med 77:977–991, 1972
14. Holland JF, Senn H, Banerjee T: Quantitative studies of localized leukocyte mobilization in acute leukemia. Blood 37:499–511, 1971
15. Craig JM, Farber S: Development of disseminated visceral mycosis during therapy for acute leukemia. Am J Pathol 29:601, 1953.
16. Fidransky H, Friedman L: The effects of cortisone and antibiotic agents on experimental pulmonary aspergillosis. Am J Pathol 35:169–185, 1959
17. Johnson HD, Johnson WW: *Pneumocystis carinii* pneumonia in children with cancer: Diagnosis and treatment, JAMA 214:1067–1073, 1970
18. Frenkel JK, Good JJ, Shultz JA: Latent Pneumocystis infection of rats, relapse, and chemotherapy. Lab Invest 15:1559–1577, 1966
19. Schatz M, Patterson R, Kloner R, et al: The prevalence of tuberculosis and positive tuberculin skin tests in a steroid-treated asthmatic population. Ann Intern Med 84:261–265, 1976
20. Canada RO, Carr DT, Ebert RH: The effect of cortisone and/or corticotropine on tuberculosis infection in man: A statement prepared by the Committee on Therapy. Am Rev Tuber 66:254–256, 1952
21. Koernoer HJ, Sun DI: Mediastinal lipomatosis secondary to steroid therapy. Am J Roentogenol Radium Ther Nucl Med 98:461–464, 1966
22. Clarysse AM, Cathey WJ, Cartwright GE, et al: Pulmonary disease complicating intermittent therapy with methotrexate. JAMA 209:1861–1864, 1969
23. Sostman HD, Matthay RA, Putman CE, et al: Methotrexate-induced pneumonitis. Medicine 55:371–388, 1976
24. Goldman GC, Moschella SL: Severe pneumonitis occurring during methotrexate therapy. Arch Dermatol 103:194–197, 1971
25. Yagoda A, Mukherji, B, Young C, et al: Bleomycin, an antitumor antibiotic. Ann Intern Med 77:861–870, 1972
26. Heard BE, Cooke RA: Busulfan lung. Thorax 23:187–193, 1968
27. Topilow AA, Rothenberg SP, Cottrell TS: Interstitial pneumonia after prolonged treatment with cyclophosphamide. Am Rev Respir Dis 108:114–117, 1973
28. Rodin AE, Haggard ME, Travis LB: Lung changes and chemotherapeutic agents in childhood. Am J Dis Child 120:337–340, 1970
29. Codling BW, Chakera TMH: Pulmonary fibrosis following therapy with melphalan for multiple myeloma. J Clin Pathol 25:668–673, 1972

30. Farney RJ, Morris AH, Armstrong JD, et al: Diffuse pulmonary disease after therapy with nitrogen mustard, vincristine, procarbazine and prednisone. Am Rev Respir Dis 115:135–145, 1977
31. DeVita VT, Serpick AA, Carbone PP: Combination chemotherapy in the treatment of advanced Hodgkin's disease. Ann Intern Med 73:881–895, 1970
32. Lokich JJ, Moloney WC: Allergic reactions to procarbazine. Clin Pharmocol Ther 13:573–574, 1972
33. Lehrer RI, Cline MJ: Leukocyte candidacidal activity and resistance to systemic candidiasis in patients with cancer. Cancer 27:1211–1217, 1971
34. Buckley M, Sathe YS, Freireich EJ: Quantitative relationships between circulating leukocytes and infections in patients with acute leukemia. Ann Intern Med 64:328–340, 1966
35. Baker RD: Leukopenia and therapy in leukemia as predisposing to fatal mycoses. Am J Clin Pathol 37:358, 1962
36. Klatte C, Yardley J, Smith EB, et al: The pulmonary manifestations and complications of leukemia. Am J Roentgen 89:598–609, 1963
37. Green RA, Nichols NJ: Pulmonary involvement in leukemia. Am Rev Respir Dis 80:833–844, 1959
38. Robbins LL: The roentgenological appearance of parenchymal involvement of the lung in malignant lymphoma. Cancer 6:80–88, 1953
39. Miller SP, Shanbron E: Infectious syndromes of leukemias lymphomas. Am J Med Sci 246:420–428, 1963
40. Levine AS, Graw RG, Young RC: Management of infections in patients with leukemia and lymphoma: Current concepts and experimental approaches. Semin Hematol 9:141–179, 1972
41. Cohen R, Roth FJ, Delgado E, et al: Fungal flora of the normal human small and large intestine. N Engl J Med 280:638–641, 1969
42. Clayton YM, Nobel WC: Observation on the epidemiology of *Candida albicans*. J Clin Pathol 76:19, 1966
43. Williams DM, Krick JA, Remington JS: Pulmonary infections in the compromised host. Am Rev Respir Dis 114:359, 1976
44. Hart PD, Russell E Jr, Remington, JS: The compromised host and infections. II Deep fungal infections. J Infect Dis 120:169–191, 1969
45. Young RC, Bennett JE, Geelhold GW, et al: Fungemia with compromised host resistance: A study of 70 cases. Ann Intern Med 80:605–612, 1974
46. Marier R, Andriole VT: Usefulness of CIE in detection of *Candida albicans* antigen and antibody. Clin Res 23:588, 1975
47. Aigello L: A comparative study of the pulmonary mycoses of Canada and the United States. Pub Health Rep 84:869–877, 1969
48. Young RC, Bennett JE, Vogel CL, et al: Aspergillosis: The spectrum of the disease in 98 patients. Medicine (Baltimore) 49:147–173, 1970
49. Comstock GW, Palmer CE, Stone RW, et al: Fungi in the sputum of normal men. Mycopathol Mycol Appl 54:55–62, 1974
50. Bodey GP: Fungal infections complicating acute leukemia. J Chronic Dis 19:667–687, 1966
51. Bartrum RJ, Watnick M, Herman PG: Roentgenographic findings in pulmonary mucormycosis. Am J Roentgenol Radium Ther Nucl Med 117:810–815, 1973
52. Parker F Jr, Jackson H Jr, Fitzhugh G, et al: Studies of diseases of lymphoid and myeloid tissues: IV. Skin reactions to avian and human tuberculin. J Immunol 22:277–282, 1932

53. Young R, Corder M, Haynes H, et al: Delayed hypersensitivity in Hodgkin's disease. Am J Med 52:63–72, 1972
54. Aisenberg AC, Leskowitz S: Antibody formation in Hodgkin's disease. N Engl J Med 268:1269–1272, 1963
55. Ravry M, Maldonado N, Velez-Garcia E, et al: Serious infection after splenectomy for the staging of Hodgkin's disease. Ann Intern Med 77:11–14, 1972
56. Fisher AMH, Kendall B, Van Leuven BD: Hodgkin's disease: A radiological survey. Clin Radiol 13:115, 1962
57. Leading Article, Outlook in Hodgkin's disease. Br Med J 2:328–329, 1967
58. Strickland B: Intra-thoracic Hodgkin's disease: Part II. Peripheral manifestations of Hodgkin's Disease in the chest. Br J Radiol 40:930–938, 1967
59. Moolten S: Hodgkin's disease of the lung. Am J Cancer 21:253–294, 1934
60. Casazza AR, Duvall CP, Carbone PP: Summary of infectious complications occurring in patients with Hodgkin's disease. Cancer Res 26:1290–1296, 1966
61. Armstrong D, Young LS, Meyer RD, et al: Infectious complication of neoplastic disease. Med Clin North Am 55:729–745, 1971
62. Littman ML, Walter JE: Cryptococcosis: Current status. Am J Med 45:922–932, 1968
63. Wolfe JN, Jacobson G: Roentgen manifestation of torulosis (cryptococcosis). Am J Roentgen 79:216–227, 1958
64. Bonmati J, Rogers JV Jr, Hopkins WA: Pulmonary cryptococcosis. Radiology 66:188–194, 1956
65. Campbell GD: Primary pulmonary cryptococcosis. Am Rev Respir Dis 94:236–243, 1966
66. Warr W, Bates JH, Stone A: The spectrum of pulmonary cryptococcosis. Ann Intern Med 69:1109–1116, 1968
67. Buechner HA, Seabury JH, Campbell CC, et al: The current status of serolgic immunologic, and skin tests in the diagnosis of pulmonary mycosis: Report of the Committee of Fungus Disease and Subcommittee on Criteria for Clinical Diagnosis, American College of Chest Physicians. Chest 63:259–270, 1973
68. Casazza AR, Duvall CP, Carbone PP: Infection in lymphoma. JAMA 197:710–716, 1966
69. Miller DG: Patterns of immunological deficiency in lymphomas and leukemias. Ann Intern Med 57:703–716, 1962
70. Rosenberg SA, Diamond HD, Jaslowitz B, et al: Lymphosarcoma: A review of 1296 cases. Medicine 40:31–84, 1961
71. Samuels ML, Howe CD, Dodd CD Jr, et al: Endobronchial malignant lymphoma: Report of five cases in adults. Am J Roentgenol 85:87, 1961
72. Dammin CJ, Couch, NP, Murray JE: Prolonged survival of skin homografts in uremic patients. Ann NY Acad Sci 64:967–976, 1957
73. Bach MC, Adler JL, Breman J, et al: Influence of rejection therapy on fungal and nocardial infections in renal transplant recipients. Lancet 1:180–184, 1973
74. Goodell B, Jacobs JB, Powell RD, et al: *Pneumocystis carinii:* The spectrum of diffuse interstitial pneumoniae in patients with neoplastic disease. Ann Intern Med 72:337–340, 1970
75. Rifkind D, Faris TD, Hill RB: *Pneumocystis carinii* pneumonia: Studies on the diagnosis and treatment. Ann Intern Med 65:943–956, 1966
76. Hughes WT, Price RA, Sisko F, et al: Protein-calories malnutrition, a host determinant for *Pneumocystis carinii* infection. Am J Dis Child 44:128, 1974

77. Singer C, Armstrong D, Rosen PP, et al: *Pneumocystis carinii* pneumonia: A cluster of eleven cases. Ann Intern Med 82:772–777, 1975
78. Thomas SF, Dutz W, Khodadad EJ: *Pneumocystis carinii* pneumonia (plasma cell pneumonia): Roentgenographic, pathologic and clinical correlation. Am J Roentgen 98:318–322, 1966
79. Price RA, Hughes WT: Histopathology of *Pneumocystis carinii* infestation in malignant disease in childhood. Hum Pathol 5:737–752, 1974
80. Schultz MG: *Pneumocystis carinii* pneumonia in the United States: Epidemiologic, diagnostic and clinical features. Ann Intern Med 80:83–93, 1974
81. Vietzke WM, Gelderman AH, Grimley PM, et al: Toxoplasmosis complicating malignancy. Cancer 21:816–827, 1968
82. Williams DM, Krick JA, Remington JS: Pulmonary infection in the compromised host. Am Rev Respir Dis 114:593–627, 1976
83. Kanich RE, Craighead JE: Cytomegalovirus infection and cytomegalic inclusion disease in renal homotransplant recipients. Am J Med 40:874–882, 1966
84. Ho M, Suwansirikul S, Dowling JN, et al: The transplanted kidney as a source of cytomegalovirus infection. N Engl J Med 293:1109–1112, 1975
85. Fiala M, Payne JE, Berne TV, et al: Epidemiology of CMV infection after transplantation and immunosuppression. J Infect Dis 132:421–433, 1975.
86. Rifkind D, Goodman N, Hill RB: The clinical significance of CMV infection in renal transplant recipients. Ann Intern Med 66:1116, 1967
87. Craighead JE: Pulmonary cytomegalovirus infection in the adult. Am J Pathol 63:487–504, 1971
88. Neiman PE, Thomas ED, Reeves W, et al: Opportunistic infection and interstitial pneumoniae following marrow transplantation for aplastic anemia and hematologic malignancy. Transplant Proc 8:663, 1976
89. UCLA Bone Marrow Transplantation Group: Bone marrow transplantation with intensive combination chemotherapy/radiation therapy (SCARI) in acute leukemia. Ann Intern Med 86:155–161, 1977
90. Remington JS, Gaines JD, Griepp RB, et al: Further experience with infection after cardiac transplantation. Transplant Proc 4:699–705, 1972
91. Ruskin J, Remington JS: Toxoplasmosis in the compromised host. Ann Intern Med 84:193–199, 1976
92. Greenman, RL, Goodall PT, King D: Lung biopsy in immunocompromised hosts. Am J Med 59:488–496, 1975
93. Scheinhorn DJ, Joyner LR, Whitcomb ME: Transbronchial forceps lung biopsy through the fiberoptic bronchoscope in *Pneumocystis carinii* pneumonia. Chest 66:294–295, 1974
94. Finley R, Kieff E, Thomsen S, et al: Bronchial brushing in the diagnosis of pulmonary disease in patients at risk for opportunistic infections. Am Rev Respir Dis 109:379–387, 1974
95. Cunningham JH, Zavala DC, Corry RJ, et al: Trephine air drill, bronchial brush, and fiberoptic transbronchial lung biopsies in immunosuppressed patients. Am Rev Respir Dis 115:213–220, 1977
96. Bandt PD, Blank N, Castellino RA: Needle diagnosis of pneumonitis: Value in high risk patients. JAMA 220:1578–1580, 1972
97. Aisner J, Kvols LK, Sickles EA, et al: Transtracheal selective bronchial brushing for pulmonary infiltrates in patients with cancer. Chest 69:367–371, 1976.

98. Bartlett JG, Alexander J, Mayhew J, et al: Should fiberoptic bronchoscopy aspirates be cultured? Am Rev Respir Dis 114:73–78, 1976
99. Arnet FC, Whelton JC, Zizic TM, et al: Methotrexate therapy in polymyositis. Ann Rheum Dis 32:536, 1973
100. Gendel RR, Ende M, Norman SL: Cryptococcosis. A review with special reference to apparent association with Hodgkin's disease. Am J Med 9:343–355, 1950
101. Mills SA, Seigler HF, Walfe WG: The incidence and management of pulmonary mycosis in renal allograft patients. Am Surg 182:617, 1975
102. Gage AA, Dean DC, Schimert G, et al: Aspergillus infection after cardiac surgery. Arch Surg 101:384, 1970
103. Herzig, RH, Herzig GP, Graw RG, et al: Successful granulocyte transfusion therapy for gram negative septicemia. N Engl J Med, 296:701–705, 1977
104. Alavi JB, Root RK, Djerassi I, et al: A randomized clinical trail of granulocyte transfusion for infection in acute leukemia. N Engl J Med 296:706–711, 1977
105. Greene WH, Schimpff SC, Young VM, et al: Empiric carbenicillin, gentamicin, and cephalothin therapy for presumed infection in patients with granulocytopenia and cancer. Ann Intern Med 78:825–826, 1973
106. Valdivieso M, Gil-Extremera B, Zornoza J, et al: Gram negative bacillary pneumonia in the compromised host. Medicine 56:241–254, 1977

Stanley S. Siegelman, M.D.
Frederick P. Stitik, M.D.
Warren R. Summer, M.D.

14

Management of the Patient with a Localized Pulmonary Lesion

In this chapter we shall set forth our current ideas on the proper management of the patient with a solitary lesion in the lung which may represent cancer. Much of the material upon which our final conclusions are based has already been set forth in Chapters 2, 5, 6, 7, 8, 9, and 10. Although some of the directives in this presentation will echo the reasoning of prior contributors, we offer a patient-oriented approach to supplement the earlier material which was primarily focused on technique.

THE SOLITARY PULMONARY NODULE

The solitary pulmonary nodule is the prototype of the localized mass lesion in the lung. Various authors have applied different restrictions on what constitutes a solitary nodule. In general any patient whose chest roentgenogram shows a single rounded or ovoid lesion in the lung parenchyma which is not associated with obvious adenopathy, atelectasis, or pneumonia is considered to have a solitary pulmonary nodule. The term "coin lesion" was first offered by O'Brien et al. to describe the focal mass.[1] The use of the term enjoyed a short-lived popularity but has since been disparaged as the description implies a flattened object while we are actually dealing with a spherical mass. Solitary pulmonary nodule is currently the most appropriate designation for such lesions.[2–7]

WHAT DOES A SOLITARY PULMONARY NODULE REPRESENT?

Excision of the solitary pulmonary nodule including resection of the involved lobe if necessary became a commonly accepted technique in the early 1950s. As data on such cases accumulated it became apparent that a significant percentage of solitary nodules actually represented lung cancer. Steele summarized the results of nine separate series of resected solitary nodules which had been published in the 1950s.[5] Each series contained more than 100 cases. The incidence of malignant disease ranged from 10 to 68 percent and exceeded 40 percent in 6 of the 9 studies. In Tables 14-1 and 14-2, we have summarized the results of 5 surveys of solitary pulmonary nodules. Criteria for inclusion in these series varied as outlined in Table 14-1. Despite the variation in case selection, the nature of the resected nodules was very similar in all 5 series. As may be seen from Table 14-2, the commonest lesions by far are granulomas and bronchogenic cancer. Hamartoma, metastases, bronchial adenoma, bronchogenic cysts, benign pleural tumor, chronic pneumonia and bronchopulmonary sequestration follow in order of decreasing frequency. The series also included examples of arteriovenous fistula, pulmonary infarct, subpleural lymph nodes, localized anthrosilicosis and neurofibroma.

ASSESSMENT OF THE NATURE OF THE SOLITARY PULMONARY NODULE

As a result of the extensive experience with *resected* pulmonary nodules, the message became clear: the patient with a solitary mass as detected on a chest roentgenogram has a moderate likelihood of harboring a lung cancer. French et al., in a typical 1950s response, advocated an aggressive approach with early exploratory thoracotomy for *all* solitary pulmonary nodules.[8] Many other thoracic surgeons firmly agreed with such a philosophy. Opponents of this aggressive approach reasoned that *selection* was responsible for the high incidence of cancer in the published series of patients subjected to thoracotomy. Solitary pulmonary nodules constitute a heterogeneous mixture. Solitary nodules detected during mass screenings of the general population proved to be malignant in only 3–6 percent of the cases.[9,10] The patients selected for operation in the series with a 40+ percent incidence of malignancy were those referred to the surgeon because of some concern about the size, the appearance, or the growth rate of their lesion. Therefore, it is possible to develop diagnostic criteria by means of which each individual case can be analyzed.

OTHER EXPERIENCES WITH ASSESSMENT

The late doctor L. Henry Garland championed the concept that accurate nonoperative assessment of solitary pulmonary nodules was feasible.

Table 14-1
Criteria for Inclusion of Cases in Series of Solitary Pulmonary Nodules

	Davis et al.[2]	Good et al.[14]	Steele[27]	Taylor et al.[6]	Walske[7]
1. Total Number of Cases	215	156	887	236	217
2. Sex	135 males 80 females	89 males 67 females	Males only	208 males 25 females	Males only
3. Size	6 cm or less	No restriction	6 cm or less	1–6 cm	1–5 cm
4. Shape	"Minimal lobulation tolerated"	No restriction	No restriction	"Slight lobulation tolerated"	"Slight lobulation tolerated"
5. Calcification	Calcified lesions excluded	32 Calcified 25 Granulomas 7 Hamartomas	No restriction	58 Calcified 57 Granulomas 1 Scar tumor	No restriction
6. Cavitation	No restriction	No restriction	Excluded	No restriction	No restriction
7. Symptoms	No restriction	No restriction	Excluded	No restriction	Excluded
8. Other Features	Minimal pleural component tolerated	—	—	Sputum positive cases excluded	—

Table 14-2
The Nature of Solitary Pulmonary Nodules

	Davis et al.[2]	Good et al.[14]	Steele[27]	Taylor et al.[6]	Walske[7]	Total	
1. Granulomas	82	65	474	183	118	922	53.9%
2. Bronchogenic carcinoma (or other primary malignancy)	82	26	285	18	74	485	28.3%
3. Hamartoma	9	25	65	8	6	113	6.6%
4. Metastasis	10	17	26	2	5	60	3.5%
5. Bronchial adenoma	9	12	7	3	3	34	2.0%
6. Bronchogenic cyst	3	—	7	8	3	21	1.2%
7. Chronic pneumonitis or abscess	6	—	2	4	6	18	1.1%
8. Benign pleural tumor	6	3	6	2	0	17	1.0%
9. Bronchopulmonary sequestration	3	—	1	4	0	8	0.5%
10. Other benign conditions	5	8	14	4	2	33	1.9%
TOTAL NUMBER OF CASES	215	156	887	236	217	1711	

He reported his own experience in evaluating 115 consecutive cases of solitary pulmonary nodules. In 106 of the 115 cases he was able to make a decision concerning the nature of the nodule; 68 were classified as benign and 38 were called probably malignant. Among the 68 lesions designated as benign there were two proven cancers. Thirty-four of the 38 cases designated probably malignant were verified as malignant.[3] In a separate study Dr. Garland and his associates presented roentgenograms of 50 patients with solitary pulmonary nodules to a panel of 5 radiologists. The majority of the radiologists correctly identified all 8 malignant lesions and classified all 42 benign lesions as benign.[11] Taylor et al. concluded after a review of 236 cases of resected solitary nodules including 23 maligant lesions that "if all cases which had fuzzy borders or were greater than 4.0 cm in diameter had exploratory thoracotomy *every* malignant tumor would have been discovered."[6]

It is our current policy to make an assessment of the nature of the localized pulmonary mass based upon the age of the patient and the radiographic appearance of the lesion. This assessment plays a significant role in directing patient management. The five key factors in the evaluation are:

1. The growth rate of the lesion.
2. The presence of calcification.
3. The patient's age.
4. The contour of the lesion and the sharpness of the margin.
5. The size of the mass.

The factors have been listed in the order of their general significance but in the individual case, any one of the factors may prove decisive in judging a solitary pulmonary nodule as probably benign or probably malignant. The avoidance of unnecessary thoracotomy is an important basic principle guiding the diagnostic work-up. Every effort is made to employ methods or procedures which will establish a diagnosis of benign disease.

Growth Rate

The absence of detectable growth over a long period of observation is probably the single most reliable criterion for establishing that a pulmonary nodule is benign. Review of prior chest roentgenograms is thus an important factor in the evaluation of the patient with a solitary nodule. If a lesion is unchanged in size and appearance over a two-year period, no tests are indicated other than a series of periodic yearly follow-up chest roentgenograms. What about the application of the growth rate principle to the solitary pulmonary nodule without prior chest roentgenograms? Should the nature of a pulmonary lesion be determined by serial observations at brief intervals? Nathan, Collins, and Adams directed their attention to this question by a study of the growth rate of 177 malignant nodules and 41 benign nodules.[12] The authors reached a series of interesting conclusions. In patients under age 40, it was found that malignant neoplasms grow rapidly. Among 27 such patients, the longest doubling time was 199 days. Included in this group were 8 patients with solitary nodules, all of which exhibited a doubling time of 49 days or less with a single exception having a doubling time of 102 days.[11] Among patients of all age groups, pulmonary nodules enlarging more slowly than one doubling every 18 months are invariably benign.* In practice, Nathan et al. measured the diameter of the lesion by tracing the circumference of each nodule and then choosing the diameter of the best-fitting reference circle.[12] Therefore, Nathan has proposed that growth rate be employed as a primary tool in the evaluation of solitary pulmonary nodules in patients 30–45 years old.[4] Rather than an immediate thoracotomy for the undiagnosed nodule, Nathan advises a two-week delay to obtain a follow-up chest roentgenogram. If no growth of the nodule is detected, a second delay of four weeks is proposed. If again no growth is detected, chest x-rays are advised at continually increasing intervals up to two years, at which point the nodule may be deemed benign. If any definite growth of the nodule is observed at any point, immediate surgery is advised. Wise et al. studied 19 patients with lung cancer in whom serial chest roentgenograms were available for study and found that the doubling times ranged from 1.8 to 10 months.[13] Growth rate monitoring is contrary to recommendations of C. Allen Good, a distinguished radiologist at the Mayo Clinic. Dr. Good, who has devoted his attention to the solitary pulmonary nodule for many years, is opposed to any policy of watchful waiting.[14,15] On the basis of his experience, he has advocated immediate thoracotomy for all patients with noncalcified lesions without prior roentgenograms.[16]

Calcification

The presence of calcification within a lesion is generally a reliable sign that the lesion is benign. As mentioned in Chapter 9, when pulmonary nodules contain definite calcium deposits as detected by plain chest roentgenography or tomography, we assume that the lesion is benign and we follow the patient with a limited series of annual chest radiographs. The prudence of the policy of watchful waiting for calcified pulmonary nodules was illustrated by the experiences of Holin et al. and McClure et al.[9,10] Each group followed over 200 patients with calcified solitary nodules for over five years and no instances of lung cancer occurred in either study.

The best documentation of the distribution and the nature of calcifications within solitary pulmonary nodules was carried out at the Mayo Clinic and reported in a series of articles in the 1950s.[14,15,17] In the period from 1940 to 1951, 156 solitary masses were resected including 32 lesions with obvious calcium content. Each of the 32 calcified lesions proved to be benign, 25 were granulomas and 7 were hamartomas. This series included

* Doubling time refers to doubling of volume. Since the volume of a sphere is equal to $\frac{4}{3}\pi r^3$, a two-fold increase in the diameter of a nodule yields an eight-fold increase in volume.

26 carcinomas, 17 metastases, and 12 bronchial adenomas, none of which were calcified.[14] In the period from 1951 to 1954, 705 patients with solitary pulmonary nodules were analyzed. In 294 cases, the masses exhibited calcium deposits by chest roentgenography or tomography (in 36 suspicious cases, tomography confirmed the presence of calcification, in 5 cases tomography revealed unsuspected calcium deposits). Surgical exploration was undertaken in only 16 of the 294 cases and again, all proved to be benign lesions.[15] In a separate study, specimen radiography was obtained on 207 solitary pulmonary masses (including 149 of the 156 lesions resected in the period 1940–1951, and 58 additional specimens obtained in 1951 and 1952). Four different patterns of calcification were noted:

1. A laminated pattern with calcium deposited in concentric layers, between rings of fibrous tissue. The laminated pattern is a reliable indication of the existence of a granuloma.
2. The dense central nidus.
3. Diffuse and irregular nodular deposits—the popcorn type of calcification which is very suggestive of hamartoma.
4. Punctate calcification.

In addition, studies showed that 6 of 38 bronchogenic carcinomas, 2 of the 14 bronchial adenomas, and 2 of the 20 metastatic lesions also contained evidence of calcification. The malignant lesions generally had eccentric focal areas of punctate calcification.[17] Calcifications within pulmonary neoplasms are frequently present within areas of old inflammatory disease engulfed by the enlarging tumor, but they may also represent actual tumor necrosis. On occasion, calcium in the lung anterior or posterior to a malignant lesion may appear to be within the mass.

If one accepts the principle that nodules with calcium detectable by chest roentgenography or tomography are benign, the number of patients with granulomas subjected to thoracotomy will decrease. This point is illustrated in Tables 14-1 and 14-2. Davis et al. did not operate on calcified nodules and hence, resected 82 granulomas versus 82 carcinomas. In the series reported by Good et al. and by Taylor et al., calcified lesions were removed and the ratio between granulomas and carcinomas resected was correspondingly higher.

The actual incidence of detectable calcium within lung cancers is probably less than 1%. Theros found 7 examples of radiologically detected calcification in 1267 lung cancers.[18] Sporadic cases have been reported in which a false sense of security engendered by the presence of calcium within the lung cancer had led to mismanagement.[19] Fortunately, however, such cases are extremely unusual.

As indicated by Bloch, the term "calcification" as used in radiologic diagnoses is arbitrary, since lesions may contain considerable amounts of calcium which are not identified by roentgenograms.[20] Methods of detecting calcium within the lung vary greatly in sensitivity. Calcium deposits which are overlooked on 70 mm minifilms will often be identified in 14 × 17 chest roentgenograms.[9] Tomography will show calcification not detected in plain chest roentgenography. Specimen radiography will reveal calcification which was not appreciated on tomography.[17] Finally, microscopic examination will disclose additional calcium deposits which are not seen on specimen radiography.

Moderate variations in density are observed among pulmonary nodules which do not qualify for classification as "calcified." As a possible extension of the concept that calcified lesions are benign, there is some indication that density may be a useful parameter for determining the nature of a small lesion. Small nodules which are dense are more apt to be benign. Vivas and Crabtree developed a classification of solitary lung lesions based upon radiographic density.[21] The "heavy density" category referred to lesions which equalled or exceeded the density of the heart shadow. Lesions which were inconspicuous because they were considerably less dense than the heart were classified as "light density." The "moderate density" category was for lesions which were fairly obvious but definitely less dense than the heart shadow. All 10 lesions which were 3 cm or smaller in the light density category were malignant. All 7 lesions which were 1 cm or less in diameter and which were classified as heavy density (5) or moderate density (2) proved to be benign. Among 16 lesions, 1–3 cm in diameter which were classified as heavy or moderate density, 13 were benign and 3 were malignant. Davis et al. were in general agreement with the guidelines that for lesions 2 cm or less in size, the definitely dense nodules were granulomas whereas the less dense nodules could be considered carcinomas.[2] One of the difficulties with this concept is that apparent density on a chest roentgenogram is an imprecise parameter. CT number as determined by computed tomography is a much more precise means of assessing the density of a nodule (see Chapter 5). There is some indication that computed tomography may provide more precise information on the calcium content of solitary nodules.

Age

Solitary pulmonary nodules are almost invariably benign in patients under age 30. Taylor et al. resected 81 nodules in patients aged 20–29 and found one bronchogenic carcinoma, one bronchial adenoma, and 79 benign lesions including 67 granulomas.[6] Bateson collected 100 cases of solitary circumscribed bronchogenic carcinoma and his series contained no patients under age 30.[22] Solitary nodules in patients under age 30 may be presumed to be benign, but should be followed with serial chest roentgenograms for at least 2 years. Pulmonary malignancies should not be considered rare in the 30–39 year old age group. Among 39 lesions resected in this age group, Davis et al. found 9 bronchogenic carcinomas.[2] There is increasing concern about the possibility of malignancy in any newly discovered pulmonary nodule encountered in the fifth and sixth decades.

Contour of the Lesion and Sharpness of the Margin

Most authors agree that malignant solitary nodules are much more apt to have an irregular contour and an ill-defined or irregular margin. The lesion with a perfectly round or oval contour and a sharply defined edge is usually benign. There is no claim that the converse of this generalization is valid (that benign lesions invariably have a sharply defined contour), since it is not rare for a granuloma to present with an ill-defined margin.[23] Most authors have confirmed the validity of these observations but have concluded that evaluation of the contour and of the margin are not sufficiently reliable means to separate malignant and benign lesions.[2,14,24] Rigler, who has been interested in the radiologic manifestations of lung cancer, has emphasized the "notch sign" of malignancy.[25] He has indicated that notching or umbilication of any portion of the border of a spherical nodule should cause concern for malignancy.[26] The notch sign is an example of irregular contour. The margin of the lesion, which represents the junction between the neoplasm and the surrounding lung parenchyma was described by Steele as poorly defined or shaggy or infiltrated in 89% of the malignant lesions he studied.[5] Taylor et al. found that 94% of bronchogenic cancers appearing as solitary nodules had definite irregularities or fuzziness of borders.[6] Bateson, in his study of 100 cases of solitary circumscribed bronchogenic carcinoma, found that 71 percent of cases had a poorly defined margin. Each of the remaining 29 cases with a well-defined margin had a lobular contour. Thus, no single case in this series had both a well-defined margin and a circular or oval contour.[22] We believe that the perfectly round or oval lesion with an exquisitely sharp margin is almost invariably benign.

Size

It is universally agreed that for solitary pulmonary nodules the likelihood of malignancy is a direct function of the size of the lesion. The best data to document this principle is from the Veteran's Administration Cooperative Study; figures are presented in Table 14-3. Our conclusion from this data is that lesions larger than 3.5 cm in diameter must be regarded as highly suspicious for malignancy. Although small lesions less than 1.5 cm in diameter are statistically much more likely to be benign, we do not think it is prudent to use small size as a significant factor in planning patient management. Small carcinomas, especially one cm or less in size, are difficult to detect on a roentgenogram presumably because they are less dense and less well defined than granulomas. However, by dint of excellent radiographic technique and skillful film interpretation, it is possible to detect 1-cm carcinomas. The reward for skillful detection of the small lesion is improved patient survival. Steele et al. reported a 53 percent four-year survival following resection in 85 patients with bronchogenic carcinoma which were 2 cm or less in diameter. The corresponding figures were 41 percent survival for 177

Table 14-3
Size of Lesion Benign versus Malignant

Size	Hamartomas & Granulomas	Malignancy	Ratio Benign/Malignant
1 cm or less	104	8	13:1
1.5–2.0 cm	225	78	3:1
2.5–3.0 cm	91	105	1:1
3.5–4.0 cm	20	59	1:3
4.5–5.0 cm	8	36	1:4.5
5.5–6.0 cm	1	20	1:20
Total	450	306	

Adapted from Steele.[27]

patients with nodules 2.5 to 4 cm in diameter and 29 percent four-year survival for 46 patients with nodules 4.5 to 6 cm in diameter.[27] It is interesting that there is a paucity of data on lesions 1.5 cm or less in size in many of the early studies of resected solitary pulmonary nodules. The prevailing opinion in the early 1950s in many centers was that thoracotomy was not indicated for such lesions. Good and Wilson, for example, reported on the outcome of 705 cases of pulmonary nodules encountered between 1951 and 1954 at the Mayo Clinic. Fifth-two nodules 1.0 cm or less in size were discovered but only 2 such lesions were removed surgically.[15] Apparently the chief reason for eschewing surgery in most cases was that the physician responsible for the patient's care had decided that the likelihood of granuloma was so great that thoracotomy was not justified. We would not follow such reasoning today. Since 1973, The Johns Hopkins University has conducted a screening program for lung cancer among a high risk population of male volunteers who are at least 45 years of age. Among the first 63 cases of lung cancer detected, 17 were 2 cm or less in diameter including 6 lesions which were 1 cm or smaller.[28]

ADDITIONAL FACTORS IN THE ASSESSMENT OF THE PATIENT WITH A LOCALIZED PULMONARY LESION

Hemoptysis

Hemoptysis portends the presence of an aggressive lesion. The series reported by Davis et al. included 11 patients with documented hemoptysis. Eight patients had bronchogenic carcinoma, one had a bronchial adenoma, and there were 2 benign lesions.[2] Bronchial adenomas are widely recognized as potentially malignant lesions. The previously cited series of Good et al. included 18 patients with a history of hemoptysis. Only 3 of the patients proved to have benign lesions. The other 15 cases included 8 bronchogenic carcinomas, 4 bronchial adenomas, and 3 other varieties of malignancy.[14]

Prior History of Malignancy

As was noted in Table 14-2, metastatic cancer is the fourth commonest cause for a solitary pulmonary nodule. Fairly good results may be obtained if such lesions are resected. Thomford et al. reported a 30 percent three-year survival following removal of pulmonary metastases.[29] More recently, a 50 percent five-year survival has been obtained at the National Institutes of Health.[30] Metastatic nodules are often less aggressive in appearance than primary cancers. In Bateson's series, half the solitary metastases had a smooth contour and a well-defined edge.[23] History of prior surgical removal of a primary cancer, therefore, must raise our suspicions that a pulmonary lesion is malignant.

In a group of patients with a previous malignancy, not all solitary lesions will be metastatic. Cahan et al. found and removed malignant lesions from 54 patients with a prior history of colon cancer. In 25 cases, the lesions were metastases but in 29 cases there was a primary lung cancer.[31] Atkins et al. found that of 31 patients with prior cancer who presented with solitary nodules, 22 were metastases, 7 were benign and 2 were primary lung cancers.[32] The rules of thumb derived from experiences at Memorial Hospital in New York are as follows:

1. If a patient has had a prior squamous cancer elsewhere, the new lung nodule is apt to be a second primary cancer.
2. If the patient has had a previous adenocarcinoma, the lung lesion has an equal chance for representing metastasis or a new primary.
3. If the first lesion was a melanoma or sarcoma of bone or soft tissue, the pulmonary nodule is probably metastatic.[31]

SEARCHING FOR A POSSIBLE PRIMARY LESION

Since metastatic disease is a serious consideration in every patient with a solitary pulmonary nodule, how vigorously should one search for a possible occult extrapulmonary primary lesion? Should all such patients have a preoperative work-up which includes a gastrointestinal series, barium enema, and intravenous urogram? Lawhorne et al. addressed this question by analyzing the various factors involved.[33] They concluded that the combination of all of the aforementioned diagnostic procedures will produce a very low yield of useful information. The majority of patients with a manifest pulmonary metastasis are already known to have a primary tumor. Occult primary cancers are responsible for only 20–25 percent of the cases of solitary metastatic pulmonary nodules. Among a thousand cases of solitary nodules, one can therefore anticipate 25 potential cases (2.5 percent) of metastasis from occult extrapulmonary cancer. In some of these patients, the screening tests may not detect the primary lesion. Moreover since resection of a metastatic pulmonary nodule contributes to control of disease, it is more expedient to search for the primary lesion after the pathology report indicates that the resected nodule was metastatic. Our present standard evaluation, therefore, includes a careful physical examination, and examination of the urine and stool for blood on three separate occasions. Abnormalities are pursued with additional studies, but if the preliminary tests are negative, no extensive search for extrapulmonary cancer should be carried out.[34] The policy of avoiding such screening tests has also been espoused by many other experienced groups.[5,7,24]

Final Assessment

In Table 14-4 we have itemized the key factors which contribute to our final assessment of the probable nature of the solitary pulmonary nodule. Points have been assigned to each factor. The ten-point items take precedence. When a lesion satisfied one of the ten-point features for benign disease, the patient is followed without a tissue diagnosis. If a lesion rates ten or more points on the malignancy scale, thoracotomy is indicated. If the nodule receives a net score (malignant points minus benign points) below ten points, a decision is made to obtain a tissue diagnosis without resorting to thoracotomy. Examples follow:

1. A 50-year-old man (4 malignant points) with a 2.5 cm (0 points) uncalcified nodule (4 malignant points) and a history of hemoptysis (5 malignant points). Total, 4 plus 4 plus 5 equals 13 malignant points. Such a patient would have bronchoscopy, evaluation for operability, and staging for resectability. If the patient were operable and resectable, a thoracotomy would be performed.
2. A 58-year-old female (4 malignant points) with a 3.0 cm (0 points) uncalcified (4 malignant points) smooth oval sharply defined (5 benign points) nodule in the lung. No history of hemoptysis or prior malignancy. Total 4 plus 4 malignant points minus 5 benign points minus 3 malignant points; decision needle biopsy.
3. 59-year-old male (4 malignant points) with 3 cm calcified lesion (10 benign points). The patient has prior history of cancer of the colon (6 malignant points). No x-rays are available for the past three years. Decision: follow patient, calcified lesion takes priority.

PERSPECTIVES

Discussion in this chapter has focused on the solitary pulmonary nodule as a prototype of the localized pulmonary lesion. The solitary pulmonary nodule is the single most common presenting manifestation of lung

Table 14-4
Factors Influencing Assessment of Solitary Pulmonary Nodules

Factor	Favors Benign	Points	Favors Malignant	Points
1. Growth rate	No growth for 2 yrs.	10	Definite growth on serial roentgenograms	10
2. Calcification	(a) laminated	10	Uncalcified	4
	(b) dense central core	10		
	(c) diffuse nodular	10		
	(d) punctate central	10		
3. Age	Under 30	9	Over 40	4
4. Contour & margin	Smooth oval or perfect circle and sharply defined	5	Lobulated-irregular or spiculated-ill defined	5
5. Size	Not a useful factor	0	Larger than 3.5 cm	5
	Dense lesion <2 cm	4	Low density lesion <2 cm	4
6. History of prior malignancy	None	0	Positive	5
7. Documented hemoptysis	None	0	Positive	5

cancer.[18,35,36] Bateson surveyed the literature and found that lung cancer was initially evidence as a peripheral parenchymal mass in 20 to 40 percent of the cases.[22] In an excellent analysis by Theros of the material from the Armed Forces Institute of Pathology, peripheral masses accounted for 40 percent (507) of 1267 cases of lung cancer.[18] Rigler estimated recently that 60 percent of lung cancers are initially manifest as solitary nodules.[37] In the Johns Hopkins early lung cancer detection study, 71 percent of the lesions discovered have been located in the periphery or mid zone of the lung.[28]

The salient objectives of any system for managing patients with localized pulmonary lesions are: (1) to avoid the false-negative diagnosis, i.e., a malignancy is present but the patient is not treated for cancer, (2) to lower the number of false-positive diagnoses, i.e., thoracotomy is performed for possible malignancy but benign disease is present. The system of management which includes thoracotomy for all noncalcified newly discovered lesions produces too many false-positive cases. The approach which employs the policy of watchful waiting to assess the growth rate of newly discovered lesions yields too many temporary false-negative diagnoses. The strategy employed at The Johns Hopkins Hospital includes: (1) thoracotomy for operable and resectable lesions assessed as probably malignant, (2) obtaining tissue diagnosis, including use of needle biopsy for lesions which are assessed as probably benign, (3) closely following patients with successful but nondiagnostic needle biopsy. This management system avoids thoracotomy for the group of patients with benign lesions diagnosed by successful needle biopsy. The only false-negative category are those patients with malignancies who are assessed as benign and are followed without thoracotomy because of an unsuccessful attempt at needle biopsy. Our experience in the last five years includes 20 patients with a diagnosis of benign disease established by needle biopsy. Nine other patients had needle biopsies which were inconclusive; but on follow-up the lesions either decreased in size or remained stable for 2 years. Finally eight other patients are being followed with presumed benign lesions after unsuccessful needle biopsy (see Table 9-3). We have not had a single case of cancer in any patient who had been followed for presumed benign disease after needle biopsy.

OTHER LOCALIZED RADIOGRAPHIC PRESENTATIONS OF LUNG CANCER

By virtue of local growth and distant spread to lymph nodes, lung cancer produces intrathoracic alterations which become evident on chest roentgenograms:

1. Unilateral hilar enlargement which may be due to either direct visualization of a tumor growing in a major bronchus (usually an epidermoid carcinoma) or the presence of lymph node metastases from a small unre-

cognized primary cancer (especially a small cell carcinoma). Isolated unilateral hilar enlargement in an adult should be considered due to pulmonary malignancy until proven otherwise.[24]

2. Bronchial obstruction and its consequences. All bronchogenic carcinomas originate in the conducting airways. Local growth of the lesion compromises the bronchial lumen and frequently produces collapse of distal lung. Roentgenograms in such cases reveal segmental atelectasis often associated with obstructive pneumonitis.
3. Other signs of intrathoracic spread. Central spread of the tumor may produce mediastinal widening due to lymphadenopathy. Pleural effusion can be due to direct spread by tumor or may reflect mediastinal lymphatic obstruction.

As a general rule, the ominous nature of the radiologic manifestations beyond the coin lesion is readily recognized and the clinician is immediately alerted to the probable existence of a bronchogenic cancer. To some extent the cell type of the tumor is related to the nature of the abnormality detected in the chest roentgenogram. The majority of adenocarcinomas and large cell undifferentiated carcinomas present as peripheral lesions whereas squamous cell cancers are much more apt to involve proximal bronchi and produce unilateral hilar enlargement or bronchial obstruction and its consequences.[35]

PLAN OF ACTION

The plan of action for the patient with a localized pulmonary lesion is set forth in Figure 14-1. A number of amplifying comments are offered; in each instance the number preceding the comment refers to the number in Figure 14-1.

1. Examination of the sputum for cytopathologic diagnosis as discussed in Chapter 6 is a routine part of the evaluation. The highest yield is from central bronchogenic carcinomas arising in primary or secondary bronchi. Cytology is less rewarding for peripheral lesions and is rarely helpful with benign tumors or bronchial adenomas. A diagnosis of undifferentiated large cell carcinoma is an indication for subsequent mediastinoscopy.
2. Bronchoscopy is the single most helpful diagnostic procedure in the evaluation of a possible lung cancer. Bronchoscopic examination may reveal unsuspected proximal spread of a peripheral lung tumor. The yield of a definite diagnosis is highest for lesions of the primary or secondary bronchi. The best results are obtained when multiple samples are submitted including microbiopsies, brushings, curettings, and lavage. In three situations, we occasionally bypass bronchoscopy and proceed directly to needle biopsy: (a) a peripheral solitary nodule which

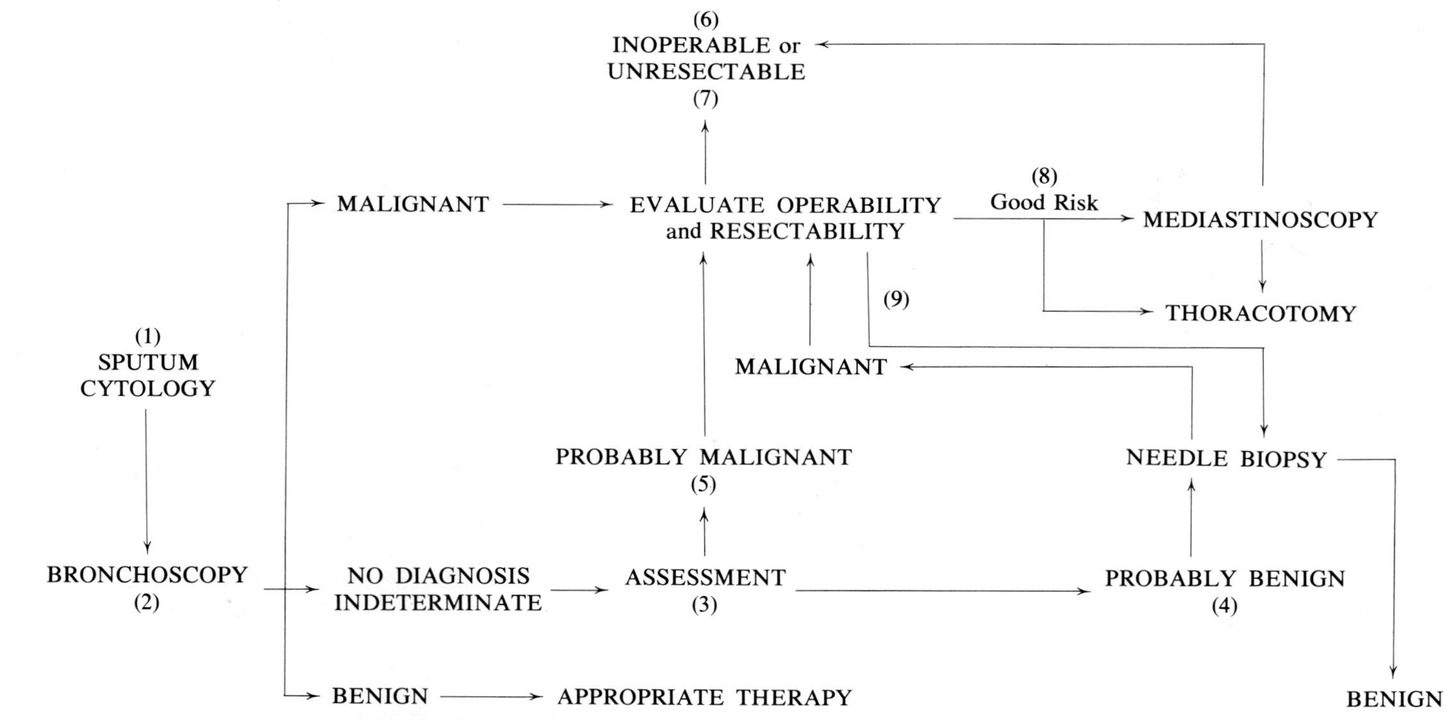

Fig. 14-1. Evaluation of the patient with a localized pulmonary lesion

is assessed as benign and is readily accessible to needle biopsy, (b) lesions which are probably metastatic, and (c) Pancoast tumors. One can anticipate a relatively low yield from bronchoscopy in these three situations.

3. An assessment of each case as probably benign or probably malignant is based upon criteria set forth in Table 14-4.
4. At this point in the evaluation we have a patient with a localized lesion and no diagnosis from cytology or bronchoscopy. For a solitary nodule assessed as benign by the criteria in Table 14-4, the next step would be to perform a needle biopsy. If the abnormality is a localized infiltrate rather than a nodule and if there is a consensus that the lesion represents an inflamatory process, then a follow-up chest x-ray would be obtained in four to six weeks. Needle biopsy would be performed if there were no resolution.
5. At this stage in the work-up a lesion has been assessed as probably malignant but no tissue diagnosis has been obtained. All such patients are evaluated for operability and resectability.
6. An inoperable patient is one who is unlikely to tolerate general anesthesia, thoracotomy, and pulmonary resection. The determination of operability involves judgment based upon the patient's age, general medical condition, and an estimation of his cardiac and pulmonary functional capacity. Cardiac disqualifications are severe angina, uncontrolled congestive heart failure, and recent myocardial infarction. Surgery is undesirable in subjects with one second forced expiratory volume (FEV_1) of less than one liter, hypercapnia with a Pco_2 greater than 44 mm Hg, or a resting mean pulmonary artery pressure greater than 30 mm Hg.[34] If the projected removal of pulmonary tissue will leave the patient with an absolute FEV_1 of less than 0.8 liters, surgery is contraindicated. Exercise tolerance tests may be performed in borderline cases. As a general rule, the most vigorous evaluations for resectability are bestowed upon the patients with the most questionable operability.
7. Resectability. Thoracotomy with its attendant morbidity and mortality should not be undertaken if the bronchogenic carcinoma is already unresectable. The entire lesion cannot be successfully removed if the tumor has extended to involve: (a) extrathoracic structures such as the liver or the brain, (b) the trachea, the heart, or the proximal pulmonary artery or vein, (c) the carina, (d) the parietal pleura, (e) lymph nodes in the anterior mediastinum or the aortopulmonary window, (f) contralateral hilar lymph nodes, (g) the extranodal soft tissues of the mediastinum, (h) ipsilateral mediastinal lymph nodes if the tumor is an adenocarcinoma or an undifferentiated large cell carcinoma. All undifferentiated small cell (oat cell) carcinomas are considered unresectable.

As previously mentioned the most vigorous investigations for resectability are carried out in those patients with borderline operability.

For more detailed information on preoperative staging of lung cancer, the reader is referred to a previous publication by Baker, Stitik, and Summer.[34] In brief, the evaluation consists of: (a) screening liver function tests followed by radionuclide liver scanning if LFT are abnormal, followed by liver biopsy if liver scan is positive; (b) perfusion lung scanning (see Chapter 3) (gross underperfusion of the lung containing the lesion makes resectability doubtful); pulmonary angiography may be performed to confirm vascular invasion; (c) bone scanning for patients with anaplastic epidermoid carcinomas and undifferentiated carcinomas; (d) barium swallow and fluoroscopy to search for posterior mediastinal adenopathy; (e) superior venacavography and angiography of the azygous vein in patients with right peritracheal lesions; (f) pleural biopsy and aspiration of pleural fluid for cytological study; and (g) computed tomography for problem cases of tumor staging.

8. Good risk patients who are obviously operable and probably resectable have chest surgery. Thoracotomy may be preceded by mediastinoscopy. Our indications for mediastinoscopy are as follows: (a) all central and midlung lesions known to be cancer, (b) all lesions larger than 3 cm, (c) all patients with hilar enlargement, (d) all patients with mediastinal widening, and (e) all patients in whom sputum cytology shows undifferentiated large cell carcinoma. Left parasternal exploration is also carried out in all patients with left upper lobe lesions or left hilar lesions in whom transcervical exploration has revealed no evidence of inoperability.
9. Needle biopsy of the lesion is the next step in a group of patients with no tissue diagnosis. The indications for needle biopsy at this juncture are (see Chapter 9): (a) the patient has a known extrathoracic malignancy; (b) the patient has known extrapulmonary metastases; (c) the patient refuses surgery; (d) the lesion is probably unresectable (a tissue diagnosis is required since radiation therapy may be indicated); (e) the lesion is probably inoperable (poor risk patient with resectable lesion); and (f) Pancoast tumor.

REFERENCES

1. O'Brien EJ, Tuttle WM, Ferkaney JE: The management of the pulmonary "coin" lesion. S Clin North America 28:1313, 1948
2. Davis EW, Peabody JE, Jr, Katz S: The solitary pulmonary nodule. J Thoracic Surg 32:728, 1956
3. Garland LH: A three-step method for the diagnosis of solitary pulmonary nodules. Canad MAJ 83:1079, 1960
4. Nathan MH: Management of solitary pulmonary nodules. An organized approach based on growth rate and statistics. JAMA 227:1141–1144. 1974
5. Steele JD: The solitary pulmonary nodule. Report of a cooperative study of

resected asymptomatic solitary pulmonary nodules in males. J Thoracic and Cardiovas Surg 46:21, 1963
6. Taylor RR, Rivkin LN, Salyer JM: The solitary pulmonary nodule. Ann Surg 147:197, 1958
7. Walske BR: The solitary pulmonary nodule. Dis Chest 49:302, 1966
8. French SW, Pfotenhauer MA, Jr, Castagno J, Mathewson C, Jr: Surgical implications of solitary pulmonary coin lesions. Am J Surg 92:300, 1956
9. Holin SM, Dwork RE, Glaser S, Rikli AE, Stocklen JB: Solitary pulmonary nodules found in a community-wide chest roentgenographic survey: A five year follow-up study. Am Rev Tuberc 79:427, 1959
10. McClure CD, Boucot KE, Shipman GA, Gilliam AG, Milmore BK, Lloyd JW: The solitary pulmonary nodule and primary lung malignancy. Arch Environ Health 3:127, 1961
11. Edwards WM, Cox RS, Garland H: The solitary nodule (coin lesion) of the lung. Am J Roentgenol 88:1020, 1962
12. Nathan MH, Collins VP, Adams RA: Differentiation of benign and malignant pulmonary nodules by growth rate. Radiology 79:221, 1962
13. Weiss W, Boucot KE, Cooper DA: Survival of men with peripheral lung cancer in relation to histologic characteristics and growth rate. Amer Rev Resp Dis 98:75, 1968
14. Good CA, Hood RT, Jr, McDonald JE: Significance of a solitary mass in the lung. Amer J Roentgenol 70:543, 1953
15. Good CA, Wilson TW: The solitary circumscribed pulmonary nodule. JAMA 166:210, 1958
16. Good CA: The solitary pulmonary nodule: A problem of management. Radiol Clin North Am 1:429, 1963
17. O'Keefe ME, Jr, Good CA, McDonald JE: Calcification in solitary nodules in the lung. Amer J Roentgenol 77:1023, 1957
18. Theros EG: Varying manifestations of peripheral pulmonary neoplasms: A radiologic-pathologic correlative study. Am J Roentgenol 128:893, 1977
19. London SB, Winter WJ: Calcification within carcinoma of the lung. Arch Int Med 94:161, 1954
20. Bloch RG: Tuberculous calcification. A clinical and experimental study. Am J Roentgenol 59:853, 1948
21. Vivas JE, Crabtree SF: The significance of size and radiographic density of solitary lesions in the lungs. Amer Prac 4:857, 1955
22. Bateson EM: The solitary circumscribed bronchogenic carcinoma. A radiological study of 100 cases. Brit J Radiol 37:598, 1964
23. Bateson EM: An analysis of 155 solitary lung lesions illustrating the differential diagnosis of mixed tumors of the lung. Clin Radiol 16:51, 1965
24. Seybold WD: Solitary "coin" lesions of the lung. Analysis of 2,258 recorded cases. Postgrad Med 36:424, 1964
25. Rigler LG: The roentgen signs of carcinoma of the lung. Amer J Roentgenol 74:415, 1955
26. Rigler LG, Heitzman EF: Planigraphy in the differential diagnosis of the pulmonary nodule. Radiology 65:692, 1955
27. Steele JD, Kleitsch WP, Dunn JE, Buell P: Survival in males with bronchogenic carcinomas resected as asymptomatic solitary pulmonary nodules. Ann Thorac Surg 2:368, 1966

28. Stitik FP, Tockman MS: Radiographic screening in the early detection of lung cancer. Radiol Clin N America (in press)
29. Thomford NE, Woolner LB, Clagett OT: The surgical treatment of metastatic tumors in the lung. J Thoracic and Cardiovas Surg 49:357, 1965
30. Neifield JP, Michaelis LL, Doppman JL: Suspected Pulmonary Metastases. Cancer 39:383, 1977
31. Cahan WG, Castro EB, Hajdu SI: The significance of a solitary lung shadow in patients with colon carcinoma. Cancer 33:414, 1974
32. Atkins PC, Wesselhoeft CW, Jr., Newman W, Blades B: Thoracotomy on the patient with previous malignancy: metastasis or new primary. J Thorac & Cardiovas Surg 56:351, 1968
33. Lawhorne TW, Jr., Baker RR, Carter D: Adenocarcinoma of the lung presenting as a solitary pulmonary nodule. Johns Hopkins Med J 133:82, 1973
34. Baker ER, Stitik FP, Summer WR: Preoperative evaluation of patients with supected bronchogenic carcinoma. Current Problems in Surgery. Year Book Publishers, Chicago, Illinois, Dec. 1974
35. Lehar TJ, Carr DT, Miller WE, Payne WS, Woolner LB: Roentgenographic appearance of bronchogenic adenocarcinoma. Amer Rev Resp Dis 96:245, 1967
36. Byrd RB, Miller WE, Carr DT, Payne WS, Woolner LB: The roentgenographic appearance of squamous cell carcinoma of the bronchus. Mayo Clin Proc 43:327, 1968
37. Rigler GG: An overview of cancer of the lung. Semin Roentgenol 12:161, 1977

Index

a b c d e f 9 g 0 h 1 i 8 2 j